S0-CQT-446

Advances in Cardiovascular Pharmacology

Edited by
Philippe R. Housmans, MD, PhD
Professor of Anesthesiology
Department of Anesthesiology
Mayo Clinic, Rochester, MN

and

Gregory A. Nuttall, MD
Professor of Anesthesiology,
Department of Anesthesiology
Mayo Clinic, Rochester, MN

with 21 contributors

Wolters Kluwer Health | Lippincott Williams & Wilkins

Advances in Cardiovascular Pharmacology

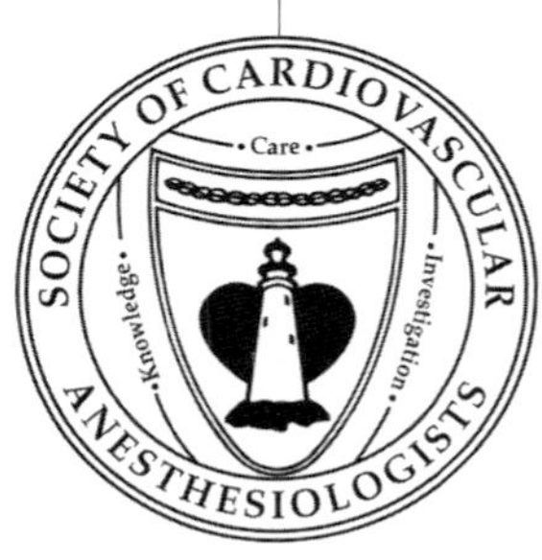

A Society of Cardiovascular Anesthesiologists Monograph

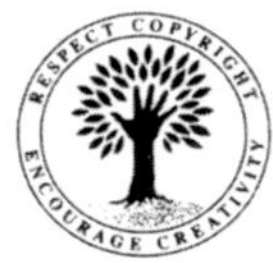

Accurate indications, adverse reactions, and dosage schedules for drugs are provided in this book, but it is possible that they may change. The reader is urged to review the package information data of the manufacturers of the medications mentioned.

Printed in the United States of America
ISBN-10: 1605470600
ISBN-13: 9781605470603

Publication Committee of the
Society of Cardiovascular Anesthesiologists

Preface

Pharmacology plays a pivotal role in the practice of cardiovascular anesthesiology. The perioperative management of cardiovascular surgical patients involves the regulation of the cardiovascular, endocrine, coagulation, fluid, and ionic homeostasis and other systems. In this monograph selected topics in pharmacology are discussed. It is not intended to be a comprehensive textbook of pharmacology, but rather a collection of carefully selected reviews of recent advances in inotropic therapy, β-adrenoreceptor antagonists, myocardial preconditioning, modulators of vascular tone, cardiac electrophysiology, coagulation management, diuretics, statins, and glucose management in cardiovascular surgery. Each of these topics has broad implications for cardiology, cardiac and vascular surgery, cardiac anesthesiology, and intensive care medicine.

Contributors

John P. Abenstein, M.S.E.E., M.D.
Associate Professor of Anesthesiology
Department of Anesthesiology
Mayo Clinic
Rochester, MN

Sylvia Archan, M.D.
Resident
Department of Anesthesiology and Intensive Care Medicine
Medical University of Graz
Graz, Austria

Antoine G. M. Aya, M.D., Ph.D.
Department of Anesthesiology, Pain Management, Emergency and Critical Care Medicine
University of Nimes
Nimes, France

Roxann D. Barnes, M.D.
Assistant Professor of Anesthesiology
Department of Anesthesiology
Mayo Clinic
Rochester, MN

Dan Berkowitz, M.D.
Associate Professor of Anesthesiology
Departments of Anesthesiology, Critical Care Medicine and Biomedical Engineering
The Johns Hopkins Medical Institutions
Baltimore, MD

Daniel R. Brown, M.D., Ph.D., F.C.C.M.
Assistant Professor of Anesthesiology
Department of Anesthesiology
Mayo Clinic
Rochester, MN

Pierre-Géraud Claret, M.D., M.Sc.
Department of Anesthesiology, Pain Management, Emergency and Critical Care Medicine
University of Nimes
Nimes, France

Pierre Coriat, M.D.
Professor of Anesthesiology
Department of Anesthesiology and Critical Care
University Hospital La Pitié-Salpêtrière
Paris, France

Jean-Emmanuel de La Coussaye, M.D., Ph.D.
Professor of Anesthesiology
Department of Anesthesiology, Pain Management, Emergency and Critical Care Medicine
University of Nimes
Nimes, France

James D. Hannon, M.D.
Assistant Professor of Anesthesiology
Department of Anesthesiology
Mayo Clinic
Rochester, MN

Philippe R. Housmans, M.D., Ph.D.
Professor of Anesthesiology
Department of Anesthesiology
Mayo Clinic
Rochester, MN

Roy Kan, M.B.B.S. (Singapore), M.Med. (Anesthesia)
Postdoctoral Fellow
Departments of Anesthesiology, Critical Care Medicine and Biomedical Engineering
The Johns Hopkins Medical Institutions
Baltimore, MD

Daryl J. Kor, M.D.
Instructor in Anesthesiology
Department of Anesthesiology
Mayo Clinic
Rochester, MN

Yannick Le Manach, M.D.
Department of Anesthesiology and Critical Care
University Hospital La Pitié-Salpêtrière
Paris, France

James J. Lynch, M.D.
Instructor in Anesthesiology
Department of Anesthesiology
Mayo Clinic
Rochester, MN

William J. Mauermann, M.D.
Instructor in Anesthesiology
Department of Anesthesiology
Mayo Clinic
Rochester, MN

Gregory A. Nuttall, M.D.
Professor of Anesthesiology
Department of Anesthesiology
Mayo Clinic
Rochester, MN

Juan N. Pulido, M.D.
Fellow, Cardiovascular Anesthesia
Department of Anesthesiology
Mayo Clinic
Rochester, MN

Jacob Raphael, M.D.
Assistant Professor of Anesthesiology
Department of Anesthesiology
University of Virginia Health Sciences Center
Charlottesville, VA

Paul E. Stensrud, M.D.
Assistant Professor of Anesthesiology
Department of Anesthesiology
Mayo Clinic
Rochester, MN

Wolfgang G. Toller, M.D.
Associate Professor of Anesthesiology
Department of Anesthesiology and Intensive Care Medicine
Medical University of Graz
Graz, Austria

Contents

Preface

Contributors

1 1

Inotropic Therapy
James D. Hannon, M.D. and Philippe R. Housmans, M.D., Ph.D.
Department of Anesthesiology
Mayo Clinic, Rochester, MN

2 17

Levosimendan
Wolfgang G. Toller, M.D. and Sylvia Archan, M.D.
Department of Anesthesiology and Intensive Care Medicine
Medical University of Graz
Graz, Austria

3 43

β-Adrenergic Receptor Antagonists
Juan N. Pulido, M.D. and Daryl J. Kor, M.D.
Department of Anesthesiology
Mayo Clinic, Rochester, MN

4 67

Modulators of Vascular Tone: Implications for New Pharmacological Therapies
Roy Kan, M.B.B.S., M.Med. and Dan Berkowitz, M.D.
Departments of Anesthesiology, Critical Care Medicine and Biomedical Engineering
The Johns Hopkins Medical Institutions
Baltimore, MD

5 91
Physiology and Pharmacology of Myocardial Preconditioning
Jacob Raphael, M.D.
Department of Anesthesiology
University of Virginia Health Sciences Center
Charlottesville, VA

6 115
Cardiac Electrophysiology: Pharmacological Applications
Antoine G.M. Aya, M.D., Ph.D., Pierre-Géraud Claret, M.D., M.Sc., and Jean-Emmanuel de La Coussaye, M.D., Ph.D.
Department of Anesthesiology, Pain Management, Emergency and Critical Care Medicine
University of Nimes
Nimes, France

7 157
Procoagulant Agents
James J. Lynch, M.D. and Gregory A. Nuttall, M.D.
Department of Anesthesiology
Mayo Clinic, Rochester, MN

8 183
Pharmacology of Antifibrinolytic Agents
Paul E. Stensrud, M.D. and Gregory A. Nuttall, M.D.
Department of Anesthesiology
Mayo Clinic, Rochester, MN

9 205
Diuretics and Cardiovascular Anesthesia
William J. Mauermann, M.D. and Roxann D. Barnes, M.D.
Department of Anesthesiology
Mayo Clinic, Rochester, MN

10 227
Statins in the Perioperative Period
Yannick Le Manach, M.D. and Pierre Coriat, M.D.
Department of Anesthesiology and Critical Care
University Hospital La Pitié-Salpêtrière
Paris, France

11 251
Perioperative Glycemic Control
John P. Abenstein, M.S.E.E., M.D. and
Daniel R. Brown, M.D., Ph.D., F.C.C.M.
Department of Anesthesiology
Mayo Clinic, Rochester, MN

James D. Hannon, MD
Philippe R. Housmans, MD, PhD

1 Inotropic Therapy

INTRODUCTION

Intravenous positive inotropic agents are often used in the perioperative period for relatively short periods of time to maintain or enhance perfusion of vital organs during general anesthesia in patients having noncardiac surgery and in cardiac surgical patients after separation from cardiopulmonary bypass. During cardiac surgery, aortic cross-clamping and reperfusion can result in transient contractile dysfunction post-bypass, especially in patients with a history of congestive heart failure (CHF) or low ejection fraction preoperatively (1–3).

Outside the perioperative environment, inotropic agents are often used to treat acute heart failure syndromes with congestive symptoms. In this setting, they do provide rapid hemodynamic and symptomatic relief, but a growing body of evidence in patients hospitalized with acute heart failure points toward an association with increased mortality, even after short-term use, due to increased ventricular ectopy, tachyarrhythmias, and ischemia (4–6). Obviously these findings raise concerns that inotropic agents may actually be harmful to patients, but it is difficult to advocate withholding this therapy in the setting of hypotension, and therefore it is easy to understand why they continue to be used, albeit at progressively lower rates (7). It is also important to keep in mind that these agents are probably best used as a temporizing measure until a definitive treatment such as revascularization or transplant can take place or until intrinsic contractility improves.

Advances in Cardiovascular Pharmacology, edited by Philippe R. Housmans, MD, PhD and Gregory A. Nuttall, M.D.
Lippincott Williams & Wilkins, Baltimore © 2008.

A working knowledge of the fundamental determinants of cardiac contractility and how inotropic agents affect them is key to understanding how the desirable effects are intimately linked to the undesirable side-effects. This type of awareness is essential to the judicious use of the available agents, as well as the rapid but enlightened adoption of new agents as they become available. In the failing heart, myocardial contraction results from a sequence of events that includes depolarization of the plasma membrane, release and sequestration of Ca^{2+} by the sarcoplasmic reticulum (Ca^{2+} transient), Ca^{2+} binding to troponin C, and crossbridge cycling. Myocardial contractility is defined as the potential to do work, and is the manifestation of many factors that influence the interactions between intracellular Ca^{2+} and the contractile proteins. It can be expressed as any change in the ability of myocardial tissue to develop tension or shorten that is not caused by a change in initial fiber length. Pressure, as well as its rate of change (dP/dt), and velocity of shortening are frequently used as indices of contractility.

A key element of this discussion is that each time the heart beats the intracellular [Ca^{2+}] transiently increases and decreases about 10-fold (Ca^{2+} transient), and that this Ca^{2+} signal drives the system by binding to troponin C and allowing actin and myosin to interact and produce force and shortening. One useful way to classify inotropic mechanisms, then, is according to their ability to (1) increase the intracellular Ca^{2+} transient ("upstream" mechanisms), (2) increase the affinity of troponin C for Ca^{2+} ("central" mechanisms), and (3) increase the response of the myofibrillar proteins to a given level of Ca^{2+} ("downstream" mechanisms) (8). With the notable exception of levosimendan, which works via the central mechanism (Ca^{2+} sensitization), all clinically useful inotropic agents primarily work via upstream mechanisms that increase intracellular Ca^{2+}. Therefore, it is not surprising that they have been found to cause Ca^{2+} overload, the underlying substrate for arrhythmias, myocardial cell injury and, ultimately, cell death (9). In addition, they tend to increase cellular metabolism and alter the cellular oxygen supply–demand relationship unfavorably. Consequently, the higher mortality associated with positive inotropic drugs in decompensated congestive heart failure trials is also really no surprise. However, emerging therapeutic agents evoke optimism that the deleterious effects of currently available inotropic drugs will eventually be overcome (10).

Physiology

Ultimately positive inotropic drugs affect the contractile mechanisms by which the heart produces force and shortening, also known as cardiac excitation-contraction coupling, so an appreciation for the underlying

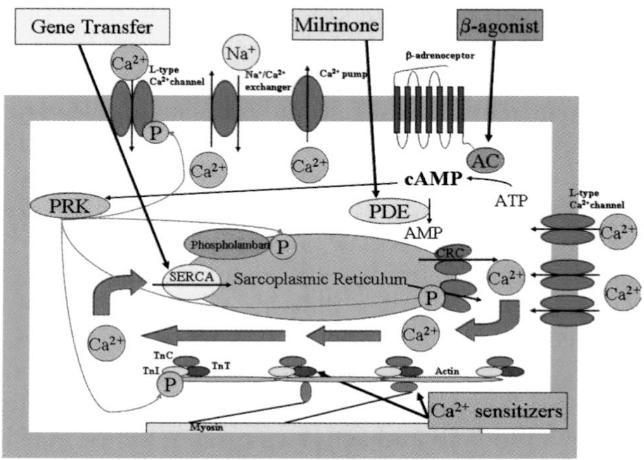

FIGURE 1–1. **Simplified model of the effects of positive inotropic agents on intracellular Ca^{2+} and crossbridge cycling. SERCA2a: sarcoplasmic reticulum calcium ATPase type 2a; CRC: Ca^{2+} release channel; AC: adenylyl cyclase; PDE: phosphodiesterase; PRK: protein kinase A; P: phosphorylation site.**

physiology will help to explain how the various agents are similar and different in this respect.

A relatively small number of proteins are intimately involved in producing the Ca^{2+} transient each time the heart beats (Figure 1–1). First, the surface membrane depolarizes, opening voltage-gated surface membrane Ca^{2+} channels and allowing a small amount of Ca^{2+} to enter the cell. Next, the large capacity Ca^{2+} release channels located in the sarcoplasmic reticulum membrane sense this Ca^{2+} entry, opening briefly and releasing large quantities of Ca^{2+} stored in the sarcoplasmic reticulum (SR) (11). The Ca^{2+} released from the SR then raises the intracellular Ca^{2+} concentration over 10-fold, leading to activation of troponin C, a regulatory protein located in the contractile apparatus, and switching on crossbridge formation between actin and myosin (12). All the while, a Ca^{2+}-ATPase located in the SR (SERCA2a) pumps the majority of Ca^{2+} back into the SR, causing the myocyte to relax. Two other proteins, the Na^{+}-Ca^{2+} exchanger (NCX) (13) and the sarcolemmal Ca^{2+}-ATPase (PMCA) (12, 14) are, for the most part, involved in extruding calcium from the cell and compete with SERCA for intracellular Ca^{2+}. To summarize, during steady-state contractions in the heart, Ca^{2+} entry across the surface membrane through L-type Ca^{2+} channels (I_{Ca}) is balanced by an equal efflux of Ca^{2+} from the cell via the NCX and PMCA proteins. At the same time SERCA competes with NCX and PMCA, sequestering Ca^{2+} in the intracellular reservoir called the SR for release in subsequent beats.

The normal heart has tremendous reserve in terms of pumping ability, increasing cardiac output during intense exercise to 35–40 liters per minute in some trained endurance athletes (15). Much of the augmentation is due to increased heart rate and more favorable ventricular filling, but a significant amount also results from a non-length dependent biochemical cascade that increases pressure development and stroke volume (16). The effects of β-adrenergic stimulation provide an example of how such augmentation can occur (Figure 1–1). For example, when epinephrine binds to the β1-adrenergic receptor, it causes a conformational change in the receptor complex allowing it to bind to a G-protein that subsequently converts GTP to GDP (17). This conversion results in dissociation of the $G\alpha_s$ and $G\beta\gamma$ subunits, activation of membrane bound adenylyl cyclase (AC type V) by $G\alpha_s$, and increased intracellular cAMP (18). cAMP then binds to and activates protein kinase A (PKA) which modulates cardiac contractility by phosphorylating several proteins, including the voltage-gated surface membrane Ca^{2+} channel (increases calcium entry), troponin I (decreases duration of contraction, enhances relaxation), phospholamban (activates SERCA, enhancing relaxation and increasing sarcoplasmic reticulum Ca^{2+} content), and the cardiac ryanodine receptor (also known as the Ca^{2+} release channel; enhances channel opening, releasing more stored Ca^{2+}) (12, 19). The sum of these effects is to produce an increase in the peak intracellular Ca^{2+} transient as well as an increase in the rate of its decline. The heart therefore produces significantly greater force and systole is relatively shorter, even at high heart rates, allowing more time for myocardial perfusion.

Phosphodiesterase (PDE) inhibition (milrinone) can also produce a dramatic increase in contractility because cAMP is exclusively hydrolyzed by PDE in the heart, and therefore plays a key role in regulating the signal conveyed by cAMP (20). Under normal conditions, PDE activity determines the basal level of cAMP by continuously hydrolyzing cAMP produced by constitutively active adenylyl cyclases and by controlling the amplitude and duration of increases in cAMP concentration due to external stimulation (21). The various isoforms of PDE apparently play a role in the spatial regulation of cAMP by virtue of their unique distribution patterns within the cell. For example, the differential effects of β_1 and β_2 receptor stimulation on contractility appear to be due, at least in part, to the activity of PDE4 on β_2-generated cAMP (21).

Epinephrine

Epinephrine is a potent catecholamine that stimulates both α and β receptors throughout the body, but seems to have limited popularity as an inotropic agent. It has a powerful stimulant effect on the heart that results predominantly from activation of β_1 receptors, but it also activates β_2, β_3, α_1, and α_2 receptors, producing widespread effects on various organ systems.

Epinephrine increases systolic blood pressure by increasing the strength of ventricular contraction (β_1), increasing heart rate (β_2), and constricting vascular beds in the skin, mucosa, and kidney, as well as the venous system in general (α_1). Chronically over-stimulated β_1 and β_2 receptors, as in heart failure, undergo downregulation due to their phosphorylation, producing a decreased contractile response to subsequent stimulation (22). In addition, β_3 receptors in the heart produce a negative inotropic effect and are not downregulated, potentially decreasing inotropy further due to their relative abundance (23).

Cerebral perfusion increases in direct relation to the arterial blood pressure because the cerebral circulation has very little constrictor response. Epinephrine increases coronary perfusion, even when systemic blood pressure is unaffected, due to the relatively longer duration of diastole and due to increased release of adenosine from more metabolically active cells. At usual doses (Table 1–1), cardiac output increases, venous return increases, and diastolic blood pressure tends to decrease due to greater sensitivity to activation of vasodilator β_2 than constrictor α_1 receptors in skeletal muscle. Myocardial work and oxygen consumption can increase dramatically. Epinephrine increases the rate of diastolic depolarization of the pacemaker cells in the SA node as well as in Purkinje fibers, and shortens the refractory period of the AV node.

TABLE 1–1. Principle mechanism of action and dosage for frequently used positive inotropic agents.

Drug	Mechanism	Dose	Half Life
Dopamine	β Agonist	Infusion: Low: <2 mcg/kg/min Intermediate: 2–5 mcg/kg/min High: 5–15 mcg/kg/min	3 min
Dobutamine	β Agonist	Infusion: 2–15 mcg/kg/min	3 min
Epinephrine	β Agonist	Infusion: 0.1–1 mcg/kg/min	3 min
Levosimendan[a]	Ca^{2+} Sensitizer	Load: 6–24 mcg/kg Infusion: 0.05–0.2 mcg/kg/min	1 hr
Milrinone	PDE III Inhibitor	Load: 50mcg/kg[b] Infusion: Minimum: 0.375 mcg/kg/min Standard: 0.5 mcg/kg/min Maximum: 0.75 mcg/kg/min	2 hr

[a] Not available in USA.
[b] Loading dose often avoided due to tendency to produce hypotension.

Insulin secretion tends to be inhibited, leading to hyperglycemia. Hypertriglyceridemia results from stimulation of β_3 receptors in fat cells and increased lipolysis. Epinephrine causes increased uptake of K^+ into skeletal muscle, resulting in decreased plasma K^+ concentrations.

In a relatively small study of coronary artery bypass patients comparing epinephrine with milrinone on left ventricular compliance post-cardiopulmonary bypass, milrinone, but not epinephrine, increased compliance to pre-bypass levels, possibly due to more favorable effects of milrinone on myocardial oxygen demand (24). However, in a later study of coronary artery bypass patients with good systolic and only mildly impaired diastolic function, no difference was seen (25). Similarly, in a study of patients having aortic valve replacement for aortic stenosis, there was no difference in the effects of epinephrine, milrinone, or placebo on left ventricular compliance, although both inotropic agents produced favorable hemodynamics (26).

Norepinephrine

Norepinephrine is a potent catecholamine and the biochemical precursor to epinephrine. It, too, stimulates both α and β receptors, but with a different relative affinity profile. Norepinephrine stimulates primarily α_1 receptors, producing constriction of arterial and venous capacitance vessels and increasing systemic blood pressure and coronary blood flow. It also acts on β_1 receptors, but relatively less so than epinephrine. At low doses the cardiac stimulant effect predominates, and with higher doses the vasoconstrictor effect becomes predominant.

Norepinephrine increases total peripheral resistance and systolic and diastolic blood pressure, but cardiac output does not change or decreases. Heart rate tends to slow due to compensatory vagal output, and stroke volume usually increases. Norepinephrine constricts mesenteric vessels and reduces splanchnic and hepatic blood flow. Coronary flow increases due to metabolite-induced coronary dilation and to elevated blood pressure. The metabolic effects of norepinephrine are similar to epinephrine, but tend to be less pronounced.

Norepinephrine is most commonly used in patients with low systemic vascular resistance due to sepsis or post-cardiotomy hypotension (27, 28). A recently completed prospective randomized trial of norepinephrine plus or minus dobutamine against epinephrine in patients with septic shock showed no difference in clinical outcomes (29).

Dopamine

Dopamine is a naturally occurring catecholamine and is the precursor for norepinephrine and epinephrine. It is produced in the proximal tubule epithelial cells in the kidney and plays a key role in the regulation of salt balance, causing diuresis and natriuresis via direct effects (30). Stimulation of the D_1 receptor in the kidney also causes renin release and angiotensin gene expression (31).

The cardiovascular effects of dopamine are mediated by several types of receptors, including dopaminergic and adrenergic, that vary in their affinity for dopamine. At low infusion rates ($<$2 mcg/kg/min), dopamine interacts with D_1-dopaminergic receptors in the renal, mesenteric, and coronary vascular beds, raising intracellular cAMP and causing vasodilation. At somewhat higher doses (2–5 mcg/kg/min), dopamine acts on β_1 receptors in the heart, producing a positive inotropic response. Systolic and mean arterial blood pressure usually increase somewhat, while diastolic blood pressure remains unchanged. At high doses (5–15 mcg/kg/min), dopamine causes generalized vasoconstriction by interacting with α_1 receptors in the vasculature.

Dopamine continues to be used, primarily at low doses, in the hopes of preserving renal function in patients at risk. Surprisingly, there are no large, randomized, controlled trials studying the effects of short-term or long-term dopamine infusion in heart failure. In a small non-randomized study in 9 patients with chronic severe HF, renal blood flow nearly doubled and cardiac index increased by 21% at a dose of 2.1 μg/kg/min, whereas at a dose of 4.0 μg/kg/min, cardiac index increased maximally with no further augmentation of renal blood flow (32). A recent meta-analysis of selected parallel group randomized and quasi-randomized controlled trials, including cardiac and vascular surgery patients, of low dose ($<$5 μg/kg/min) dopamine versus control showed that dopamine increased urine output by 24% only on the first day of treatment but did not increase adverse events (33).

Dobutamine

Dobutamine is a racemic mixture that stimulates both β_1- and β_2-adrenergic receptors, and is most often used for short-term support of cardiac output in patients with heart failure. At clinically useful concentrations most of its effect is due to action at the β_1-adrenergic receptor, although it also stimulates β_2 and α-adrenergic receptors. Dobutamine activates the β_1 cardiac receptor and, like epinephrine, increases contractility by phosphorylating several proteins, including the voltage-gated surface membrane Ca^{2+} channel, troponin I, phospholamban, and the cardiac ryanodine receptor.

Therefore, dobutamine increases myocardial contractility and accelerates relaxation. Stroke volume also increases, but dobutamine affects heart rate relatively little unless doses in the high range are used (see

Table 1–1). Dobutamine also produces a mild decrease in systemic vascular resistance and filling pressures due to a greater influence at β_2-adrenergic receptors as compared to α-adrenergic receptors in the vasculature. In patients who have been receiving a β-adrenergic antagonist, the response may be attenuated.

Which inotropic agent is used clinically is often based more on familiarity than on hard science, but dobutamine seems to be the standard against which new drugs are tested, based on its well-known and predictable hemodynamic effects. In a randomized study comparing the effects of dobutamine and milrinone on hemodynamics in cardiac surgical patients with low cardiac index post-cardiopulmonary bypass, dobutamine caused greater increases in cardiac index and HR, but not stroke index, and greater increases in MAP and left ventricular SWI than milrinone (34). Dobutamine was also associated with a significantly higher incidence of hypertension and rhythm changes. However, De Hert et al. found that cardiac output was better preserved in cardiac surgical patients with low preoperative ejection fraction when a combination of dobutamine plus levosimendan was compared to dobutamine plus milrinone, suggesting that adding agents with significantly different mechanisms of action may be beneficial (35).

Outcome studies in patients receiving dobutamine and other inotropic agents have largely focused on nonsurgical patients hospitalized for acute exacerbations of heart failure. An early meta-analysis of randomized studies comparing dobutamine with placebo in patients with heart failure showed a non-significant trend for dobutamine (and other inotropic agents as well) to be associated with excess mortality (36). In a large, multicenter, randomized and controlled study of dobutamine compared to levosimendan, the LIDO study, dobutamine was associated with less satisfactory hemodynamics (the primary endpoint of the study) and excess mortality up to 180 days after the infusion (37). However, the more recent SURIVE trial comparing dobutamine to levosimendan in nonsurgical patients with acute decompensated heart failure indicated that short-term dobutamine administration was not associated with increased mortality at 180 days when compared with to levosimendan (primary endpoint) (5).

Milrinone

Milrinone is used for short-term support of cardiac output in patients with heart failure. It inhibits phosphodiesterase type III (PDE3) found in cardiac muscle, leading to a prolonged increase in the concentration of cAMP. Milrinone increases cardiac contractility and accelerates myocardial relaxation. Milrinone causes balanced relaxation of arterial and venous smooth muscle and produces a fall in both the systemic and pulmonary vascular resistances. Cardiac output increases because of the increase in contractility and the decrease in afterload, with relatively little effect on heart rate and, apparently, myocardial oxygen demand.

Despite these seemingly favorable effects on hemodynamics, clinical trials have yielded disappointing results. One of the earliest randomized trials to examine the efficacy of milrinone was the PROMISE trial, a randomized, double-blinded, placebo-controlled study that examined the effects of oral milrinone plus conventional therapy in over 1,000 patients with severe CHF. Overall there was a 34% increase in cardiovascular mortality, and the mortality difference was greatest in the patients with the most severe symptoms (4).

More recently completed, the OPTIME-CHF study was a multicenter, randomized, double-blinded, placebo-controlled trial of the short-term IV administration of milrinone to patients who had been hospitalized for no more than 48 hours for exacerbation of known systolic chronic heart failure (38). Although the subjective health status improved markedly and by a similar degree both in the milrinone and placebo group, with 90% of the patients feeling better at discharge, the 48 hr infusion of milrinone was associated with increased early treatment failures, particularly caused by new atrial arrhythmias and significant hypotension. This study also showed a tendency toward increased mortality in the milrinone group, both in the inpatient phase and at 60 days, even though the medication was used for only 48–72 hours. This result adds to the mounting evidence that short-term use of inotropic agents can have long-term effects on morbidity and mortality.

In a post hoc analysis of the OPTIME-CHF data, the relationship between CHF etiology (ischemic vs. nonischemic) and milrinone treatment was examined. In patients with ischemic CHF, milrinone treatment was associated with higher mortality and prolonged hospitalization. In patients with nonischemic CHF, however, there appeared to be some benefit to treatment with milrinone in terms of lower in-hospital mortality and rehospitalization at 60 days (39).

Levosimendan

Levosimendan is a relatively new positive inotropic agent that works primarily by increasing the Ca^{2+} sensitivity of the contractile apparatus (positive inotropy) and by activating ATP sensitive potassium channels in vascular smooth muscle (vasodilation). The positive inotropic action is apparently due to calcium-dependent binding of levosimendan to troponin C (40). It is receiving a great deal of attention due to the hope that it will provide a much-needed safer positive inotropic agent, and therefore is reviewed in great detail in a separate chapter.

EVOLVING THERAPIES

SERCA Expression

SR function appears to be critical to maintaining normal contractility in the heart, and although there is a wide variation in SERCA protein levels in failing human hearts, there may be an inverse relationship between diastolic chamber size and SERCA expression (41). SERCA is a 110 kD transmembrane protein located intracellularly in the SR. The pumping of Ca^{2+} is an energy-dependent process as SERCA pumps two molecules of Ca^{2+} per ATP hydrolyzed. The level of SERCA2a (cardiac subtype) expression in the heart is apparently not fixed. The level of expression increases with development and later decreases with senescence and is known to vary with thyroid hormone status. Ventricular hypertrophy and heart failure reduce the density of SERCA pumps and Ca^{2+} release channels (ryanodine receptors) in the SR membrane (41–43). These changes are characterized by a prolongation of the intracellular Ca^{2+} transient and slowing of the mechanics of the twitch (44–46). It has been suggested that this slowing of the intracellular Ca^{2+} transient is an adaptive process that slows crossbridge attachment and detachment to increase the efficiency of hypertrophied myocardium.

Nevertheless, adenoviral mediated gene transfer of SERCA2a has been used to restore the function of the SR in human ventricular myocytes from patients with heart failure (47). This treatment resulted in increased expression of SERCA2a that was accompanied by greater contraction and relaxation velocities as well as decreased diastolic and increased systolic [Ca^{2+}]. However this approach is still somewhat controversial since decreased SR function may be an adaptive process and up-regulation of SERCA might be expected to increase energy demands and accelerate progression of heart failure. In addition, SERCA overexpression could produce adverse outcomes similar to treatment with positive inotropic drugs. In partial answer to these questions, increased expression of SERCA2a seems to compare favorably with adrenergic agonists in terms of decreased arrhythmic after-contractions and increased survival of cultured myocytes (48). Notably, overexpression of SERCA in normal hearts has recently been reported to increase contractility and relaxation with no increase in oxygen consumption (49).

Myosin Activators

Myosin activators are small molecule drugs that have been designed to activate cardiac myosin directly, without increasing the concentration of intracellular Ca^{2+} (10). They are postulated to shift the actin-myosin enzymatic cycle in favor of the strongly bound, force-producing state of myosin. This mechanism apparently does not change the velocity of shortening, but does increase the extent of shortening and lengthens the duration of contraction resulting in increased cardiac contractility.

The effects of myosin activators on diastolic function are difficult to predict. Based on the mechanism of action, one might predict an unfavorable lusitropic effect. An example of this type of drug that has just begun to undergo testing in humans is CK-1827452. Animal studies presented in abstract form indicate that CK-1827452 is effective in heart failure, producing greater increases in stroke volume and cardiac output. It is reported to increase the force of contraction without increasing intracellular Ca^{2+}. A phase 1 clinical trial has been completed with CK-1827452 administered as an intravenous formulation in healthy volunteers. Doses above the maximum tolerated dose produced prolonged ejection time and decreased diastolic filling. Phase 2 clinical trials are currently underway (50).

Theoretically, this type of drug should be able to increase the contractile performance of the heart without causing arrhythmias and with minimal effect on energy balance. Yet a note of caution is in order until large-scale randomized and controlled clinical studies are completed.

CONCLUSION

Inotropic agents continue to be used to support cardiac output in situations where vital organs are at risk of hypoperfusion. This is relatively commonplace in the perioperative and intensive care settings, because it is estimated that over 5 million patients in the United States have been diagnosed with CHF. Unfortunately, it appears that positive inotropes, especially those that increase intracellular cAMP, even when used for short periods of time, do not improve survival and may actually worsen it. This leads to a clinical dilemma that may only be resolved as newer drugs and ventricular assist devices with improved characteristics become available in the future. In addition, it would probably be wise to better define the lowest clinically acceptable blood pressure, perhaps through the development of improved monitors of tissue perfusion, in order to minimize the harmful effects of currently available positive inotropic agents (51).

References

1. Butterworth JF, Legault C, Royster RL, Hammon JW, Jr.: Factors that predict the use of positive inotropic drug support after cardiac valve surgery. Anesth Analg 1998; 86:461–7

2. Rao V, Ivanov J, Weisel RD, et al.: Predictors of low cardiac output syndrome after coronary artery bypass. J Thorac Cardiovasc Surg 1996; 112:38–51
3. McKinlay KH, Schinderle DB, Swaminathan M, et al.: Predictors of inotrope use during separation from cardiopulmonary bypass. J Cardiothorac Vasc Anesth 2004; 18:404–8
4. Packer M, Carver JR, Rodeheffer RJ, et al.: Effect of oral milrinone on mortality in severe chronic heart failure. The PROMISE Study Research Group. N Engl J Med 1991; 325:1468–75
5. Mebazaa A, Nieminen MS, Packer M, et al.: Levosimendan vs dobutamine for patients with acute decompensated heart failure: the SURVIVE Randomized Trial. JAMA 2007; 297:1883–91
6. Abraham WT, Adams KF, Fonarow GC, et al.: In-hospital mortality in patients with acute decompensated heart failure requiring intravenous vasoactive medications: an analysis from the Acute Decompensated Heart Failure National Registry (ADHERE). J Am Coll Cardiol 2005; 46:57–64
7. Fonarow GC, Heywood JT, Heidenreich PA, et al.: Temporal trends in clinical characteristics, treatments, and outcomes for heart failure hospitalizations, 2002 to 2004: findings from Acute Decompensated Heart Failure National Registry (ADHERE). Am Heart J 2007; 153:1021–8
8. Blinks JR, Endoh M: Modification of myofibrillar responsiveness to Ca^{2+} as an inotropic mechanism. Circulation 1986; 73:III85–III98
9. Endoh M, Hori M: Acute heart failure: inotropic agents and their clinical uses. Expert Opin Pharmacother 2006; 7:2179–202
10. deGoma EM, Vagelos RH, Fowler MB, Ashley EA: Emerging therapies for the management of decompensated heart failure: from bench to bedside. J Am Coll Cardiol 2006; 48:2397–409
11. Díaz MEGH, O'Neill SC, Trafford AW, Eisner DA: The control of sarcoplasmic reticulum Ca^{2+} content in cardiac muscle. Cell Calcium 2005; 38:391–6
12. Bers DM: Calcium fluxes involved in control of cardiac myocyte contraction. Circ Res 2000; 87:275–81
13. Bers DM: Measurement of calcium transport in heart using modern approaches. New Horizons 1996; 4:36–44
14. Bassani RA, Bassani JW, Bers DM: Relaxation in ferret ventricular myocytes: role of the sarcolemmal Ca ATPase. Pflugers Archiv 1995; 430:573–8
15. Ekblom B, Hermansen L: Cardiac output in athletes. J Appl Physiol 1968; 25:619–25

16. Hopkins MG, Spina RJ, Ehsani AA: Enhanced beta-adrenergic-mediated cardiovascular responses in endurance athletes. J App Physiol 1996; 80:516–21
17. Pleger STBM, Most P, Koch WJ: Targeting myocardial beta-adrenergic receptor signaling and calcium cycling for heart failure gene therapy. J Card Fail 2007; 13:401–14
18. Salazara NCCJ, Rockman HA: Cardiac GPCRs: GPCR signaling in healthy and failing hearts. Biochim Biophys Acta 2007; 1768:1006–18
19. Bers DM: Cardiac excitation-contraction coupling. Nature 2002; 415:198–205
20. Zaccolo M, Movsesian MA: cAMP and cGMP signaling cross-talk: role of phosphodiesterases and implications for cardiac pathophysiology. Circ Res 2007; 100:1569–78
21. Mongillo M, McSorley T, Evellin S, et al.: Fluorescence resonance energy transfer-based analysis of cAMP dynamics in live neonatal rat cardiac myocytes reveals distinct functions of compartmentalized phosphodiesterases. Circ Res 2004; 95:67–75
22. Brodde OE: Beta-adrenoceptors in cardiac disease. Pharmacol Ther 1993; 60:405–30
23. Gauthier C, Tavernier G, Charpentier F, et al.: Functional beta 3-adrenoceptor in the human heart. J Clin Invest 1996; 98:556–62
24. Lobato EB, Gravenstein N, Martin TD: Milrinone, not epinephrine, improves left ventricular compliance after cardiopulmonary bypass. J Cardiothorac Vasc Anesth 2000; 14:374–7
25. Lobato EB, Willert JL, Looke TD, et al.: Effects of milrinone versus epinephrine on left ventricular relaxation after cardiopulmonary bypass following myocardial revascularization: assessment by color m-mode and tissue Doppler. J Cardiothorac Vasc Anesth 2005; 19:334–9
26. Maslow AD, Regan MM, Schwartz C, et al.: Inotropes improve right heart function in patients undergoing aortic valve replacement for aortic stenosis. Anesth Analg 2004; 98:891–902
27. Kristof AS, Magder S: Low systemic vascular resistance state in patients undergoing cardiopulmonary bypass. Crit Care Med 1999; 27:1121–7
28. Landry DW, Oliver JA: The pathogenesis of vasodilatory shock. N Engl J Med 2001; 345:588–95
29. Annane D, Vignon P, Renault A, et al.: Norepinephrine plus dobutamine versus epinephrine alone for management of septic shock: a randomised trial. Lancet 2007; 370:676–84
30. Lokhandwala MF, Vyas SJ, Hegde SS: Renal dopamine and tubular DA-1 receptors in the regulation of sodium excretion. J Auton Pharmacol 1990; 10 Suppl 1:s31–9

31. Yamaguchi I, Yao L, Sanada H, et al.: Dopamine D1A receptors and renin release in rat juxtaglomerular cells. Hypertension 1997; 29:962–8
32. Maskin CS, Ocken S, Chadwick B, LeJemtel TH: Comparative systemic and renal effects of dopamine and angiotensin-converting enzyme inhibition with enalaprilat in patients with heart failure. Circulation 1985; 72:846–52
33. Friedrich JO, Adhikari N, Herridge MS, Beyene J: Meta-analysis: low-dose dopamine increases urine output but does not prevent renal dysfunction or death. Ann Intern Med 2005; 142:510–24
34. Feneck RO, Sherry KM, Withington PS, Oduro-Dominah A: Comparison of the hemodynamic effects of milrinone with dobutamine in patients after cardiac surgery. J Cardiothorac Vasc Anesth 2001; 15:306–15
35. De Hert SG, Lorsomradee S, Cromheecke S, Van der Linden PJ: The effects of levosimendan in cardiac surgery patients with poor left ventricular function. Anesth Analg 2007; 104:766–73
36. Thackray S, Easthaugh J, Freemantle N, Cleland JG: The effectiveness and relative effectiveness of intravenous inotropic drugs acting through the adrenergic pathway in patients with heart failure-a meta-regression analysis. Eur J Heart Fail 2002; 4:515–29
37. Follath F, Cleland JG, Just H, et al.: Efficacy and safety of intravenous levosimendan compared with dobutamine in severe low-output heart failure (the LIDO study): a randomised double-blind trial. Lancet 2002; 360:196–202
38. Cuffe MS, Califf RM, Adams KF, Jr., et al.: Short-term intravenous milrinone for acute exacerbation of chronic heart failure: a randomized controlled trial. JAMA 2002; 287:1541–7
39. Felker GM, Benza RL, Chandler AB, et al.: Heart failure etiology and response to milrinone in decompensated heart failure: results from the OPTIME-CHF study. J Am Coll Cardiol 2003; 41:997–1003
40. Kivikko M, Lehtonen L: Levosimendan: a new inodilatory drug for the treatment of decompensated heart failure. Curr Pharm Des 2005; 11:435–55
41. Leszek P, Korewickia J, Klisiewicza A, et al.: Reduced myocardial expression of calcium handling protein in patients with severe chronic mitral regurgitation. Eur J Cardio-Thoracic Surg 2006; 30:737–43
42. Hasenfuss G, Meyer M, Schillinger W, et al.: Calcium handling proteins in the failing human heart. Basic Res Cardiol 1997; 92:87–93
43. Hasenfuss G, Reinecke H, Studer R, et al.: Relation between myocardial function and expression of sarcoplasmic reticulum Ca^{2+}-ATPase

in failing and nonfailing human myocardium. Circ Res 1994; 75:434–42

44. Gwathmey JK, Morgan JP: Altered calcium handling in experimental pressure-overload hypertrophy in the ferret. Circ Res 1985; 57:836–43
45. Baudet S, Noireaud J, Leoty C: Effect of haemodynamic pressure overload of the adult ferret right ventricle on inotropic responsiveness to external calcium and rest periods. Pflugers Archiv 1992; 420:603–10
46. Flemal K, Qiu Z, Ablin L et al.: Ca^{2+} handling and myofibrillar Ca^{2+} sensitivity in ferret cardiac myocytes with pressure-overload hypertrophy. Am J Physiol 1994; 267:H918–H24
47. del Monte F, Harding SE, Schmidt U, et al.: Restoration of contractile function in isolated cardiomyocytes from failing human hearts by gene transfer of SERCA2a. Circulation 1999; 100:2308–11
48. Davia K, Bernobich E, Ranu HK, et al.: SERCA2A overexpression decreases the incidence of aftercontractions in adult rabbit ventricular myocytes. J Mol Cell Cardiol 2001; 33:1005–15
49. Sakata S, Lebeche D, Sakata N, et al.: Targeted gene transfer increases contractility and decreases oxygen cost of contractility in normal rat hearts: restoration of mechanical and energetic function in failing aortic-banded rat hearts by gene transfer of calcium cycling proteins. Am J Physiol Heart Circ Physiol 2007; 292:H2356–63
50. Teerlink JR: The selective cardiac myosin activator CK-1827452, a calcium-independent inotrope, increases LV systolic function by increasing ejection time: results of a first-in-human study of a unique and novel mechanism. 10th Annual Scientific Meeting of the Heart Failure Society of America. Seattle, Washington, 2006
51. Singer M: Catecholamine treatment for shock-equally good or bad? Lancet 2007; 370:636–7

Wolfgang Toller, MD
Sylvia Archan, MD

2 Levosimendan

INTRODUCTION

The support of severely impaired myocardial contractile function and peripheral hypoperfusion with positive inotropic agents represents a mainstay of therapy in critically ill patients despite the lack of evidence for efficacy or safety. The currently available positive inotropic agents are catecholamines such as dobutamine, phosphodiesterase III inhibitors (PDEI) such as milrinone, and in some countries, calcium-sensitizing agents such as levosimendan.

β_1-adrenoceptor agonists and PDEI effectively enhance contractility and improve symptoms in patients with heart failure (HF), irrespective whether used during acute decompensation of chronic HF, contractile dysfunction after myocardial infarction, or stunning after cardiac surgery. These traditional drugs, however, have substantial limitations in the treatment of myocardial contractile dysfunction (1) because they enhance myocardial contractility, but also myocardial oxygen demand and the incidence of arrhythmias (2). These side effects are particularly detrimental in the presence of concomitant ischemia, as for example in patients with ischemic cardiomyopathy (3). A possible explanation for the poor safety record of traditional inotropic agents is that, despite different primary sites of action, all of these drugs eventually enhance myocardial contractility by increasing intracellular levels of cyclic adenosine monophosphate (cAMP), either generated by an increased rate of synthesis (β_1-

Advances in Cardiovascular Pharmacology, edited by Philippe R. Housmans, MD, PhD and Gregory A. Nuttall, M.D.
Lippincott Williams & Wilkins, Baltimore © 2008.

adrenoceptor agonists) or by a decreased rate of degradation (PDEI), which ultimately results in an augmentation of free calcium in the cytosol (4).

In contrast, calcium-sensitizers increase the calcium sensitivity of contractile regulatory proteins, causing an increase in myocardial contractility. These agents are free from the risk of calcium overload and do not require an increase in activation energy. Thus, they improve hemodynamic parameters with a minimum increase in energy expenditure and a low risk of arrhythmias, even under pathological conditions, such as acidosis and stunned myocardium. The change in the sensitivity of the myofilaments can be demonstrated by plotting the intracellular calcium concentration against the generated force (Figure 2–1). Under several conditions, e.g., stunning (5), ischemia (6), hypothermia (7) and others, the response of the myofilaments to calcium is decreased, i.e., the myofilaments are desensitized and the relationship is shifted to the right. The consequence of desensitization of the myofilaments is that more calcium is needed to achieve a sufficient response with a concomitant increase of myocardial oxygen demand. In contrast, calcium-sensitizers shift this relationship to the left (8), i.e., more contractile force is generated with the same amount of calcium. Thus, a neutral effect on myocardial energy consumption is observed.

In addition, due to their site of action, no antagonistic effects are observed when β-adrenergic antagonists are used in parallel. The calcium-sensitizer and vasodilator levosimendan is the most promising agent of this drug-group to date.

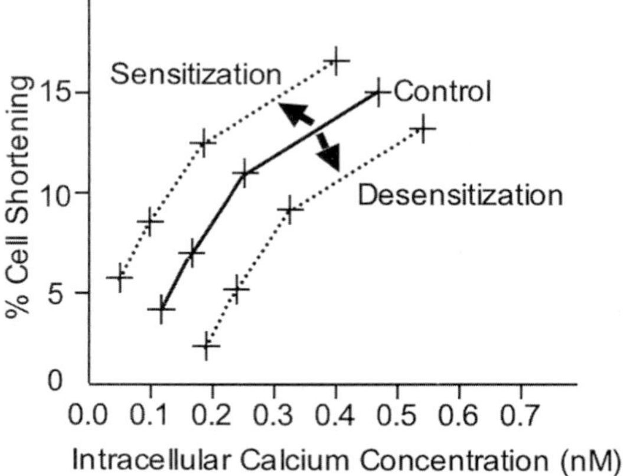

FIGURE 2–1. Relation between intracellular Ca^{2+} concentration and myocardial cell shortening.

LEVOSIMENDAN—MECHANISMS OF ACTION

Myofilament Ca^{2+} Sensitization. Levosimendan enhances myocardial contractility by binding to cardiac TnC with a high affinity (9–11) and stabilizing the Ca^{2+}-bound conformation of the regulatory protein (9). Therefore, systolic interaction of actin-myosin filaments is prolonged without alterating the rate of cross-bridge cycling. Other myofilament Ca^{2+} sensitizers are bound to the TnC-Ca^{2+} complex during both systole and diastole with improvement of systolic but possible impairment of diastolic function (12) due to facilitation of cross-bridging at diastolic Ca^{2+} levels. In contrast, binding of levosimendan to TnC is dependent on the cytosolic Ca^{2+} concentration; that is, it increases during systole but is relatively unchanged during diastole when Ca^{2+} levels decrease (13). This mechanism may be the reason for the parallel enhancement of myocardial contractility and improvement of left ventricular diastolic function (14) without promoting arrhythmogenesis or alteration of myocardial oxygen demand in experimental (13, 15, 16) and clinical (17, 18) studies.

Phosphodiesterase III Inhibition. In addition to myofilament Ca^{2+} sensitization, levosimendan inhibits cardiac PDE, predominantly PDE III (19), in muscle strips from human hearts (20) and various animal models (19, 21, 22). This effect is observed predominantly at higher concentrations (>100 ng/ml) (21, 23), but is not seen (10 ng/ml) or is less pronounced (33.33–100 ng/ml) at concentrations reflecting the clinically recommended therapeutic range of 10–100 ng/ml (24, 25). The less important impact of phosphodiesterase inhibition for the effects of levosimendan is also suggested by investigations comparing typical PDEI, e.g. milrinone with levosimendan. In this matter, levosimendan has substantially different and superior effects comparing influence on myocardial oxygen consumption (26, 27), vasodilation of pulmonary vasculature (28), incidence of ventricular arrhythmias during regional myocardial ischemia (29), improvement of diastolic function during septic conditions (30) and influence on gastric mucosal oxygenation (31) as compared with milrinone.

Opening of Potassium Channels-Vasodilation. Levosimendan produces vasodilation in several vasculatures including coronary (32–34), pulmonary (35), renal (36), splanchnic (36), cerebral (36), and systemic (27, 37) arteries as well as saphenous (38), portal (39), and systemic (27, 37) veins. An important mechanism in vascular smooth muscle of systemic, coronary (33, 40), and pulmonary (35) arteries is opening of potassium channels, including ATP-sensitive K^+ (K_{ATP}) channels in small resistance vessels and Ca^{2+}-activated K^+ and voltage-dependent K^+ channels in large conductance vessels (41, 42). Opening of these channels hyperpolarizes the membrane, inhibits inward Ca^{2+} current, and activates the Na^+-Ca^{2+} exchanger to extrude Ca^{2+}.

The resultant decrease in intracellular Ca^{2+} produces vasodilation. Attenuation of levosimendan-induced dilation of coronary arteries during concomitant administration of the K_{ATP} channel antagonist glibenclamide emphasizes the role of K_{ATP} channels in this setting (33, 40). A second mechanism involved in levosimendan-induced vasodilation is reduction of Ca^{2+} sensitivity of the (TnC-lacking) contractile proteins in vascular smooth muscle (43). This decrease in contractile force of vascular myofilaments occurs without a proportionate decrease in intracellular Ca^{2+}. In addition, PDE inhibition has been proposed to contribute to levosimendan-induced vasodilation because of increases in cAMP in vascular smooth muscle (44). This effect, however, predominantly occurs at excessive doses of levosimendan (34). Although the importance and relative contribution of each of these mechanisms of vasodilation is unclear and may be different in various vessels and dependent on the dose of levosimendan, an important role of K^+ channel opening is obvious, whereas the role of PDE inhibition remains to be defined.

Vasodilation observed with administration of levosimendan is followed by numerous consequences. Pulmonary vasodilation decreases right heart filling pressures (37), which, in context with positive inotropic effects, could explain increases in right ventricular contractility and improvement of right ventricular-vascular coupling (45) observed with administration of levosimendan (45–49). Systemic vasodilation decreases left heart filling pressures (50), enhances left ventricular-arterial coupling (27), and increases blood flow to various tissues, including myocardium, gastric mucosa (31), renal medulla, small intestine, and liver (36).

Systemic vasodilation produced by levosimendan may, identical to all vasodilators, naturally and indirectly be accompanied by hypotension and possibly arrhythmias, especially in patients who are highly dependent on a proper organ perfusion pressure, such as ischemic cardiomyopathy. While the decrease of systemic vascular resistance is a crucial target in the treatment of patients with acute HF, achievement and maintenance of an adequate perfusion pressure is also of utmost importance in these patients, because of the association of low blood pressure and negative outcome (51, 52). Therefore, a precise management of blood pressure is mandatory when levosimendan is administered, including adequate monitoring, proper mode of administration, correction of electrolytes and, if required, a transient use of vasopressors, such as norepinephrine.

K_{ATP} Channel Opening—Cardioprotection

Levosimendan opens both mitochondrial (53, 54) and sarcolemmal (55, 56) K_{ATP} channels. Although the definite relevance of these actions is unknown, opening of mitochondrial K_{ATP} channels has repeatedly been implicated in mediation of anti-ischemic actions (57). Prevention of mitochondrial Ca^{2+} overload, restoration and stabilization of mitochondrial membrane potential, preservation of high-energy phosphates, and regulation of mitochondrial matrix volume have been proposed as underlying mechanisms (58).

Levosimendan protected ischemic myocardium (59, 60) in isolated guinea pig and rabbit hearts and decreased myocardial infarct size when administered before and during myocardial ischemia in dogs (40). Furthermore, levosimendan started before coronary artery occlusion reduced the metabolic response as compared with administration of the drug during regional ischemia in pigs, suggesting a preconditioning effect (61). Beneficial effects in terms of survival, cardioprotection, antiarrhythmic activity, and metabolic status were also observed both after levosimendan pretreatment and ischemic preconditioning in rabbits. Consistently with mitochondrial K_{ATP} channel opening, these effects of levosimendan were abolished after administration of 5-HD, a mitochondrial K_{ATP} channel antagonist (62). In addition to K_{ATP} channel opening, a role of nitric oxide was proposed in mediating the cardioprotective effects of levosimendan because inhibition of nitric oxide synthase also antagonized cardioprotection by the drug (62). Consistently with cardioprotection, levosimendan-treated patients during cardiac surgery had lower postoperative troponin I concentrations than control patients without production of adverse effects (63).

Opening of sarcolemmal K_{ATP} channels has been implicated in both mediating cardioprotective effects (64) and exerting a theoretical proarrhythmic potential (65) initiated by the large outward repolarizing K^+ current. Subsequent hyperpolarization of resting membrane potential and shortening of action potential duration decreases the effective refractory period (66) of the tissue and thereby increases the susceptibility to reentrant arrhythmias. Although levosimendan indeed hyperpolarized membrane potential (55), shortened action potential duration in isolated cells (56), and slightly shortened effective refractory period in patients (67), experimental and clinical studies so far have demonstrated a neutral effect of this drug on heart rhythm rather than proarrhythmic potential (59, 67, 68).

Because levosimendan does not increase myocardial oxygen demand and possibly exerts anti-ischemic effects (40, 60, 69), efficacy and safety of this substance have been intensively tested before, during, and after ischemia-reperfusion injury in experimental and clinical studies. Levosimendan did not promote ischemia-reperfusion arrhythmias compared with dobutamine in guinea pig hearts (59) and in patients with stable moderate-to-severe ischemic cardiomyopathy when used in recommended clinical concentrations (6–24 μg/kg loading dose over 10 min, followed by an infusion of 0.05–0.2 μg/kg/min) in a double-blind, placebo-controlled, randomized, multicenter study (25). Furthermore, the incidence of arrhythmias was not increased when levosimendan was compared with placebo in patients with acute myocardial infarction (70) or administered perioperatively in patients with coronary artery bypass grafting (71). Although obviously having a neutral profile on heart rhythm, levosimendan consistently improved contractile function in the setting of global ischemia-reperfusion injury in experimental (59, 60, 72, 73) and clinical studies (17, 70, 71).

In contrast, experimental studies using regional myocardial ischemia demonstrated detrimental effects of levosimendan during ischemia, i.e., increase in the rate of ventricular arrhythmias (74) and worsening of the myocardial contractile function in the ischemic area (75). In addition, an increased frequency of ventricular arrhythmias was observed with very high doses of levosimendan in patients with stable ischemic cardiomyopathy (25) and in patients with acutely decompensated HF when a low blood pressure, additional vasodilators, and low serum potassium were present (51, 76). These diverse findings concerning heart rhythm may be related to indirect rather than direct proarrhythmic effects of levosimendan because of a vasodilation-mediated decline in coronary perfusion pressure. Therefore, as with any other vasodilator, caution is advised with the use of levosimendan, especially in high doses, in patients who have a risk for myocardial ischemia and are critically dependent on an adequate perfusion pressure. In these patients, modification of the mode of administration, reduction of the dose, and/or temporary administration of vasopressors are advisable.

CLINICAL TRIALS EVALUATING POSSIBLE INDICATIONS FOR LEVOSIMENDAN

The guidelines of the European Society of Cardiology recommend levosimendan as a second-line therapy for patients with AHF (Figure 2–2), when the initial therapy with continuous positive airway pressure, loop diuretics, and vasodilators had not been successful and the patient has adequate blood pressure (systolic blood pressure between 85 and 100 mm Hg) (class of recommendation IIa, level of evidence B) (77). Even though the drug has been on the market in several countries in Europe and South America for several years, it has not yet been approved in the USA, Germany, France, and the UK.

Acute Decompensation of Chronic Heart Failure

A comparison between the effects of levosimendan and dobutamine in 203 patients with acute decompensated low-output HF was performed

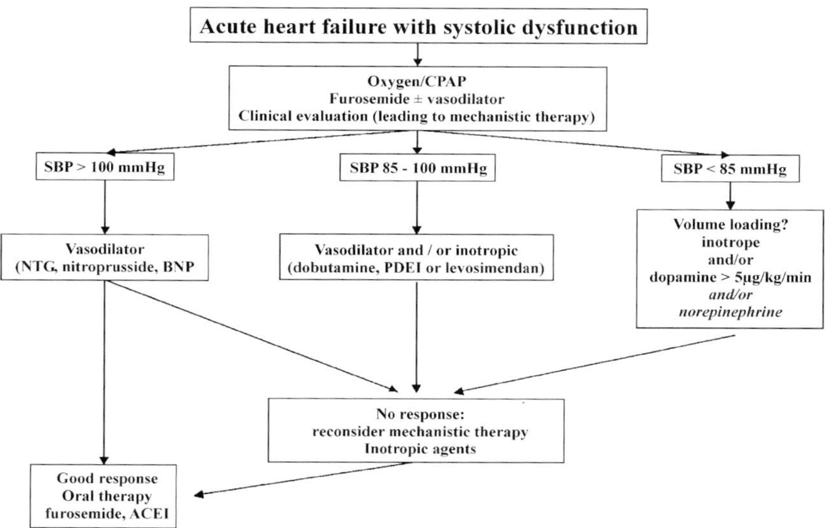

FIGURE 2–2. **Diagram of guidelines for treatment of acute heart failure.**

in a randomized, double-blind, multicenter trial (78). These patients had a left ventricular ejection fraction of less than 35%, a cardiac index of less than 2.5 L/min/m(2), and a pulmonary capillary wedge pressure (PCWP) of 15 mm Hg or greater on the basis of deterioration of severe chronic HF, HF after cardiac surgery, or acute HF related to a cardiac or noncardiac disorder of recent onset. A loading dose of levosimendan of 24 μg/kg was infused over 10 minutes, followed by a continuous infusion of 0.1 μg/kg/min for 24 hours. Dobutamine was infused for 24 hours at an initial dose of 5 μg/kg/min without a loading dose. The infusion rate of each drug was doubled if the response was inadequate at 2 hours. The primary endpoint was the proportion of patients with hemodynamic improvement (i.e., increase of cardiac output of 30% or more and decrease of PCWP of 25% or more) at 24 hours. All-cause mortality was assessed prospectively at 31 days and retrospectively at 180 days after randomization. Levosimendan treatment was superior to dobutamine in increasing cardiac output and decreasing PCWP, and a significantly greater proportion of patients in the levosimendan group achieved the primary endpoint compared with the dobutamine group (28% vs. 15%; $P = 0.022$). Although overall frequency of adverse events was similar, headache tended to be associated more frequently with levosimendan, whereas rhythm disorders and myocardial ischemia were more common with dobutamine. Administration of levosimendan was associated with both a significantly lower 31-day (8% vs. 17%; $P = 0.049$) and

180-day (26% vs. 38%; $P = 0.029$) mortality. Levosimendan was equally effective in patients with concurrent β_1-adrenoceptor blocker therapy, whereas the actions of dobutamine were attenuated, as expected.

Beneficial hemodynamic effects of levosimendan were also observed in a 6-h short-term treatment of 146 patients with acute decompensated ischemic or dilated cardiomyopathy in a multicenter, double-blind, placebo-controlled trial (37). In these patients with NYHA functional class III or IV symptoms of HF and ejection fractions of 30% or less, levosimendan therapy was initiated with a loading dose of 6 μg/kg, followed by an continuous infusion of 0.1 μg/kg/min. At hourly intervals, a repeat bolus of 6 μg/kg was given, and the infusion rate was up-titrated by increments of 0.1 μg/kg/min until a maximum rate of 0.4 μg/kg/min was achieved or a dose-limiting event occurred. The primary endpoint was the proportion of patients with an increase in stroke volume or a decrease in PCWP of 25% or more at 6 h. Levosimendan dose-dependently increased LV stroke volume (maximum 28% with the highest dose), cardiac index (maximum 39%), and heart rate (maximum 8%), and decreased PCWP (maximum 6 ± 1 mm Hg) when compared with placebo.

Due to the encouraging results of these and other moderate-size randomly controlled multicenter trials (70, 78), recently larger trials were performed to test the hypothesis that levosimendan might improve survival of patients with decompensated HF compared to placebo or to dobutamine.

The Randomized Multicenter Evaluation of Intravenous Levosimendan Efficacy (REVIVE-2) trial (76), evaluated the clinical course of 600 patients hospitalized for worsening HF, with a left ventricular ejection fraction ≤35% and dyspnea at rest despite intravenous administration of diuretics. All patients received current standard of care and placebo or levosimendan (loading dose of 6 or 12 μg/kg with a maintenance dose of either 0.1 or 0.2 μg/kg/min). Changes in symptoms, worsening HF, or death over 5 days were assessed as primary composite endpoints. Secondary endpoints included BNP levels, patient global and dyspnea assessment, days alive and out of hospital, death or worsening HF over 31 days, and all-cause mortality over 90 days. Patient characteristics were well matched between treatment groups, and similar proportions of patients in each group received ACE inhibitors, angiotensin receptor II blockers, β_1-adrenoceptor blockers, and intravenous vasodilators or inotropes. At day 5, more patients in the levosimendan group had improved (33%) and fewer had worsened as compared with the placebo group ($P = 0.015$ for both differences). Furthermore, 43% fewer patients needed rescue therapy for worsening HF. BNP levels were significantly reduced after 24 hours in levosimendan-treated patients compared with placebo ($P < 0.001$) and remained significantly lower at day

5 ($P = 0.001$). Ninety-day all-cause mortality, however, was higher in the levosimendan treatment arm (15.1% vs. 11.6%). Importantly, the risk of death was increased up to 10-fold in those with baseline systolic blood pressure <100 mm Hg receiving levosimendan. In contrast, when patients with baseline hypotension were excluded from the analysis, no excess mortality was seen with levosimendan.

The Survival of Patients with Acute Heart Failure in Need of Intravenous Inotropic Support (SURVIVE) study was a prospective, randomized trial to monitor long-term survival in 1327 patients with AHF (51). All patients had an ejection fraction of 30% or less and required intravenous inotropic support, as evidenced by an insufficient response to intravenous diuretics and/or vasodilators, and at least 1 of the following at screening: (1) dyspnea at rest or mechanical ventilation for acute decompensated HF; (2) oliguria not as a result of hypovolemia; or (3) PCWP of 18 mm Hg or higher and/or cardiac index of 2.2 L/min/m(2) or less. A loading dose of levosimendan (12 μg/kg) or placebo was administered over 10 minutes, followed by an infusion (0.1 μg/kg/min) for 50 minutes; the rate was increased to 0.2 μg/kg/min for an additional 23 hours as tolerated. The infusion of dobutamine or placebo was initiated at a rate of 5 μg/kg/min and could be increased at the discretion of the investigator to a maximum rate of 40 μg/kg/min. The infusion was maintained as long as clinically appropriate (minimum of 24 hours) and was tapered according to each patient's clinical status. The primary endpoint of the study was all-cause mortality during the 180 days. Secondary endpoints included all-cause mortality during 31 days, change in BNP level from baseline to 24 hours, number of days alive and out of the hospital during the 180 days, change in patient-assessed dyspnea at 24 hours, patient-assessed global assessment at 24 hours, and cardiovascular mortality through 180 days. The groups were well matched for cardiovascular history and other baseline characteristics: 86% and 85%, respectively, were in NYHA class IV, and mean left ventricular ejection fraction was 24% in both groups. In each group approximately 70% were receiving either ACE inhibitors or angiotensin receptor II blockers and approximately 54% were on β_1-adrenoceptor blockers. There was no significant difference between groups in the proportion of patients receiving other vasodilators or inotropes following randomization. Despite a marked initial decrease in plasma BNP level in patients in the levosimendan group, the results revealed no significant difference between levosimendan and dobutamine in all-cause mortality at 31 and 180 days after study drug infusion. A post-hoc analysis revealed that, in both treatment groups, a higher mortality was observed at all time points in patients whose baseline systolic blood pressure was <100 mm Hg.

Apart from the greater number of patients included, several possible explanations for the differences between the results of earlier trials and the REVIVE-2 and SURVIVE studies were subsequently discussed. First, the volume status of the patients in these studies obviously was different compared to earlier trials. While the initial studies with levosimendan included only "wet" patients according to the hemodynamic classification of HF patients (79), the REVIVE-2 and SURVIVE protocols also allowed "dry" patients to be included. Moreover, patients in REVIVE-2 and SURVIVE were not invasively monitored. A second possible explanation for these diverse findings related to the suggestion that levosimendan may have exerted beneficial survival effects only in a subgroup of AHF patients. Especially in patients receiving β_1-adrenoceptor antagonists, levosimendan outperformed dobutamine in earlier studies and also in a subanalysis of the SURVIVE trial (51). Similarly, treatment differences in favor of levosimendan were more apparent in patients with a history of HF as compared to those with a recent onset of HF (80). The individualized dosing strategy adopted for dobutamine in the SURVIVE trial offered a third possible explanation for the lack of differences between dobutamine and levosimendan. While patients received an average low dose of 6 µg/kg/min dobutamine, a high dosing regime of levosimendan was mandated, suggesting comparison of a low-dose dobutamine group with a high-dose levosimendan group of patients. Importantly, the high loading dose and rapid forced up-titration of levosimendan used in SURVIVE and REVIVE-2 did not reflect clinical practice in countries with the experience of thousands of administrations of levosimendan. Finally, major differences between countries in patient survival suggested that variable treatment practices may have influenced patient outcomes (81).

Combination with Catecholamines

Although there are no clinical data evaluating specific combinations of positive inotropic drugs, numerous reports suggest the efficacy and benefit of levosimendan in combination with dobutamine in patients with decompensated HF that is refractory to dobutamine alone (82–84).

Myocardial Ischemia and Cardioprotection

Safety, efficacy, and effects on mortality of various doses of levosimendan were investigated in the RUSSLAN (Randomized Study on Safety and Effectiveness of Levosimendan in Patients with Left Ventricular Failure due to an Acute Myocardial Infarct) study, when this drug or placebo was administered in 504 patients with LV failure complicating acute myocardial infarction in a randomized, double-blind, multicenter trial (70). In this investigation, four different dosing regimens of levosimendan were tested (6–24 μg/kg loading dose infused over a period of 10 minutes, followed by 6 hour infusions of 0.1–0.4 μg/kg/min). At the time of levosimendan administration, most patients were using nitrates and diuretics, approximately 40% were using ACE inhibitors or β_1-adrenoceptor blockers, and 17% had received thrombolysis. None of the patients had received percutaneous transluminal coronary angioplasty or coronary artery bypass grafting. In the highest dosing group (24 μg/kg loading dose followed by 0.4 μg/kg/min), a trend toward higher frequency of ischemia and hypotension was observed, but these effects were not evident at lower doses (6 μg/kg loading dose; 0.1–0.2 μg/kg/min). Importantly, this study suggests that levosimendan in low loading doses of 6 μg/kg and infusions of 0.1–0.2 μg/kg/min are favorable compared with higher doses, because they combine a low potential of side effects with a maintained positive effect on survival in patients with LV failure complicating acute myocardial infarction. In addition to the confirmation of a safe use of levosimendan in this study in patients with acute myocardial infarction, levosimendan-treated patients in general experienced a lower risk of death and worsening HF than patients receiving placebo during both the 6-hour infusion (2.0% vs. 5.9%) and over 24 hours (4.0% vs. 8.8%; $P = 0.044$). Furthermore, all-cause mortality among levosimendan-treated patients was significantly lower than with placebo for the 14-day period after the start of treatment (11.7% vs. 19.6%; $P = 0.031$) and exhibited a trend toward reduced mortality after 180 days of follow-up (22.6% vs. 31.4%; $P = 0.053$). However, an important limitation of the RUSSLAN study is that is was not prospectively designed and not adequately powered to show a difference in mortality as an end-point.

In addition to these beneficial effects in patients with acute myocardial infarction, a direct cardioprotective effect was suggested from earlier experimental studies due to opening of myocardial ATP-sensitive potassium channels by levosimendan. Accordingly, in a recent pilot study (63), 24 patients with stable angina undergoing elective CABG surgery were randomized to receive either placebo or levosimendan (24 μg/kg) infused intravenously over a 10-minute period just before placing the patient on cardiopulmonary bypass. Levosimendan-treated patients showed evidence of less myocardial damage, as manifested by lower postoperative troponin I concentrations, than control patients without production of adverse effects. Though statistical significance was not achieved because of the small sample size, these data are consistent with a preconditioning effect in humans.

Similarly, several reports of a successful use of levosimendan in the setting of myocardial stunning (17, 85, 86) suggest an important role of this drug especially in the setting of myocardial ischemia. This is also underlined by the fact that levosimendan improves ventriculo-arterial coupling and cardiovascular performance in coronary patients with LV dysfunction both by enhancing myocardial contractility and reducing arterial elastance (87).

Cardiogenic Shock

Despite its vasodilatory effects, successful and effective administration of levosimendan has been frequently reported, both as single substance or especially in combination with other catecholamines (85, 86, 88–92) during cardiogenic shock. These findings suggest an important role of the different mechanism of action as compared to other inotropes in this setting.

AREAS OF INTEREST FOR POTENTIAL FUTURE APPLICATION

Experience with levosimendan in several other clinical settings is encouraging due to its unique mechanisms of action that considerably differ from those of the traditional inotropes.

Right Ventricular Dysfunction

In addition to the beneficial effects on left-sided hemodynamics, levosimendan improved right ventricular performance and pulmonary hemodynamics in several experimental and clinical studies (48, 49, 93). Compared to dobutamine, levosimendan was superior in patients with depressed right ventricular function and elevated pulmonary arterial pressures because of similar inotropic effects, but additional pulmonary vasodilatory action (49).

In a clinically relevant porcine model of ischemia-reperfusion induced right ventricular dysfunction, Missant et al. demonstrated that levosimendan optimized right ventriculovascular coupling by moderately increasing right ventricular contractility and reducing right ventricular afterload (45). Importantly, levosimendan did not affect normal pulmonary vascular tone while effectively counteracting pulmonary vasoconstriction during pathologic conditions. In the perioperative period, several small studies report beneficial effects of levosimendan on severe right ventricular dysfunction following mitral valve replacement (94) or heart transplantation (95, 96).

Sepsis

Based on the pathophysiology of myocardial contractile dysfunction during sepsis, i.e. desensitization of myocardial myofilaments, administration of levosimendan theoretically may be an excellent alternative for hemodynamic optimization and improvement of splanchnic perfusion in septic shock. Accordingly, in a rabbit model of sepsis-induced myocardial dysfunction, levosimendan but not milrinone or dobutamine improved both systolic and diastolic cardiac function (30). Similarly, in a model of endotoxic shock, both levosimendan and dobutamine increased cardiac output and maintained whole body oxygen delivery, but only levosimendan prevented a decrease in mesenteric oxygen delivery (97). Superiority of levosimendan over milrinone and dobutamine in increasing gastric mucosal oxygenation in dogs (31) indicated redistribution of perfusion towards splanchnic organs by this drug. Although the clinical evidence for a benefit of levosimendan at the moment is restricted to case reports (98, 99), this drug in the future may become a prophylactic or therapeutic option to support the integrity of the gastrointestinal mucosa and to preserve or restore its barrier function with a subsequent attenuation of the onset or severity of organ failure.

Finally, experimental evidence suggests that levosimendan exerts beneficial effects on the kidneys during sepsis because of a substantial protection against endotoxemic acute renal failure in a rodent model (100).

Uptitration of β_1-adrenoceptor Blockade

The neutral effects of concomitant β_1-adrenoceptor blockade on the actions of levosimendan as compared to dobutamine (51, 78) suggest an interesting and important role during uptitration of β_1-adrenoceptor blockade in patients with severe contractile dysfunction. A prospective, randomized, open, parallel group trial of monthly 24-hour infusions with levosimendan and chronic infusion with prostaglandin E1, both facilitated uptitration of β_1-adrenoceptor blocker therapy in previously intolerant advanced CHF patients. Prostaglandin E1 treatment, however, allowed uptitration in more patients and resulted in a better clinical outcome compared to levosimendan (101). Whether shorter time intervals between levosimendan infusions might be more effective remains to be elucidated.

PRACTICAL USE OF LEVOSIMENDAN

Dosage and Prerequisites for Optimal Effect and Safety

While administration of a 6–24 mcg/kg loading dose delivered in 10 min followed by a 24-hour infusion at 0.05–0.2 mcg/kg/min was considered the optimal dosing regimen (25), the results of recent large clinical studies and the experience of many users suggest omission of the loading dose, especially in case of a low blood pressure before start of the infu-

TABLE 2–1. Prerequisites for optimal effect and safety before treatment with levosimendan

- Correct volume
- Correct electrolytes ($K^+ \geq 4, 5 \leq 5, 5$ mmol/L, $Mg^{2+} \geq 1, 0 \leq 1, 3$ mmol/L)
- Tight BP monitoring (especially during the first hours)
- Administer norepinephrine, if systolic blood pressure <90 mmHg
- Optimize diuretics (decrease dose or stop, then re-adapt)
- Continue β-Blockers (whenever possible)

sion (51, 76). Also, the dose should be reduced in patients with severe renal insufficiency, as the half-life of the levosimendan metabolites was prolonged 1.5-fold in patients with severe chronic renal failure and end-stage renal disease patients undergoing hemodialysis (102). The use of levosimendan (Table 2–1) should always be performed with a proper monitoring (invasive arterial blood pressure measurement, ECG, assessment of volume status such as central venous pressure) and should be preceded by a correction of the volume status and electrolytes (e.g. potassium and magnesium). β_1-adrenoceptor blockers should be continued whenever possible and diuretics discontinued or reduced in dose. In patients with a low blood pressure before the initiation of levosimendan, temporarily norepinephrine should be used in parallel to avoid further blood pressure drops until a steady state plasma concentration of levosimendan is reached.

Safety

At present, there is more controlled clinical data available on levosimendan than on any other intravenous inotropic drug. Levosimendan is generally well tolerated in moderate to severe HF patients, with an overall frequency of adverse events of 17%–29%, which is similar to that of placebo (17%–20%) (25, 37, 70). The most common adverse events reported in randomized placebo- or dobutamine-controlled clinical trials were hypotension, headache, ventricular tachycardia, and atrial fibrillation (51, 70, 78, 81). In the SURVIVE study, levosimendan was associated with a higher incidence of hypotension compared with dobutamine (16% vs. 14%) (51). In most clinical trials, no serious interactions with other routine HF drugs including angiotensin-converting enzyme (ACE) inhibitors, β_1-adrenoceptor blockers, digoxin, furosemide, and spironolactone have been reported (51, 81). Interestingly, a recent study demonstrated inhibitory effects of levosimendan on platelet function in an in vitro model at clinically relevant doses (103). Although the clinical relevance of this action is currently unknown, no detrimental effects on hemostasis in terms of increased bleeding during levosimendan treat-

TABLE 2–2. Recommendation for mode of administration of levosimendan

- Typically administer no bolus
- Typically start with continuous infusion (0,1 μg/kg/min)
- Time for first effects 2–4 hours
- Adapt dose after 2–4 hours (0,05 – 0,2 μg/kg/min)
- Bolus may be used if immediate effect necessary
- Bolus may be used if patient has high initial blood pressure
- Bolus may be used if patient is volume overloaded
- Typically administer 1 vial of levosimendan (costs)
- Second (or third) vial only if clinically necessary

ment so far have been reported. On the other hand, inhibitory effects on platelet aggregation might be beneficial particularly before or during states of myocardial ischemia. As suggested on the label of levosimendan, the drug should not be used in the presence of a glomerular filtration rate of less than 30 ml/min. While in the presence of renal dysfunction the dose of levosimendan clearly should be reduced (102), recent studies however also demonstrated improvements in renal function in patients awaiting heart transplantation (104) or hospitalized with decompensated HF (105). Therefore, the definitive role of levosimendan during renal dysfunction remains to be defined.

Perioperative Administration of Levosimendan

The clinical data on the perioperative administration of levosimendan are not as extensive as concerning the treatment of HF and are primarily restricted to cardiac surgery (106), but the efficacy of levosimendan during states of ischemia, myocardial stunning, and postoperative low-output states suggests that levosimendan in general might be a useful drug before, during, and after surgery (Table 2–2).

The rationale of preoperative administration of levosimendan is related to both possible preconditioning effects (63, 107) and the preparation of high-risk cardiomyopathic patients to the frequent hemodynamic derangements during surgery both in patients with preoperative low-output syndrome (108) and those with low-gradient low-output aortic stenosis (109, 110). Although these effects have not been investigated in a large number of patients, this concept appears very attractive and promising, because outcome of such patients is known to be poor, strategies for therapy lacking and administration of levosimendan can be performed without the necessity of a loading dose. At our institution, such patients are transferred to the PACU 4–12 hours preoperatively and receive levosimendan 0.1 μg/kg/min without a loading dose. Standard monitoring including ECG, pulsoxymetry, and invasive blood pressure measurement is performed and electrolytes including potassium and magnesium are corrected. Using this strategy, no serious adverse events have occurred so far.

Although levosimendan is also beneficial when started intraoperatively (83, 106, 111, 112) administration during this time is more challenging and requires the clinician to have some experience with the use of this drug because of its pharmacological profile. As intraoperatively, the requirement for a positive inotropic drug is mostly urgent and effects are needed within a few minutes, levosimendan typically has to be administered with a loading dose. While rapid positive inotropic effects can be achieved by such a strategy, the concomitant vasodilatory effects can produce hypotension in this situation due to additional anesthesia-related vasodilation and possibly relative hypovolemia. Consequently, parallel administration of a vasoconstrictor such as norepinephrine is frequently necessary in this situation. Despite the fact that levosimendan is sometimes started intraoperatively at our institution, we believe more easily titratable positive inotropic drugs with a short elimination half-life like dobutamine or epinephrine are preferable in this situation.

In contrast, most evidence regarding the perioperative use of levosimendan relates to the postoperative period including treatment of postcardiotomy low-cardiac output (28, 106, 113–117), acute graft failure after heart transplantation (96), weaning from postcardiotomy mechanical assist device (118), or intraaortic balloon counterpulsation (119). Compared to the intraoperative period, hemodynamic derangements, blood losses, and the effects of anesthesia are substantially lower in the postoperative period and therefore suggest a prudent and safe administration of levosimendan in this setting both as addition to or as replacement of other positive inotropic therapy. In our institution, we postoperatively administer levosimendan early without a loading dose in the situation of anticipated duration of standard catecholamine therapy for more than 3 days or existing combination of several catecholamines and PDEI. Administration of levosimendan in this setting is always a supplement to the existing positive inotropic therapy with a subsequent weaning and removal of other inotropic therapy. If another drug has to be added in rare cases of insufficient inotropic support by levosimendan alone, a combination of levosimendan with dobutamine is more effective than a combination of milrinone with dobutamine (83).

SUMMARY

Recent large-scale randomized trials have demonstrated a potential of levosimendan to decrease blood pressure and thereby produce arrhythmias, which in high-risk patients may be accompanied by detrimental effects on outcome. Importantly, although there seems to be no ideal inotropic agent at present, the differing mechanisms of action of levosimendan in comparison to other cardiotonic drugs provide a new approach in the management of cardiac failure; many other investigators have reported beneficial effects of levosimendan in various fields. From the positive experience of many users in the countries where the drug is approved, the necessity of precise monitoring and management has to be underlined in order to utilize the beneficial effects of the drug without producing avoidable side effects in these sick patients. The beneficial effects of levosimendan in patients receiving β_1-adrenoceptor blockers especially indicate that in general, low doses of inotropes and vasodilators should be used. Combinations of low doses of inotropes may be superior to a higher dose of a single drug. Derived from the practical experience with levosimendan, the drug can be effectively and safely used in these severely sick patients, but adequate circumstances similar to the treatment of other severe illnesses should be present.

References

1. Thackray S, Easthaugh J, Freemantle N, et al.: The effectiveness and relative effectiveness of intravenous inotropic drugs acting through the adrenergic pathway in patients with heart failure—a meta-regression analysis. Eur J Heart Fail 2002; 4:515–29
2. Burger AJ, Horton DP, LeJemtel T, et al.: Effect of nesiritide (B-type natriuretic peptide) and dobutamine on ventricular arrhythmias in the treatment of patients with acutely decompensated congestive heart failure: the PRECEDENT study. Am Heart J 2002; 144:1102–8
3. Felker GM, Benza RL, Chandler AB, et al.: Heart failure etiology and response to milrinone in decompensated heart failure: results from the OPTIME-CHF study. J Am Coll Cardiol 2003; 41:997–1003
4. Toller WG, Stranz C: Levosimendan, a new inotropic and vasodilator agent. Anesthesiology 2006; 104:556–69
5. Perez NG, Marban E, Cingolani HE: Preservation of myofilament calcium responsiveness underlies protection against myocardial stunning by ischemic preconditioning. Cardiovasc Res 1999; 42:636–43
6. Gao WD, Atar D, Backx PH, et al.: Relationship between intracellular calcium and contractile force in stunned myocardium. Direct evidence for decreased myofilament Ca^{2+} responsiveness and altered diastolic function in intact ventricular muscle. Circ Res 1995; 76:1036–48

7. Nakae Y, Fujita S, Namiki A: Isoproterenol enhances myofilament Ca^{2+} sensitivity during hypothermia in isolated guinea pig beating hearts. Anesth Analg 2001; 93:846–52
8. Haikala H, Nissinen E, Etemadzadeh E, et al.: Troponin C-mediated calcium sensitization induced by levosimendan does not impair relaxation. J Cardiovasc Pharmacol 1995; 25:794–801
9. Haikala H, Kaivola J, Nissinen E, et al.: Cardiac troponin C as a target protein for a novel calcium sensitizing drug, levosimendan. J Mol Cell Cardiol 1995; 27:1859–66
10. Pollesello P, Ovaska M, Kaivola J, et al.: Binding of a new Ca^{2+} sensitizer, levosimendan, to recombinant human cardiac troponin C. A molecular modelling, fluorescence probe, and proton nuclear magnetic resonance study. J Biol Chem 1994; 269:28584–90
11. Sorsa T, Pollesello P, Rosevear PR, et al.: Stereoselective binding of levosimendan to cardiac troponin C causes Ca^{2+}-sensitization. Eur J Pharmacol 2004; 486:1–8
12. Hajjar RJ, Schmidt U, Helm P, et al.: Ca^{++} sensitizers impair cardiac relaxation in failing human myocardium. J Pharmacol Exp Ther 1997; 280:247–54
13. Haikala H, Levijoki J, Linden IB: Troponin C-mediated calcium sensitization by levosimendan accelerates the proportional development of isometric tension. J Mol Cell Cardiol 1995; 27:2155–65
14. Givertz MM, Andreou C, Conrad CH, et al.: Direct myocardial effects of levosimendan in humans with left ventricular dysfunction: alteration of force-frequency and relaxation-frequency relationships. Circulation 2007; 115:1218–24
15. Sato S, Talukder MA, Sugawara H, et al.: Effects of levosimendan on myocardial contractility and Ca^{2+} transients in aequorin-loaded right-ventricular papillary muscles and indo-1-loaded single ventricular cardiomyocytes of the rabbit. J Mol Cell Cardiol 1998; 30:1115–28
16. McGough MF, Pagel PS, Lowe D, et al.: Effects of levosimendan on left ventricular function: correlation with plasma concentrations in conscious dogs. J Cardiothorac Vasc Anesth 1997; 11:49–53
17. Sonntag S, Sundberg S, Lehtonen LA, et al.: The calcium sensitizer levosimendan improves the function of stunned myocardium after percutaneous transluminal coronary angioplasty in acute myocardial ischemia. J Am Coll Cardiol 2004; 43:2177–82
18. Lilleberg J, Nieminen MS, Akkila J, et al.: Effects of a new calcium sensitizer, levosimendan, on haemodynamics, coronary blood flow and myocardial substrate utilization early after coronary artery bypass grafting. Eur Heart J 1998; 19:660–8

19. Szilagyi S, Pollesello P, Levijoki J, et al.: The effects of levosimendan and OR-1896 on isolated hearts, myocyte-sized preparations and phosphodiesterase enzymes of the guinea pig. Eur J Pharmacol 2004; 486:67–74
20. Hasenfuss G, Pieske B, Castell M, et al.: Influence of the novel inotropic agent levosimendan on isometric tension and calcium cycling in failing human myocardium. Circulation 1998; 98:2141–7
21. Edes I, Kiss E, Kitada Y, et al.: Effects of levosimendan, a cardiotonic agent targeted to troponin C, on cardiac function and on phosphorylation and Ca^{2+} sensitivity of cardiac myofibrils and sarcoplasmic reticulum in guinea pig heart. Circ Res 1995; 77:107–13
22. Boknik P, Neumann J, Kaspareit G, et al.: Mechanisms of the contractile effects of levosimendan in the mammalian heart. J Pharmacol Exp Ther 1997; 280:277–83
23. Lancaster MK, Cook SJ: The effects of levosimendan on $[Ca^{2+}]_i$ in guinea-pig isolated ventricular myocytes. Eur J Pharmacol 1997; 339:97–100
24. Jonsson EN, Antila S, McFadyen L, et al.: Population pharmacokinetics of levosimendan in patients with congestive heart failure. Br J Clin Pharmacol 2003; 55:544–51
25. Nieminen MS, Akkila J, Hasenfuss G, et al.: Hemodynamic and neurohumoral effects of continuous infusion of levosimendan in patients with congestive heart failure. J Am Coll Cardiol 2000; 36:1903–12
26. Kaheinen P, Pollesello P, Levijoki J, et al.: Effects of levosimendan and milrinone on oxygen consumption in isolated guinea-pig heart. J Cardiovasc Pharmacol 2004; 43:555–61
27. Pagel PS, Hettrick DA, Warltier DC: Comparison of the effects of levosimendan, pimobendan, and milrinone on canine left ventricular-arterial coupling and mechanical efficiency. Basic Res Cardiol 1996; 91:296–307
28. Al-Shawaf E, Ayed A, Vislocky I, et al.: Levosimendan or milrinone in the type 2 diabetic patient with low ejection fraction undergoing elective coronary artery surgery. J Cardiothorac Vasc Anesth 2006; 20:353–7
29. Papp JG, Pollesello P, Varro AF, et al.: Effect of levosimendan and milrinone on regional myocardial ischemia/reperfusion-induced arrhythmias in dogs. J Cardiovasc Pharmacol Ther 2006; 11:129–35
30. Barraud D, Faivre V, Damy T, et al.: Levosimendan restores both systolic and diastolic cardiac performance in lipopolysaccharide-treated rabbits: comparison with dobutamine and milrinone. Crit Care Med 2007; 35:1376–82

31. Schwarte LA, Picker O, Bornstein SR, et al.: Levosimendan is superior to milrinone and dobutamine in selectively increasing microvascular gastric mucosal oxygenation in dogs. Crit Care Med 2005; 33:135–42
32. Michaels AD, McKeown B, Kostal M, et al.: Effects of intravenous levosimendan on human coronary vasomotor regulation, left ventricular wall stress, and myocardial oxygen uptake. Circulation 2005; 111:1504–9
33. Kaheinen P, Pollesello P, Levijoki J, et al.: Levosimendan increases diastolic coronary flow in isolated guinea-pig heart by opening ATP-sensitive potassium channels. J Cardiovasc Pharmacol 2001; 37:367–74
34. Gruhn N, Nielsen Kudsk JE, Theilgaard S, et al.: Coronary vasorelaxant effect of levosimendan, a new inodilator with calcium-sensitizing properties. J Cardiovasc Pharmacol 1998; 31:741–9
35. De Witt BJ, Ibrahim IN, Bayer E, et al.: An analysis of responses to levosimendan in the pulmonary vascular bed of the cat. Anesth Analg 2002; 94:1427–33
36. Pagel PS, Hettrick DA, Warltier DC: Influence of levosimendan, pimobendan, and milrinone on the regional distribution of cardiac output in anaesthetized dogs. Br J Pharmacol 1996; 119:609–15
37. Slawsky MT, Colucci WS, Gottlieb SS, et al.: Acute hemodynamic and clinical effects of levosimendan in patients with severe heart failure. Circulation 2000; 102:2222–7
38. Hohn J, Pataricza J, Petri A, et al.: Levosimendan interacts with potassium channel blockers in human saphenous veins. Basic Clin Pharmacol Toxicol 2004; 94:271–3
39. Pataricza J, Hohn J, Petri A, et al.: Comparison of the vasorelaxing effect of cromakalim and the new inodilator, levosimendan, in human isolated portal vein. J Pharm Pharmacol 2000; 52:213–7
40. Kersten JR, Montgomery MW, Pagel PS, et al.: Levosimendan, a new positive inotropic drug, decreases myocardial infarct size via activation of K_{ATP} channels. Anesth Analg 2000; 90:5–11
41. Pataricza J, Krassoi I, Hohn J, et al.: Functional role of potassium channels in the vasodilating mechanism of levosimendan in porcine isolated coronary artery. Cardiovasc Drugs Ther 2003; 17:115–21
42. Yokoshiki H, Sperelakis N: Vasodilating mechanisms of levosimendan. Cardiovasc Drugs Ther 2003; 17:111–3
43. Bowman P, Haikala H, Paul RJ: Levosimendan, a calcium sensitizer in cardiac muscle, induces relaxation in coronary smooth muscle through calcium desensitization. J Pharmacol Exp Ther 1999; 288:316–25

44. Haikala H, Linden IB: Mechanisms of action of calcium-sensitizing drugs. J Cardiovasc Pharmacol 1995; 26 Suppl 1:S10–9
45. Missant C, Rex S, Segers P, et al.: Levosimendan improves right ventriculovascular coupling in a porcine model of right ventricular dysfunction. Crit Care Med 2007; 35:707–15
46. Leather HA, Ver Eycken K, Segers P, et al.: Effects of levosimendan on right ventricular function and ventriculovascular coupling in open chest pigs. Crit Care Med 2003; 31:2339–43
47. Ukkonen H, Saraste M, Akkila J, et al.: Myocardial efficiency during levosimendan infusion in congestive heart failure. Clin Pharmacol Ther 2000; 68:522–31
48. Parissis JT, Paraskevaidis I, Bistola V, et al.: Effects of levosimendan on right ventricular function in patients with advanced heart failure. Am J Cardiol 2006; 98:1489–92
49. Kerbaul F, Rondelet B, Demester JP, et al.: Effects of levosimendan versus dobutamine on pressure load-induced right ventricular failure. Crit Care Med 2006; 34:2814–9
50. Duygu H, Ozerkan F, Nalbantgil S, et al.: Effect of levosimendan on E/E′ ratio in patients with ischemic heart failure. Int J Cardiol 2007
51. Mebazaa A, Nieminen MS, Packer M, et al.: Levosimendan vs dobutamine for patients with acute decompensated heart failure: the SURVIVE Randomized Trial. JAMA 2007; 297:1883–91
52. Gheorghiade M, Abraham WT, Albert NM, et al.: Systolic blood pressure at admission, clinical characteristics, and outcomes in patients hospitalized with acute heart failure. JAMA 2006; 296:2217–26
53. Kopustinskiene DM, Pollesello P, Saris NE: Levosimendan is a mitochondrial K_{ATP} channel opener. Eur J Pharmacol 2001; 428:311–4
54. Kopustinskiene DM, Pollesello P, Saris NE: Potassium-specific effects of levosimendan on heart mitochondria. Biochem Pharmacol 2004; 68:807–12
55. Yokoshiki H, Katsube Y, Sunagawa M, et al.: Levosimendan, a novel Ca^{2+} sensitizer, activates the glibenclamide-sensitive K^+ channel in rat arterial myocytes. Eur J Pharmacol 1997; 333:249–59
56. Yokoshiki H, Katsube Y, Sunagawa M, et al.: The novel calcium sensitizer levosimendan activates the ATP-sensitive K^+ channel in rat ventricular cells. J Pharmacol Exp Ther 1997; 283:375–83
57. Gross GJ, Fryer RM: Mitochondrial K_{ATP} channels: triggers or distal effectors of ischemic or pharmacological preconditioning? Circ Res 2000; 87:431–3
58. Gross GJ, Peart JN: K_{ATP} channels and myocardial preconditioning: an update. Am J Physiol Heart Circ Physiol 2003; 285:H921–30

59. Du Toit EF, Muller CA, McCarthy J, et al.: Levosimendan: effects of a calcium sensitizer on function and arrhythmias and cyclic nucleotide levels during ischemia/reperfusion in the Langendorff-perfused guinea pig heart. J Pharmacol Exp Ther 1999; 290:505–14
60. Rump AF, Acar D, Rosen R, et al.: Functional and antiischaemic effects of the phosphodiesterase inhibitor levosimendan in isolated rabbit hearts. Pharmacol Toxicol 1994; 74:244–8
61. Metzsch C, Liao Q, Steen S, et al.: Levosimendan cardioprotection reduces the metabolic response during temporary regional coronary occlusion in an open chest pig model. Acta Anaesthesiol Scand 2007; 51:86–93
62. Das B, Sarkar C: Pharmacological preconditioning by levosimendan is mediated by inducible nitric oxide synthase and mitochondrial K_{ATP} channel activation in the in vivo anesthetized rabbit heart model. Vascul Pharmacol 2007; 47:248–56
63. Tritapepe L, De Santis V, Vitale D, et al.: Preconditioning effects of levosimendan in coronary artery bypass grafting—a pilot study. Br J Anaesth 2006; 96:694–700
64. Gross GJ, Fryer RM: Sarcolemmal versus mitochondrial ATP-sensitive K^+ channels and myocardial preconditioning. Circ Res 1999; 84:973–9
65. Fischbach PS, White A, Barrett TD, et al.: Risk of ventricular proarrhythmia with selective opening of the myocardial sarcolemmal versus mitochondrial ATP-gated potassium channel. J Pharmacol Exp Ther 2004; 309:554–9
66. Wilde AA, Janse MJ: Electrophysiological effects of ATP sensitive potassium channel modulation: implications for arrhythmogenesis. Cardiovasc Res 1994; 28:16–24
67. Singh BN, Lilleberg J, Sandell E-P, et al.: Effects of levosimendan on cardiac arrhythmia: electrophysiologic and ambulatory electrocardiographic findings in phase II and phase III clinical studies in cardiac failure. Am J Cardiol 1999; 83:16–20
68. Lilleberg J, Ylonen V, Lehtonen L, et al.: The calcium sensitizer levosimendan and cardiac arrhythmias: an analysis of the safety database of heart failure treatment studies. Scand Cardiovasc J 2004; 38:80–4
69. Rump AF, Acar D, Klaus W: A quantitative comparison of functional and anti-ischaemic effects of the phosphodiesterase-inhibitors, amrinone, milrinone and levosimendan in rabbit isolated hearts. Br J Pharmacol 1994; 112:757–62
70. Moiseyev VS, Poder P, Andrejevs N, et al.: Safety and efficacy of a novel calcium sensitizer, levosimendan, in patients with left ventricular failure due to an acute myocardial infarction. A random-

ized, placebo-controlled, double-blind study (RUSSLAN). Eur Heart J 2002; 23:1422–32

71. Nijhawan N, Nicolosi AC, Montgomery MW, et al.: Levosimendan enhances cardiac performance after cardiopulmonary bypass: a prospective, randomized placebo-controlled trial. J Cardiovasc Pharmacol 1999; 34:219–28
72. Chen Q, Camara AK, Rhodes SS, et al.: Cardiotonic drugs differentially alter cytosolic [Ca^{2+}] to left ventricular relationships before and after ischemia in isolated guinea pig hearts. Cardiovasc Res 2003; 59:912–25
73. Eriksson O, Pollesello P, Haikala H: Effect of levosimendan on balance between ATP production and consumption in isolated perfused guinea-pig heart before ischemia or after reperfusion. J Cardiovasc Pharmacol 2004; 44:316–21
74. Du Toit E, Hofmann D, McCarthy J, et al.: Effect of levosimendan on myocardial contractility, coronary and peripheral blood flow, and arrhythmias during coronary artery ligation and reperfusion in the in vivo pig model. Heart 2001; 86:81–7
75. Tassani P, Schad H, Heimisch W, et al.: Effect of the calcium sensitizer levosimendan on the performance of ischaemic myocardium in anaesthetised pigs. Cardiovasc Drugs Ther 2002; 16:435–41
76. Packer M: REVIVEII: Multicenter placebo-controlled trial of levosimendan on clinical status in acutely decompensated heart failure. American Heart Association Scientific Sessions 2005; Late Breaking Clinical Trials II
77. Nieminen MS, Bohm M, Cowie MR, et al.: Executive summary of the guidelines on the diagnosis and treatment of acute heart failure. Eur Heart J 2005; 26:384–416
78. Follath F, Cleland JG, Just H, et al.: Efficacy and safety of intravenous levosimendan compared with dobutamine in severe low-output heart failure (the LIDO study): a randomised double-blind trial. Lancet 2002; 360:196–202.
79. Nohria A, Lewis E, Stevenson LW: Medical management of advanced heart failure. JAMA 2002; 287:628–40.
80. Cohen-Solal A, Mebazaa A, Thakkar R, et al.: Levosimendan, compared to dobutamine, reduces mortality in patients with a history of heart failure. Eur J Heart Fail 2007; 6 (Suppl):109
81. Cleland JG, Freemantle N, Coletta AP, et al.: Clinical trials update from the American Heart Association: REPAIR-AMI, ASTAMI, JELIS, MEGA, REVIVE-II, SURVIVE, and PROACTIVE. Eur J Heart Fail 2006; 8:105–10

82. Cavusoglu Y: The use of levosimendan in comparison and in combination with dobutamine in the treatment of decompensated heart failure. Expert opinion on pharmacotherapy 2007; 8:665–77
83. De Hert SG, Lorsomradee S, Cromheecke S, et al.: The effects of levosimendan in cardiac surgery patients with poor left ventricular function. Anesth Analg 2007; 104:766–73
84. Nanas JN, Papazoglou PP, Terrovitis JV, et al.: Hemodynamic effects of levosimendan added to dobutamine in patients with decompensated advanced heart failure refractory to dobutamine alone. Am J Cardiol 2004; 94:1329–32
85. Ellger BM, Zahn PK, Van Aken HK, et al.: Levosimendan: a promising treatment for myocardial stunning? Anaesthesia 2006; 61:61–3
86. Lechner E, Moosbauer W, Pinter M, et al.: Use of levosimendan, a new inodilator, for postoperative myocardial stunning in a premature neonate. Pediatr Crit Care Med 2007; 8:61–3
87. Guarracino F, Cariello C, Danella A, et al.: Effect of levosimendan on ventriculo-arterial coupling in patients with ischemic cardiomyopathy. Acta Anaesthesiol Scand 2007; 51:1217–24
88. Rokyta Jr R, Pechman V. The effects of levosimendan on global haemodynamics in patients with cardiogenic shock. Neuro Endocrinol Lett 2006; 27:121–7
89. Tsagalou EP, Nanas JN: Resuscitation from adrenaline resistant electro-mechanical dissociation facilitated by levosimendan in a young man with idiopathic dilated cardiomyopathy. Resuscitation 2006; 68:147–9
90. Delle Karth G, Buberl A, Geppert A, et al.: Hemodynamic effects of a continuous infusion of levosimendan in critically ill patients with cardiogenic shock requiring catecholamines. Acta Anaesthesiol Scand 2003; 47:1251–6
91. Lehmann A, Lang J, Boldt J, et al.: Levosimendan in patients with cardiogenic shock undergoing surgical revascularization: a case series. Med Sci Monit 2004; 10:MT89–93
92. Russ MA, Prondzinsky R, Christoph A, et al.: Hemodynamic improvement following levosimendan treatment in patients with acute myocardial infarction and cardiogenic shock. Crit Care Med 2007
93. Morelli A, Teboul JL, Maggiore SM, et al.: Effects of levosimendan on right ventricular afterload in patients with acute respiratory distress syndrome: a pilot study. Crit Care Med 2006; 34:2287–93
94. Morais RJ: Levosimendan in severe right ventricular failure following mitral valve replacement. J Cardiothorac Vasc Anesth 2006; 20:82–4

95. Petäjä LM, Sipponen JT, Hämmäinen PJ, et al.: Levosimendan reversing low output syndrome after heart transplantation. Ann Thorac Surg 2006; 82:1529–31
96. Beiras-Fernandez A, Weis FC, Fuchs H, et al.: Levosimendan treatment after primary organ failure in heart transplantation: a direct way to recovery? Transplantation 2006; 82:1101–3
97. Dubin A, Murias G, Sottile JP, et al.: Effects of levosimendan and dobutamine in experimental acute endotoxemia: a preliminary controlled study. Intensive Care Med 2007; 33:485–94
98. Powell BP, De Keulenaer BL: Levosimendan in septic shock: a case series. Br J Anaesth 2007; 99:447–8
99. Ramaswamykanive H, Bihari D, Solano TR: Myocardial depression associated with pneumococcal septic shock reversed by levosimendan. Anaesth Intens Care 2007; 35:409–13
100. Zager RA, Johnson AC, Lund S, et al.: Levosimendan protects against experimental endotoxemic acute renal failure. Am J Physiol Renal Physiol 2006; 290:F1453-F62
101. Berger R, Moertl D, Huelsmann M, et al.: Levosimendan and prostaglandin E1 for uptitration of beta-blockade in patients with refractory, advanced chronic heart failure. Eur J Heart Fail 2007; 9:202–8
102. Puttonen J, Kantele S, Kivikko M, et al.: Effect of severe renal failure and haemodialysis on the pharmacokinetics of levosimendan and its metabolites. Clin Pharmacokinet 2007; 46:235–46
103. Kaptan K, Erinc K, Ifran A, et al.: Levosimendan has an inhibitory effect on platelet function. Am J Hematol 2007
104. Zemljic G, Bunc M, Yazdanbakhsh AP, et al.: Levosimendan improves renal function in patients with advanced chronic heart failure awaiting cardiac transplantation. Journal of cardiac failure 2007; 13:417–21
105. Yilmaz MB, Yalta K, Yontar C, et al.: Levosimendan improves renal function in patients with acute decompensated heart failure: comparison with dobutamine. Cardiovasc Drugs Ther 2007
106. Raja SG, Rayen BS: Levosimendan in cardiac surgery: current best available evidence. Ann Thorac Surg 2006; 81:1536–46
107. Pollesello P, Papp Z: The cardioprotective effects of levosimendan: preclinical and clinical evidence. J Cardiovasc Pharmacol 2007; 50:257–63
108. Tasouli A, Papadopoulos K, Antoniou T, et al.: Efficacy and safety of perioperative infusion of levosimendan in patients with compromised cardiac function undergoing open-heart surgery: importance of early use. Eur J Cardiothorac Surg 2007

109. Hoefer D, Jonetzko P, Hoermann C, et al.: Successful administration of levosimendan in a patient with low-gradient low-output aortic stenosis. Wien Klin Wochenschr 2006; 118:60–2
110. Prior DL, Flaim BD, MacIsaac AI, et al.: Pre-operative use of levosimendan in two patients with severe aortic stenosis and left ventricular dysfunction. Heart Lung Circ 2006; 15:56–8
111. Akgul A, Mavioglu L, Katircioglu SF, et al.: Levosimendan for weaning from cardiopulmonary bypass after coronary artery bypass grafting. Heart Lung Circ 2006; 15:320–4
112. Barisin S, Husedzinovic I, Sonicki Z, et al.: Levosimendan in off-pump coronary artery bypass: a four-times masked controlled study. J Cardiovasc Pharmacol 2004; 44:703–8
113. Malliotakis P, Xenikakis T, Linardakis M, et al.: Haemodynamic effects of levosimendan for low cardiac output after cardiac surgery: a case series. Hellenic J Cardiol 2007; 48:80–8
114. Alvarez J, Bouzada M, Fernandez AL, et al.: Hemodynamic effects of levosimendan compared with dobutamine in patients with low cardiac output after cardiac surgery. Rev Esp Cardiol 2006; 59:338–45
115. Caimmi PP, Grossini E, Molinari C, et al.: Intracoronary infusion of levosimendan to treat postpericardiotomy heart failure. Ann Thorac Surg 2006; 82:e33–4
116. Labriola C, Siro Brigiani M, Carrata F, et al.: Hemodynamic effects of levosimendan in patients with low-output heart failure after cardiac surgery. Int J Clin Pharmacol Ther 2004; 42:204–11
117. Ploechl W, Rajek A: The use of the novel calcium sensitizer levosimendan in critically ill patients. Anaesth Intens Care 2004; 32:471–5
118. Braun JP, Jasulaitis D, Moshirzadeh M, et al.: Levosimendan may improve survival in patients requiring mechanical assist devices for post-cardiotomy heart failure. Crit Care 2006; 10:R17
119. Tokuda Y, Grant PW, Wolfenden HD, et al.: Levosimendan for patients with impaired left ventricular function undergoing cardiac surgery. Interact CardioVasc Thorac Surg 2006; 5:322–6

Juan N. Pulido, MD
Daryl J. Kor, MD

3 β-Adrenergic Receptor Antagonists

INTRODUCTION

The understanding of the sympathetic nervous system and its complex contributions to health and disease continues to evolve, underlining its importance in numerous cardiovascular diseases and perioperative medicine. It is well recognized that sympathetic over-activity plays a significant role in the genesis and progression of heart failure (1), hypertension, and ischemic heart disease, all of which comprise a major epidemiologic concern in the industrialized world.

Sympathetic stimulation induces a variety of physiological effects, such as tachycardia, augmentation of cardiac contractility, vascular tone, modulation of bronchial and gastrointestinal smooth muscle tone, and carbohydrate and lipid metabolism. These actions are mediated through a family of nine G-protein coupled receptors linked to a second-messenger system. This adrenergic receptor family is divided into five major types: α_1, α_2, β_1, β_2, and β_3 receptors. This review will focus on the β-adrenergic receptor (β-AR) subfamily, the current understanding of the β-adrenergic signal-transduction pathways and β-AR antagonists, concluding with the clinical uses and current perspectives and controversies of β-blocker therapy in perioperative medicine.

β-ADRENERGIC RECEPTORS

The β-AR were historically subdivided into β_1 and β_2 receptors on the basis of the response to epinephrine and norepinephrine in different tis-

Advances in Cardiovascular Pharmacology, edited by Philippe R. Housmans, MD, PhD and Gregory A. Nuttall, M.D.
Lippincott Williams & Wilkins, Baltimore © 2008.

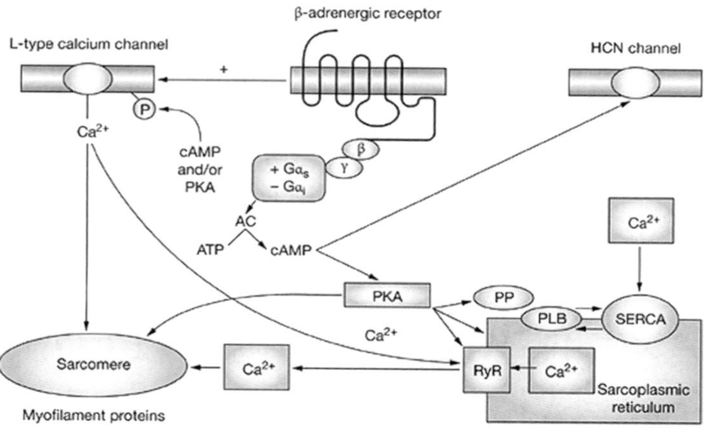

FIGURE 3–1. β-adrenergic receptor signaling.

sues (2). The receptors mediating the responses in the heart were designated β_1 and those responsible for vasorelaxation and bronchodilation were designated β_2. Current understanding is that the ratio of β_1 to β_2 receptors in a normal human heart is approximately 70:30 to 80:20 (atria vs. ventricle); this ratio varies depending on age and pathologic state (3, 4). A β_3 receptor that mediates thermogenesis and lipolysis in brown and white fat, respectively, was characterized in 1989 and probably plays a role in the failing heart (5). All β-ARs belong to the G-protein coupled receptor (GPCR) family, consisting of seven transmembrane domains with the NH_2 terminus being extracellular and glycosylated and an intracellular C-terminus with sites for phosphorylation by protein kinase A (PKA) and β-adrenoreceptor kinase (β-ARK) (6). The β-ARK-β-arrestin mechanism helps to terminate the β receptor signal by a rapid desensitization of the receptor (7). This mechanism plays a mayor role in long-term desensitization of the β-AR in heart failure.

Once a β-AR is activated, a series of intracellular events are initiated by the activation of a member of the G-protein subfamily. Depending on receptor type, this can be an inhibitory (G_i) or excitatory (G_s) pathway (Figure 3–1). β_1-ARs activate the G_s pathway with an increase in cyclic AMP (cAMP) via adenylyl cyclase (AC). Alternatively, β_2-ARs can activate either the G_i or G_s signaling pathway, depending on the type of stimuli, tissue, or cell line involved. The G_s signaling pathway stimulates AC, increasing the production of cAMP and activation of PKA. This modulates the activity of various proteins required for optimal myocyte function and calcium homeostasis (e.g., L-type calcium channels, ryanodine receptors, troponin T, phospholamban, hyperpolarization-activated cyclic nucleotide-gated (HCN) channels, and myosin-binding proteins) (8). Conversely, the G_i pathway regulates receptor signaling and nuclear transcription and decreases production of cAMP. It is important to understand that while both receptors (β_1 and β_2) bind to G_s and thereby elevate intracellular concentrations of cAMP, distinct downstream signaling pathways increase contractility in cardiac myocytes (β_1) and decrease it in smooth muscle cells (β_2). The perceived global activity of any cell is the sum of multiple serial events, the combination of which leads to cellular changes resulting in alterations in organ function, such as vasodilation, positive chronotropy, inotropy and lusitropy, and bronchodilation.

β-ARs are also present in non-myocytes cell lines in the heart. These cells can affect myocyte function via paracrine effects. It is postulated that this discrete intercellular signaling mechanism may also play a role in health and disease (8).

In addition to the complex balance of interactions that determine intracellular signaling, the β-ARs are also known to be polymorphic. There are at least two functionally important single nucleotide polymorphisms (SNPs) in the β_1-adrenergic receptor gene: at position 49 in the extracellular NH_2 terminus of the β_1-AR and at position 389 of the intracellular C terminus. In the former (Ser49Gly), glycine replaces serine at position 49, resulting in a variant that seems to exhibit faster downregulation after long-term adrenergic stimulation. The latter results from glycine replacing arginine at position 389 (Arg389Gly). This particular variant displays higher adenylyl cyclase activity (9). These SNPs exemplify how genomics can play a significant role in the genesis and progression of disease, and the variable therapeutic response with attempts at pharmacologic intervention.

Finally, enhanced activation of the β-adrenergic signaling pathway has been shown to result in myocardial cell apoptosis (10, 11). This lends credence to the potential role of excessive adrenergic stimulation in the pathogenesis of heart failure as it leads to the architectural rearrangement of myocytes, ventricular remodeling, and decreased contractile function in the failing heart. Indeed, circulating catecholamine levels are reliable markers for the severity and outcome of congestive heart failure and support the neurohormonal hypothesis of the progression of this disease (12).

β-ADRENERGIC RECEPTOR ANTAGONISTS

The pharmacologic properties of β-AR antagonists (β-blockers) are best explained by examining the various responses elicited by β-AR stimulation (Table 3–1).

These medications are competitive antagonists of the β-AR and vary in their selectivity between the two major subclasses of β-ARs (β_1 and

TABLE 3–1. Physiologic Properties of β-AR Stimulation in Various Tissues

Tissue	Receptor	Response to stimulus
Heart		
SA node	$\beta_1 > \beta_2$	Increased heart rate
Atria	$\beta_1 > \beta_2$	Increased contractility and conduction velocity
AV node	$\beta_1 > \beta_2$	Increased automaticity and conduction velocity
His-Purkinje system	$\beta_1 > \beta_2$	Increased automaticity and conduction velocity
Ventricles	$\beta_1 > \beta_2$	Increased automaticity, contractility and conduction velocity
Arteries		
Peripheral	β_2	Vasodilation
Coronary	β_2	Vasodilation
Carotid	β_2	Vasodilation
Other		
Lungs	β_2	Bronchodilation
Liver	β_2	Increased glycogenolysis
Muscle	β_2	Increased glycogenolysis
Uterus	β_2	Smooth muscle relaxation
Eyes (ciliary muscle)	β_2	Relaxation (mydriasis)
Kidney	β_1	Increased rennin secretion (juxtaglomerular apparatus)
Posterior pituitary	β_1	ADH secretion
Pancreas	β_1	Increased insulin release
Adipose tissue	β_1, β_2, β_3	Increased lipolysis

β_2). Other important differences within this class of medications include the presence or absence of intrinsic sympathomimetic activity, degree of absorption, protein binding, bioavailability, lipid solubility, and activity against α-adrenergic receptors (Table 3–2).

β-Blocker Properties

Cardioselectivity

Cardioselectivity refers to the relative antagonism of the β_1-AR located primarily in the heart compared with the β_2-AR located in numerous areas throughout the body (e.g., lungs, peripheral blood vessels, liver, and muscle).

Intrinsic Sympathomimetic Activity

Intrinsic sympathomimetic activity (ISA) refers to the presence of partial β-AR agonist activity. Agents with this property can induce a measurable sympathetic response while blocking the more potent agonist

TABLE 3–2. Pharmacologic/Pharmacokinetic Properties of β-AR Antagonists

Drug	Membrane Stabilizing Activity	ISA[£]	Lipid solubility	Absorption (%)	Oral bioavailability (%)	Plasma $t_{1/2}$ (hours)	Protein binding (%)
Non-Selective β-Blocking Agents – First Generation							
Nadolol	0	0	Low	30	30–50	20–24	30
Penbutolol	0	+	High	~100	~100	~5	80–98
Pindolol	+	+++	Low	>95	~100	3–4	40
Propranolol	++	0	High	<90	30	3–5	90
Timolol	0	0	Low to Moderate	90	75	4	<10
β1-Selective (Cardioselective) β-Blocking Agents – Second Generation							
Acebutolol	+	+	Low	90	20–60	3–4	26
Atenolol	0	0	Low	90	50–60	6–7	6–16
Bisoprolol	0	0	Low	90	80	9–12	~30
Esmolol	0	0	Low	NA	NA	0.15	55
Metoprolol	+*	0	Low to Moderate	~100	40–50	3–7	12
Non-Selective β-Blocking Agents with Additional Actions ¥ – Third Generation							
Labetalol	+	+	Low	>90	~33	3–4	~50
Carvedilol	++	0	Moderate	>90	~30	7–10	98
β1-Selective β-Blocking Agents with Additional Actions ¥ – Third Generation							
Celiprolol	0	+	Low	~74	30–70	5	4–5

*Only at high doses

£ ISA = Intrinsic sympathomimetic activity

¥ Additional actions:

- Carvedilol and labetalol are also α-AR antagonists.
- Celiprolol has additional partial β2 receptor agonism,

Modified from Goodman and Gillman's The Pharmacological basis of Therapeutics, 11th Ed, Chapter 10.

effects of endogenous catecholamines. The result is a less-pronounced decline in heart rate, contractility, and resultant cardiac output.

Lipid Solubility

As with any drug, the lipid solubility of β-blockers is a major determinant of their absorption, metabolism, and potency. Lipophilic β-blockers such as propranolol, metoprolol, and pindolol are readily absorbed from the gastrointestinal tract and metabolized predominantly by the liver. Their half-life is short, requiring at least twice-daily administration to maintain consistent pharmacologic effects. When administered intravenously, higher serum concentrations are reached. The hydrophilic β-blockers (e.g., atenolol and nadolol) are not as readily absorbed from the gastrointestinal tract and are less extensively metabolized. Their half-life is relatively long, allowing for once-daily dosing. Hydrophilic β-blockers are generally eliminated unchanged by the kidneys. Lipid-soluble agents are often preferable in patients with significant renal dysfunction for whom clearance of water-soluble agents is reduced. Greater lipid solubility is associated with greater penetration to the central nervous system and may contribute to many side effects (e.g., lethargy, depression, and hallucinations) which are not clearly related to β-blocking activity.

Structure Activity Relationships

β-AR antagonists are derivatives of the β-AR agonist agent isoproterenol. Substitutions of the benzene ring determine agonist or antagonist activity on the β-AR. The levorotatory forms of both agonists and antagonists are more potent than their dextrorotatory counterparts.

Oxidation Phenotype

The metabolism of certain β-AR antagonists (metoprolol, carvedilol, and propranolol) may be influenced by genetic polymorphisms or other medications (13). As an example, the oxidative metabolism of metoprolol and timolol occur mainly via the cytochrome P450-CYP2D6. This enzyme exhibits genetic polymorphisms rendering some individuals poor metabolizers with a resultant prolongation of the elimination half-life. In such individuals, the therapeutic target may be achieved with a single daily dose rather than the more typical twice or three times a day administration schedule (14). A similar pattern can be seen with medications that interact with CYP2D6.

Alpha Receptor Blocking Activity

Carvedilol and labetalol are the prototypes of combined adrenergic receptor antagonism. The α-blocking potency of labetalol is 20% of its β-blocking potency and approximately one-tenth the potency of phentolamine. Carvedilol has an α_1 to β blocking ratio of approximately 1:10 (15).

Clinical Effects and Physiological Actions in Different Tissues

Cardiovascular Effects

β-AR blockade reduces myocardial oxygen requirements by decreasing contractility and heart rate, which in turn increases diastolic time and coronary perfusion. Moreover, these drugs attenuate exercise-induced increases in blood pressure and contractility, providing a more favorable balance of myocardial oxygen supply and demand. This is believed critical in the face of limited myocardial viability or impaired myocardial perfusion as seen in ischemic heart disease, and provides the physiological premise of their use in perioperative medicine (see section below).

In normotensive individuals, β-AR antagonists generally do not reduce blood pressure. However, they are very effective antihypertensive agents in those with elevated blood pressure. While the precise mechanism underlying this important clinical effect is not well understood, it is likely multifactorial. Interestingly, the antihypertensive effects persist despite significant differences between β-blocker agents. For those without intrinsic sympathomimetic activity, cardiac output falls approximately 20% and renin release is reduced about 60%. Central nervous system β-AR blockade may also reduce sympathetic discharge (a characteristic more noticeable in lipid-soluble agents). Nonselective β-blockers have an antihypertensive effect with long-term use despite the initial unopposed α-receptor agonist-mediated vasoconstriction. With time, vascular resistance returns to baseline and an antihypertensive effect is noted. This is believed due to a reduction in renin secretion and a decrease in cardiac output.

Pulmonary Effects

The bronchial smooth muscle has a much greater concentration of β_2-ARs as compared with β_1-ARs. Stimulation of β_2-ARs induces bronchodilation. Nonselective β-blockers such as propranolol can antagonize the β_2-AR, leading to bronchoconstriction in patients with chronic obstructive pulmonary disease or asthma. Alternatively, little effect is seen in normal individuals. β_1-selective adrenergic blockers are less likely to produce bronchospasm in patients with reactive airway disease. Nevertheless, adverse effects can be seen in patients with moderate to severe disease. Caution should be taken with this specific patient population. Celiprolol, a specific β_1-selective blocker and partial β_2 agonist, may be an ideal agent in this scenario. However, at this point, clinical experience is limited (16).

Metabolic Effects

Catecholamines are counter-regulatory hormones that stimulate glycogenolysis and promote the mobilization of glucose in response to hypoglycemia and/or stress. β-ARs also mediate activation of hormone-sensitive lipase in adipocytes. The resultant rise in circulating free fatty acids provides an important fuel for exercising muscle. While uncommon, nonselective β-blockers can delay recovery from hypoglycemic episodes in diabetic patients. Hypoglycemic symptoms (tachycardia, tremors, anxiety, and diaphoresis) can be blunted as well. Therefore, β-AR antagonists and specifically the nonselective β-blocking agents should be used with great caution in diabetic patients with poor glucose control. β_1-selective blockers are preferred in this scenario as they are less likely to blunt the responses to hypoglycemia (17).

Potassium ion (K+) flux is also altered by the presence of β-AR antagonists. The normal physiologic response to stimulation of the β_2-AR includes activation of membrane Na-K-ATPase which results in a decrease in the plasma concentration of K+ as it shifts intracellularly, mostly into skeletal myocytes. Administration of β-AR antagonists blunts this physiologic response.

THERAPEUTIC USES OF β-BLOCKERS

Cardiovascular Diseases

β-AR antagonists are a first-line therapy for many cardiovascular disorders including ischemic heart disease, congestive heart failure, essential hypertension, supraventricular arrhythmias, hypertrophic obstructive cardiomyopathy, and aortic dissection. The benefits of early β-blocker therapy in acute myocardial infarction include reductions in infarct size, ventricular rupture, pulseless electrical activity, and mortality (18). Numerous trials have also demonstrated the long-term efficacy of β-blockade after myocardial infarction with reductions in mortality of up to 23% (19). It is suggested that more complete β-blockade results in greater benefit.

β-blockers are also important agents in the armamentarium against arterial hypertension. Due to the above-mentioned effects, mostly with secondary prevention, these agents are ideal in hypertensive patients with concomitant coronary artery disease. Patients with coexisting anxiety, heart failure, or tachyarrhythmias are also excellent candidates for this line of therapy.

The role of β_1-AR blockade in heart failure is now well-established. This class of therapeutic agents falls into the categories of neurohormonal and renin-angiotensin-aldosterone axis inhibitors. Generally, only the second- and third-generation agents (β_1 selective and β_1-α_1 antagonists) are tolerated by this population (20). A meta-analysis of more than 3,000 patients enrolled in 18 randomized trials reported that adding a β-blocker to conventional therapy for heart failure is associated with both hemodynamic and symptomatic improvement. Favorable effects on morbidity and mortality also were noted (21).

The efficacy of first- and second-generation β-blockers in hypertrophic cardiomyopathy is believed due to partial relief of the pressure gradient across the left ventricular outflow tract. Propranolol appears particularly useful for relieving angina, palpitations, and syncope in this patient population.

Another important indication for the use of β-AR antagonists is the medical management of acute and chronic aortic dissection. β-blockers are believed to reduce shear stress at the dissected aortic wall by reducing myocardial contractility and the resultant dP/dT. Moreover, propranolol may be efficacious in slowing the rate of progression of aortic dilatation in patients with Marfan's syndrome (22).

Finally, β-AR antagonists are also Class II anti-arrhythmic agents (Vaughn-Williams Classification system). Their administration has been found most useful in the management of supraventricular tachyarrhythmias, reentry tachycardia, exercise-induced ventricular tachycardia, and automatic dysrhythmias.

Endocrine Disorders

β-blockers can attenuate catecholamine-induced cardiomyopathy in patients with pheochromocytoma, and often play a role in the perioperative preparation for adrenalectomy. However, care must be taken to avoid unopposed α-adrenergic stimulation with the resultant potential for hypertensive crisis. This may be prevented by delaying β-blocker administration until adequate α-AR blockade has been obtained. This is most often achieved with the administration of the nonselective α-AR antagonist phenoxybenzamine or selective α_1-blockers (prazosin or terazosin).

Sympathetic hyperactivity is one of the hallmarks of hyperthyroidism as the excess thyroid hormone is known to increase the expression of β-ARs in some cells. It therefore follows that β-AR antagonists often control many of the cardiovascular signs and symptoms of hyperthyroidism and are useful therapeutic adjuvants. Moreover, propranolol inhibits the peripheral conversion of thyroxine to triiodothyronine, an effect that is likely independent of its nonselective β-receptor blockade activity.

Additional Therapeutic Uses

Several topical β-AR antagonists are currently used to treat chronic open angle glaucoma (both first- and second-generation agents).

Topically administered β-blockers have little or no effect on pupil size or accommodation. They are therefore devoid of the side effects of blurred vision and night blindness often seen with other medications used in glaucoma therapy.

Propranolol and nadolol are β-blockers commonly used in patients with cirrhosis and portal hypertension for their role in primary prevention of variceal bleeding (23). Additional therapeutic uses include prophylaxis against migraine headaches, panic attacks, alcohol withdrawal, anxiety, and essential tremor.

SIDE EFFECTS AND PRECAUTIONS

The majority of the adverse effects associated with β-AR antagonists are a result of their pharmacologic actions. Obtaining a thorough understanding of the physiology of the β-AR and the related effects of β-AR blockade is therefore key to understanding their side-effect profile. Not surprisingly, β-blocker therapy may exacerbate symptoms in patients with peripheral vascular disease and reactive airway disease. Nevertheless, second-generation β-AR antagonists (β_1-selective) are not contraindicated in patients with mild to moderate peripheral arterial disease (24) and do not appear to result in significant adverse respiratory effects in patients with mild to moderate COPD or reactive airway disease (25). Therefore, β_1-selective therapy should not be withheld from these populations if a strong indication for their use exists.

Caution also must be shown in patients with acutely impaired myocardial function. This group may be dependent on sympathetic activation to maintain cardiac performance and β-AR antagonist administration may induce congestive heart failure in susceptible patients. Atrioventricular conduction defects also can be of concern. Life-threatening bradyarrhythmias may occur with the administration of β-blockers, in particular when used in combination with other negative chronotropic or AV nodal conduction blocking agents such as verapamil, diltiazem, and amiodarone. Sudden discontinuation of β-blocker therapy can result in rebound hypertension, angina, or even myocardial infarction. Hence, slow and gradual discontinuation is advocated. It also is strongly recommended to avoid discontinuation in the perioperative period.

The most common side effect of β-blocker therapy is fatigue, likely secondary to decreased cardiac output and limited end-organ perfusion. The increased incidence of diabetes with β-AR antagonists is thought to be due to a decrease in insulin secretion and sensitivity. Despite this perceived risk, diabetic patients with hypertension and coronary artery disease are believed to benefit from this therapy and we would recommend administration of β-blocker therapy as it significantly impacts outcome (myocardial infarction and death) (26).The use of β-AR antagonists in brittle diabetics with frequent hypoglycemic episodes clearly warrants close monitoring and extreme caution.

While depression and erectile dysfunction have previously been reported as side effects, a clear association with β-blocker use is lacking. The use of β-AR antagonists in pregnancy has also been clouded by rare case reports of fetal abnormalities. While their use in this setting is increasing, information regarding the safety of these medications during pregnancy is limited.

SPECIFIC AGENTS

First Generation—Nonselective β-AR Antagonists

Propranolol. Propranolol is the classic, prototype β-AR antagonist. It interacts with β_1 and β_2 ARs with equal affinity, lacks intrinsic sympathomimetic activity, and does not block α-ARs. As the first β-blocker introduced clinically, propranolol is the standard to which all β-AR antagonist are compared. It is highly lipophilic with excellent oral absorption, but limited bioavailability (~30%) and significant pharmacokinetic inter-individual variation. It crosses the blood-brain barrier, has a volume of distribution of 4 L/kg and is 90% protein bound. It is extensively metabolized in the liver and some of its metabolites (4-OH propranolol) have weak β-AR antagonist activity. Its half life is approximately 4 hours. Usual dosing is 40–80 mg daily by mouth and up to a maximum dose of 360 mg. Intravenous dosing is 1–3 mg and can be repeated in 5–10 minutes to achieve the desired effect.

Nadolol. Nadolol is a non-selective β-AR antagonist without intrinsic sympathomimetic activity. It is a long-acting antagonist with a half life of 12–24 hours and a bioavailability of approximately 35%. It is a water-soluble agent with minimal inter-individual variability. It penetrates the blood brain barrier poorly when compared to more lipid soluble agents. Nadolol is excreted largely intact in the urine and therefore may accumulate in patients with renal failure. Due to its long half life, it is usually administered once daily at a dose starting at 40 mg up to 240 mg. Intravenous dosing has been described at 0.01 to 0.05 mcg/kg IV up to a total of 10 mg administered at a rate no higher than 1 mg/min.

Timolol. Timolol is a potent nonselective β-AR antagonist without intrinsic sympathomimetic or membrane stabilizing activity. It is used to treat open angle glaucoma and hypertension. This agent is highly absorbed orally and undergoes a degree of first pass hepatic metabolism. It is metabolized extensively by cytochrome P450-CYP2D6 and a small fraction is excreted unchanged in the urine. Half life is 4 hours. Usual oral dosing is twice daily and ranges from 10 mg to 60 mg a day.

Pindolol. Pindolol is a non-selective β-AR antagonist with intrinsic sympathomimetic activity, low membrane stabilizing activity and low lipid solubility. It has excellent oral absorption and high bioavailability with minimal inter-individual variation after oral administration. It is partially metabolized by the liver (~50%) and the reminder is excreted unchanged in the urine. Plasma half life is approximately 4 hours. Oral dosing ranges form 2.5 mg every 6 hours to a max of 60 mg a day; it is usually administered at 6 or 12 hour intervals.

Penbutolol. Penbutolol is another nonselective β-AR antagonist with minimal intrinsic sympathomimetic activity and no membrane stabilizing activity. It is highly lipid-soluble with excellent oral absorption and bioavailability. It readily crosses the blood brain barrier. Its elimination half life is approximately 5 hours. It is partially metabolized in the liver and 90% is excreted by the kidneys. Oral dosing regimens are usually once daily and range from 10 mg to 40 mg a day.

Second Generation—Selective β_1-AR Antagonists

Metoprolol. Metoprolol is a commonly used β_1-AR antagonist that lacks intrinsic sympathomimetic and membrane stabilizing activity. It has significant first-pass hepatic metabolism and therefore bioavailability is relatively low (~40%) despite near complete oral absorption. There is significant interindividual variability due to genetically determined differences in metabolism. Metoprolol is metabolized in the liver via cytochrome P450-CYP2D6 with only 10% recovered unchanged in the urine. Half life is 3–4 hours but can be as high as 8 hours in poor metabolizers. Depending on the formulation (metoprolol succinate vs. tartrate) oral dosing varies from 12.5 mg twice daily to 200 mg twice daily with a maximum dose of 400 mg a day. Six-hour interval dosing is advocated in the setting of an acute coronary syndrome and once daily dosing is possible when the extended release form is used. Intravenous dosing ranges from 1–5 mg every 2–5 minutes and should only be used in a monitored setting.

Atenolol. Similar to metoprolol, atenolol is a selective β_1-AR antagonist without sympathomimetic or membrane stabilizing properties. It is a hydrophilic molecule with a slightly longer half life than metoprolol (~6–7 hours). It displays minimal interindividual variation and penetrates the central nervous system poorly. It is excreted largely unchanged in the urine; therefore dosage should be adjusted in patients with renal failure.

Oral dose is 50–100 mg once daily (200 mg maximum dose). Intravenous dosing is 1–5 mg IV, which can be repeated every 10 minutes.

Esmolol. Esmolol is a rapid-onset short-acting selective β_1-AR antagonist with minimal intrinsic sympathomimetic activity and no membrane stabilizing activity. Its only route of administration is intravenous. It contains an ester linkage and the short duration of action results from rapid ester hydrolysis by erythrocyte esterases. Its half life is approximately 8 minutes. The half life of the carboxylic acid metabolite of esmolol is close to 4 hours. It is excreted in the urine and can accumulate with prolonged infusions. However, this metabolite has very low potency when compared with esmolol (1/500). The unique pharmacokinetic properties of esmolol make it a useful agent in critically ill patients or circumstances when a fast-onset short-duration agent is desired (27). The hemodynamic effects are evident within 5 minutes and disappear 10–30 minutes after an IV infusion has been stopped. Usual dose is 10–80 mg IV or 500 mcg/kg IV. This can be followed by a continuous infusion at 50–300 mcg/kg/min.

Bisoprolol. Bisoprolol is a selective β_1-AR antagonist without intrinsic sympathomimetic or membrane stabilizing activity with good oral absorption and bioavailability (80%). It is metabolized by the liver and eliminated by the kidneys (50–50%). It has an elimination half life of 9–12 hours. Usual oral dose ranges from 2.5 mg to 40 mg once daily.

Acebutolol. Acebutolol is a selective β_1-AR antagonist with partial agonist activity and membrane stabilizing effects. It has excellent oral absorption and important first-pass hepatic metabolism. Most of the pharmacologic effects are mediated via diacetolol, an active metabolite, from the first pass effect. Its elimination half life is approximately 3 hours and 8–12 hours for the active metabolite. It is typically administered orally twice daily via the oral route with dosing ranging from 400 mg to 1600 mg total daily dose.

Third Generation—β-AR Antagonist with Additional Properties

These agents do not fit well within the classic division of β-AR antagonists (cardio-selective vs. nonselective β-AR antagonists). They contain a variety of additional pharmacologic effects, the most common of which is vasodilation. These properties result from concomitant α-AR blockade, β_2-AR agonist properties, increased nitric oxide production, and antioxidant effects.

Labetalol. Labetalol is a unique anti-hypertensive agent with non-selective β-AR antagonism and α_1-AR blocking properties. It also has partial agonist activity at the β_2-AR and it inhibits neuronal uptake of norepinephrine. In humans, the β to α blocking potency ratio is 3:4 for oral labetalol to 7:1 for the intravenous formulation. Its α-blocking activity is one-fifth to one-tenth as potent as phentolamine and its β- blocking activity is one-third as potent as propranolol. Despite excellent oral absorption, the bioavailability is limited due to extensive first-pass effect (20%–40% bioavailability). The elimination half life is 5–8 hours. It is metabolized by hepatic conjugation with glucuronic acid. Minimal drug is recovered unchanged in the urine. Oral administration is twice daily and ranges from 100 mg to 800 mg total daily dose. Intravenous dosing starts with 10 mg IV repeating every 10 minutes until desired effect. Continuous infusion also has been described at 2 mg/min with a maximal dose of 300 mg.

Carvedilol. Carvedilol is a third generation β-blocker with antioxidant and antiproliferative effects in addition to nonselective β-blockade and α-blocking properties. It is highly lipid-soluble and peak plasma concentrations are reached approximately 2 hours after oral administration. It is extensively metabolized by the liver via cytochrome P 450 CYP2D6 and CYP2C9. No significant renal metabolism occurs; therefore it can be safely administered in these patients without dose adjustment. Oral administration is twice daily and the dose ranges from 3.125 mg to 50 mg per dose.

Celiprolol. Celiprolol is a third generation β_1-AR antagonist with partial β_2-AR agonist activity producing weak bronchodilation and vasodilation. It lacks membrane stabilizing activity. Celiprolol is a water-soluble agent with limited oral bioavailability (~50%). It is excreted mostly unchanged in the urine. Usual oral dosing regimens range from 200 mg to 400 mg once daily.

Antiarrhythmic Agents with β-blocker Properties

Sotalol and propafenone are antiarrhythmic agents with non-selective β-blocker properties.

PERIOPERATIVE USE OF β-ADRENERGIC RECEPTOR BLOCKERS

Rationale

Perioperative cardiac morbidity and mortality continue to be worldwide clinical and economic burdens. Recent estimates note that approximately 50,000 patients undergoing noncardiac surgery each year in the United States will have a perioperative myocardial infarction (PMI) and an estimated 1 million patients will have a perioperative cardiac complication (28, 29). Even minor increases in serum concentrations of cardiac biomarkers (troponin and creatine kinase-MB) in the early postoperative period have been associated with a significant increase in long-term mortality following vascular surgery (30).

Significant perioperative morbidity and mortality remain with cardiac surgery as well. Mortality rates up to 3% persist as do a 6% risk of PMI and a 40% risk of postoperative atrial fibrillation (31). The link between perioperative myocardial ischemia and postoperative cardiac morbidity and mortality has been well documented in both cardiac (32) and noncardiac surgery (33, 34). As a consequence of the known physiologic effects of β-AR stimulation, perioperative administration of β-AR antagonists as a means of providing perioperative cardiac protection has received great attention, particularly in the past 10 years.

Pathophysiology of Perioperative Cardiac Ischemia

The perioperative period places significant strain on patients at risk for myocardial ischemia. It is likely that multiple factors contribute to this heightened risk, and sustained increases in circulating catecholamines are believed to be intimately involved (Table 3–3) (35). The traditional theory of plaque rupture as the sentinel event leading to PMI recently has been challenged and we have begun to see a shift in emphasis toward the optimization of myocardial oxygen supply and demand. Findings that support this new paradigm include a shift away from the historic Q-wave myocardial infarction occurring between postoperative days 2 and 3 with associated mortality rates exceeding 25%. More recently, the more common clinical presentation appears to involve non-Q-wave MIs occurring earlier in the postoperative period (within the first 48 postoperative hours). These events are noted to have a much lower associated mortality (36).

Table 3-3. Perioperative Factors Associated with Increased Postoperative Cardiac Risk

Activation of the Coagulation system
Activation of the hypothalamic-pituitary-adrenal axis
Activation of the inflammatory immune response
Altered endothelial function
Anemia
Fluid shifts
Hypothermia
Pain
Sustained increase in circulating catecholamine (↑HR, ↑BP, ↑VO2, ↑free fatty acid concentration)
Sustained increased in endogenous vasoconstriction

HR = heart rate, BP = blood pressure, VO2 = oxygen consumption

Adapted from Kor DJ, et al. Contemporary Crit Care 2006 4 (1) 1–9

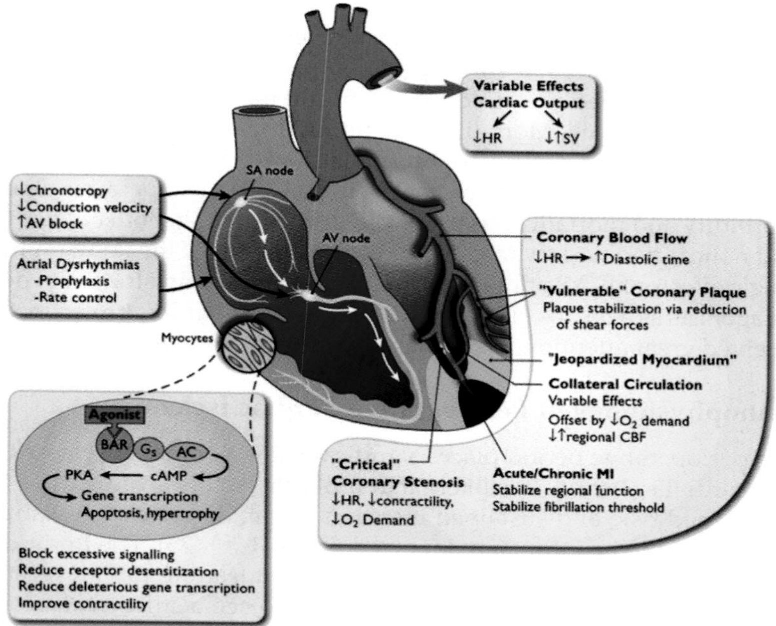

FIGURE 3–2. Potential cardiovascular effects of perioperative β-AR blockade.

Proponents of the supply-demand theory suggest that PMI is closely related to sustained elevations of heart rate and prolonged episodes of ST-segment depression (37). The administration of perioperative β-AR antagonists is thought to mitigate the unfavorable balance of myocardial oxygen supply and demand. These favorable effects are largely achieved via a reduction in heart rate and contractility (decreasing myocardial demand) and an increase in diastolic perfusion time (increasing supply). In addition, a number of other potential protective effects have been noted (Figure 3–2).

Evaluation of Clinical Efficacy

Numerous studies have been conducted in an effort to assess the efficacy of perioperative β-blockade in reducing cardiovascular morbidity and mortality after cardiac and noncardiac surgery. Despite clear pathophysiologic rationale and generalized support for this therapy, the evidence supporting widespread β-AR antagonist administration in the perioperative period is controversial (38). Supporting evidence for this practice primarily arises from two landmark trials (39, 40). Mangano et al. (39) evaluated the benefit of perioperative atenolol in patients with or at risk for coronary artery disease undergoing noncardiac surgery. The primary outcome of all cause mortality during the 2 years following hospital discharge (in-hospital mortality was not included) was significantly lower in the atenolol group (10% vs. 21%, respectively). A short time later, Poldermans et al. (40) demonstrated marked reductions in cardiac-related mortality or nonfatal MI (34% vs. 3.4% p , 0.001) with the use of perioperative bisoprolol in high-risk patients undergoing vascular surgery. Despite their limited sample sizes and small number of events, these two trials are the cornerstone of current recommendations regarding perioperative beta-blockade.

Importantly, a number of additional studies have been completed since the publication of both Mangano's and Polderman's work. The results have been mixed with at least two trials failing to show a reduction in perioperative cardiac events with the administration of β-blocker therapy (41, 42). Preliminary data from the large international, multicenter POISE trial also have been recently discussed (54). While reductions in myocardial infarction and atrial fibrillation were noted in the group randomized to metoprolol therapy, significant increases in both cerebrovascular accidents and mortality also were noted in the treatment group. We await additional details for this important study.

Furthermore, several meta-analyses have reviewed the combined evidence for perioperative β-blocker therapy. Again, the results are mixed (31, 43–46). In a meta-analysis of 21 trials evaluating pharmacologic myocardial protection in patients undergoing noncardiac surgery, 11 studies were noted to have evaluated perioperative β-blockade. The cumulative evidence showed a reduction in perioperative ischemia and nonfatal MI (44). A more recent comprehensive meta-analysis of randomized trials comparing β-blockers with either placebo or standard care in cardiac and noncardiac surgical patients also has been reported (31). Perioperative β-blocker administration was noted to reduce perioperative arrhythmias (ventricular and supraventricular) and myocardial ischemia. However, no differences in major endpoints such as death and acute myocardial infarction were noted (31) (Figures 3–3 and 3–4). Similarly, another recent meta-analysis evaluating the importance of the degree of heart rate control achieved by β-blocker therapy noted a lack of effect on mortality and nonfatal myocardial infarction with β-AR blockade (46).

Recently, the important concept of risk stratification has been discussed. Lindenauer et al. published a large retrospective multicenter study (47) in which patient outcome with the utilization of perioperative β-blockade was determined after stratification by preoperative risk. The degree of risk was determined with the Revised Cardiac Risk Index (RCRI) score. Importantly, the study noted benefit with perioperative β-

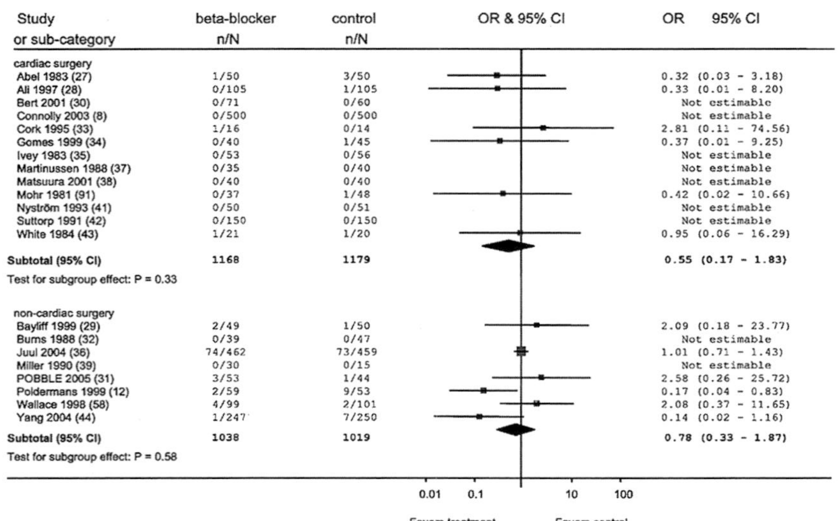

FIGURE 3–3. Effect of β-blockers on perioperative all-cause mortality.

Study or sub-category	beta-blocker n/N	control n/N	OR (95% CI)
cardiac surgery			
Abel 1983 (27)	2/50	2/50	1.00 (0.14 - 7.39)
Bert 2001 (30)	1/71	3/60	0.27 (0.03 - 2.68)
Daudon 1986 (46)	1/50	1/50	1.00 (0.06 - 16.44)
Hammon 1984 (47)	0/24	2/26	0.20 (0.01 - 4.38)
Khuri 1987 (49)	0/67	1/74	0.36 (0.01 - 9.06)
Martinussen 1988 (37)	2/35	1/40	2.36 (0.21 - 27.25)
Matangi 1985 (50)	4/82	5/82	0.79 (0.20 - 3.05)
Matangi1989 (51)	4/35	3/35	1.38 (0.28 - 6.66)
Mohr 1981 (91)	0/37	2/48	0.25 (0.01 - 5.32)
Myhre 1984 (52)	1/16	1/20	1.27 (0.07 - 21.97)
Oka 1980 (53)	0/19	4/35	0.18 (0.01 - 3.52)
Silverman 1982 (55)	5/50	6/50	0.81 (0.23 - 2.87)
Wenke 1999 (59)	8/100	4/100	2.09 (0.61 - 7.17)
White 1984 (43)	0/21	1/20	0.30 (0.01 - 7.87)
Babin-Ebell 1996 (45)	1/33	1/37	1.13 (0.07 - 18.73)
Subtotal (95% CI)	**690**	**727**	**0.89 (0.53 - 1.50)**
Test for subgroup effect: P = 0.66			
non-cardiac surgery			
Jakobsen 1997 (48)	1/18	0/17	3.00 (0.11 - 78.81)
Miller 1990 (39)	0/30	0/15	Not estimable
POBBLE 2005 (31)	3/53	5/44	0.47 (0.11 - 2.08)
Poldermans 1999 (12)	0/59	9/53	0.04 (0.00 - 0.69)
Raby 1999 (54)	0/15	1/11	0.23 (0.01 - 6.09)
Stone 1988 (56)	0/89	0/39	Not estimable
Urban 2000 (57)	1/52	3/55	0.34 (0.03 - 3.38)
Wallace 1998 (58)	10/99	5/101	2.16 (0.71 - 6.56)
Yang 2004 (44)	19/247	21/250	0.91 (0.48 - 1.74)
Zaugg 1999 (60)	0/40	3/19	0.06 (0.00 - 1.19)
Subtotal (95% CI)	**702**	**604**	**0.59 (0.25 - 1.39)**
Test for subgroup effect: P = 0.23			

0.001 0.01 0.1 10 100 1000

Favors treatment Favors control

FIGURE 3–4. The effect of β-blockers on the development of perioperative myocardial infarction. Adapted from: Wiesbauer F., et al., Anesth Analg 2007;104: 27–41

blockade only in high-risk patients (RCRI ≥3). Additionally, the potential for harm was noted in patients with low preoperative risk (RCRI score (≤1). The potential for harm in this low cardiac risk population is being recognized increasingly.

CURRENT RECOMMENDATIONS AND REMAINING QUESTIONS

The 2007 American College of Cardiology/American Heart Association (ACC/AHA) guidelines on perioperative cardiovascular evaluation and care for noncardiac surgery (48) recommends β-blockers be continued in patients undergoing surgery who are receiving β-AR antagonists to control symptoms of ischemic heart disease, symptomatic arrhythmias, hypertension, or other ACC/AHA class I guideline indications (class I recommendation, level of evidence C). A similar class I recommendation is made for patients at high cardiac risk because of the finding of ischemia on preoperative testing and who are undergoing vascular surgery. Class IIa recommendations include patients undergoing intermediate risk or vascular surgery in whom preoperative assessment identifies coronary artery disease or the presence of more than one clinical risk factor. The usefulness of perioperative β-blockade is uncertain in patients undergoing either intermediate-risk or vascular surgery with no clinical risk or a single clinical risk factor (48). The bulk of evidence to date questions the benefit of perioperative β-blockade in patients who do not have high cardiac risk (RCRI ≤2) or who are not undergoing high-risk surgery. Therefore, we currently cannot advocate routine broad use of this perioperative therapy.

Additional questions regarding patient selection include the safety and efficacy of perioperative β-AR antagonists in diabetic, elderly, and critically ill populations. While multiple trials have shown the beneficial effects of β-blocker therapy in diabetic patients with cardiac disease, a recent randomized controlled trial failed to confirm this benefit in a large cohort of diabetic patients (49). As a result, it presently would appear unwarranted to consider diabetes mellitus alone a sufficient risk factor for routine therapy. Regarding the elderly population, there is evidence of reduced analgesic and anesthetic requirements, reduced postoperative confusion, and greater hemodynamic stability in patients receiving perioperative β-blockade (50). However, the reduced ventricular compliance, lower resting heart rates, presence of cerebrovascular disease, and reduction in maximal heart rate response make routine administration of β-blocker therapy difficult in this patient population. Therefore, patients should be selected carefully. Similar concerns arise when considering perioperative β-blockade in critically ill patients with marginal hemodynamic reserve. Indeed, the POISE trial does report the potential for harm when routinely administering these agents to patients with infection or sepsis (54).

Currently, it also is unclear if a specific β-blocker should be utilized in the perioperative setting. When used for secondary prevention following MI, multiple studies have failed to show differences in outcomes between various β-blocking agents. The exception is potentially worse outcomes when utilizing agents with intrinsic sympathomimetic activity, such as pindolol (19). It has been recommended to use β_1-AR selective agents, given their lower propensity for pulmonary side effects (51, 52). Current evidence would indicate that myocardial protection is a class (β_1-AR or second generation β-AR antagonists) rather than drug-specific phenomenon. Concomitant disease such as renal failure or other conditions that alter the pharmacokinetic properties of the various medications within this class should guide the practitioner when choosing a specific agent.

The optimal duration of perioperative β-blockade is unknown. However, current literature supports the initiation of therapy prior to induction of anesthesia with continuation for at least 7 days postoperatively or until hospital discharge (39). Additional benefit may be seen when initiated up to 1 month prior to the planned surgery and continued for 30 postoperative days (40). In patients with clear indications for β-AR antagonists, therapy should be continued indefinitely.

In summary, perioperative β-blockade reduces the risk of perioperative cardiac complications in high cardiac risk patients undergoing high-risk surgeries. Appropriate lower risk patient populations and therapeutic endpoints require further investigation, particularly as statements and recommendations regarding PBB have begun to emerge from organizations such as the Leapfrog Group, the Agency for Healthcare Research and Quality, and the National Quality Forum. At the present time, utilization of a form of risk stratification (e.g. the RCRI) would appear most prudent in these lower risk populations. We hope to better refine our understanding regarding perioperative β-blockade from additional studies such as the Perioperative Ischemic Evaluation (POISE) trial.

References

1. Kaye DM, Lefkovits J, Jennings GL, et al.: Adverse consequences of high sympathetic nervous activity in the failing human heart. J Am Coll Cardiol 1995; 26:1257–63
2. Lands AM, Arnold A, McAuliff JP, et al.: Differentiation of receptor systems activated by sympathomimetic amines. Nature 1967; 214:597–8

3. Brodde OE, Michel MC: Adrenergic and muscarinic receptors in the human heart. Pharmacol Rev. 1999; 51:651–90
4. Cerbai E, Guerra L, Varani K, et al.: beta-adrenoceptor subtypes in young and old rat ventricular myocytes: a combined patch-clamp and binding study. Br J Pharmacol 1995; 116:1835–42
5. Emorine LJ, Marullo S, Briend-Sutren MM, et al.: Molecular characterization of the human beta 3-adrenergic receptor. Science 1989; 245:1118–21
6. Skeberdis VA: Structure and function of beta3-adrenergic receptors. Medicina (Kaunas) 2004; 40:407–13
7. Hall RA, Lefkowitz RJ: Regulation of G protein-coupled receptor signaling by scaffold proteins. Circ Res 2002 18; 91:672–80
8. Lohse MJ, Engelhardt S, Eschenhagen T: What is the role of beta-adrenergic signaling in heart failure?. Circ Res. 2003; 93:896–906
9. Brodde OE, Bruck H, Leineweber K: Cardiac adrenoceptors: physiological and pathophysiological relevance. J Pharmacol Sci 2006; 100:323–37
10. Zaugg M, Xu W, Lucchinetti E, et al.: beta-adrenergic receptor subtypes differentially affect apoptosis in adult rat ventricular myocytes. Circulation 2000; 102:344–-50
11. Saucerman JJ, McCulloch AD: Cardiac beta-adrenergic signaling. from subcellular microdomains to heart failure. Ann N York Acad Sci 2006; 1080:348–61
12. Cohn JN, Levine TB, Olivari MT, et al.: Plasma norepinephrine as a guide to prognosis in patients with chronic congestive heart failure. N Engl J Med 1984; 311:819–23
13. Flockhart DA, Tanus-Santos JE: Implications of cytochrome P450 interactions when prescribing medication for hypertension. Arch Intern Med. 2002; 162:405–12
14. Lennard MS: The polymorphic oxidation of beta-adrenoceptor antagonists. Pharmacol Ther 1989; 41:461–77
15. Frishman WH. Carvedilol. N Engl J Med 1998; 339:1759–65
16. Pujet JC, Dubreuil C, Fleury B, et al.: Effects of celiprolol, a cardioselective beta-blocker, on respiratory function in asthmatic patients. Eur Respir J 1992; 5:196–200
17. Dunne F, Kendall MJ, Martin U: Beta-blockers in the management of hypertension in patients with type 2 diabetes mellitus: is there a role? Drugs 2001; 61:429–35
18. Anonymous. Mechanisms for the early mortality reduction produced by beta-blockade started early in acute myocardial infarction: ISIS-1. ISIS-1 (First International Study of Infarct Survival) Collaborative Group. Lancet 1988; 1:921–3. [Erratum appears in Lancet 1988; 2:292].

19. Freemantle N, Cleland J, Young P, et al.: beta blockade after myocardial infarction: systematic review and meta regression analysis. BMJ 1999; 318:1730–7
20. Eichhorn EJ, Bristow MR: Practical guidelines for initiation of beta-adrenergic blockade in patients with chronic heart failure. Am J Cardiol 1997; 79:794–8
21. Abdulla J, Kober L, Christensen E, Torp-Pedersen C: Effect of beta-blocker therapy on functional status in patients with heart failure—a meta-analysis. Eur J Heart Fail 2006; 8:522–31
22. Shores J, Berger KR, Murphy EA, Pyeritz RE: Progression of aortic dilatation and the benefit of long-term beta-adrenergic blockade in Marfan's syndrome. N Engl J Med 1994; 330:1335–41
23. Chalasani N, Boyer TD: Primary prophylaxis against variceal bleeding: beta-blockers, endoscopic ligation, or both? Am J Gastroenterol 2005; 100:805–7
24. Heintzen MP, Strauer BE: Peripheral vascular effects of beta-blockers. Eur Heart J 1994; 15 Suppl C:2–7
25. Salpeter SR, Ormiston TM, Salpeter EE: Cardioselective beta-blockers in patients with reactive airway disease: a meta-analysis. Ann Intern Med 2002; 137:715–25
26. Sawicki PT, Siebenhofer A: Beta-blocker treatment in diabetes mellitus. J Intern Med 2001; 250:11–7
27. Helfman SM, Gold MI, DeLisser EA, Herrington CA: Which drug prevents tachycardia and hypertension associated with tracheal intubation: lidocaine, fentanyl, or esmolol? Anesth Analg; 72:482–6
28. Mangano DT, Goldman L: Preoperative assessment of patients with known or suspected coronary disease. N Engl J Med 1995; 333:1750–6
29. Mangano DT: Perioperative cardiac morbidity. Anesthesiology 1990; 72:153–84
30. Landesberg G, Mosseri M, Wolf Y, et al.: Perioperative myocardial ischemia and infarction: identification by continuous 12-lead electrocardiogram with online ST-segment monitoring. Anesthesiology 2002; 96:264–70
31. Wiesbauer F, Schlager O, Domanovits H, et al.: Perioperative β-blockers for preventing surgery-related mortality and morbidity: a systematic review and meta-analysis. Anesth Analg 2007; 104:27–41
32. Reich DL, Bodian CA, Krol M, et al.: Intraoperative hemodynamic predictors of mortality, stroke, and myocardial infarction after coronary artery bypass surgery. Anesth Analg 1999; 89:814–22
33. Mangano DT, Browner WS, Hollenberg M, et al.: Association of perioperative myocardial ischemia with cardiac morbidity and mortality in men undergoing noncardiac surgery. The Study of Perioperative Ischemia Research Group. N Engl J Med 1990; 323:1781–8.

34. Raby KE, Barry J, Creager MA et al.: Detection and significance of intraoperative and postoperative myocardial ischemia in peripheral vascular surgery. JAMA 1992; 268:222–7
35. Kor DJ, Brown DR. Update on the status of perioperative beta-blockade. Contemporary Critical Care 2006;4(1):1–9
36. Badner NH, Gelb AW: Postoperative myocardial infarction (PMI) after noncardiac surgery. Anesthesiology 1999; 90:644
37. Priebe HJ: Perioperative myocardial infarction-aetiology and prevention. Br J Anaesth 2005; 95:3–19
38. Devereaux PJ, Yusuf S, Yang H, et al.: Are the recommendations to use perioperative beta-blocker therapy in patients undergoing noncardiac surgery based on reliable evidence? CMAJ 2004; 171:245–7
39. Mangano DT, Layug EL, Wallace A, Tateo I: Effect of atenolol on mortality and cardiovascular morbidity after noncardiac surgery. Multicenter Study of Perioperative Ischemia Research Group. N Engl J Med 1996; 335:1713–20
40. Poldermans D, Boersma E, Bax JJ, et al.: The effect of bisoprolol on perioperative mortality and myocardial infarction in high-risk patients undergoing vascular surgery. Dutch Echocardiographic Cardiac Risk Evaluation Applying Stress Echocardiography Study Group. N Engl J Med 1999; 341:1789–94
41. Yang H, Raymer K, Butler R, et al.: Metoprolol after vascular surgery (MaVS). Can J Anesth 2004; 51:A7.
42. Brady AR, Gibbs JS, Greenhalgh RM, et al.: Perioperative beta-blockade (POBBLE) for patients undergoing infrarenal vascular surgery: results of a randomized double-blind controlled trial. J Vasc Surg 2005; 41:602–9
43. Auerbach AD, Goldman L: β-blockers and reduction of cardiac events in noncardiac surgery: scientific review. JAMA 2002; 287: 1435–44
44. Stevens RD, Burri H, Tramer MR: Pharmacologic myocardial protection in patients undergoing noncardiac surgery: a quantitative systematic review. Anesth Analg 2003; 97:623–33
45. McGory ML, Maggard MA, Ko CY: A meta-analysis of perioperative beta blockade: what is the actual risk reduction? Surgery 2005; 138:171–9
46. Biccard BM, Sear JW, Foex P: Meta-analysis of the effect of heart rate achieved by perioperative beta-adrenergic blockade on cardiovascular outcomes. Br J Anaesth 2008; 100:23–8
47. Lindenauer PK, Pekow P, Wang K, et al.: Perioperative beta-blocker therapy and mortality after major noncardiac surgery. N Engl J Med 2005; 353:349–61

48. Fleisher LA, Beckman JA, Brown KA, et al.: ACC/AHA 2007 guidelines on perioperative cardiovascular evaluation and care for noncardiac surgery: a report of the American College of Cardiology/American Heart Association Task Force on Practice Guidelines (Writing Committee to Revise the 2002 Guidelines on Perioperative Cardiovascular Evaluation for Noncardiac Surgery) developed in collaboration with the American Society of Echocardiography, American Society of Nuclear Cardiology, Heart Rhythm Society, Society of Cardiovascular Anesthesiologists, Society for Cardiovascular Angiography and Interventions, Society for Vascular Medicine and Biology, and Society for Vascular Surgery. J Am Coll Cardiol 2007; 50:e159–241
49. Juul AB, Wetterslev J, Gluud C, et al.: Effect of perioperative beta blockade in patients with diabetes undergoing major non-cardiac surgery: randomised placebo controlled, blinded multicentre trial. BMJ 2006; 332:1482
50. Zaugg M, Tagliente T, Lucchinetti E, et al.: Beneficial effects from beta-adrenergic blockade in elderly patients undergoing noncardiac surgery. Anesthesiology 1999; 91:1674–86
51. Bayliff CD, Massel DR, Inculet RI, et al.: Propranolol for the prevention of postoperative arrhythmias in general thoracic surgery. Ann Thorac Surg 1999; 67:182–6
52. van Zyl AI, Jennings AA, Bateman ED, Opie LH: Comparison of respiratory effects of two cardioselective beta-blockers, celiprolol and atenolol, in asthmatics with mild to moderate hypertension. Chest 1989; 95:209–13
53. Devereaux PJ, Yang H, Guyatt GH, et al.: Rationale, design, and organization of the PeriOperative ISchemic Evaluation (POISE) trial: a randomized controlled trial of metoprolol versus placebo in patients undergoing noncardiac surgery. Am Heart J 2006; 152:223–30
54. Devereaux PJ, et al. The Perioperative Ischemic Evaluation (POISE) Trial: A randomized controlled trial of metoprolol vs. placebo in patients undergoing non-cardiac surgery. AHA Meeting 2007; Abstract LBCT-20825

Roy Kan, MBBS, MMed
Dan Berkowitz, MD

4 Modulators of Vascular Tone: Implications for New Pharmacological Therapies

INTRODUCTION

Our understanding of vascular biology has burgeoned during the past 4 decades. This has been fuelled in part by our understanding of the role of the endothelium and its interaction with the underlying vascular smooth muscle. The implementation of cell, molecular biologic, and imaging techniques in combination with in vitro vascular bioassays has led to accelerated and significant drug discovery. In fact, the majority of drugs currently used in cardiovascular medicine are targeted to, or have profound effects on the vasculature. This chapter reviews a few of the more recent novel ideas regarding vascular signalling and the implication for newer vascular pharmacologic agents that have and are becoming a part of our armamentarium.

The discovery of the human circulatory system dates back to the 4th century BC. However, blood vessel function was poorly understood. Since blood pools in the veins after death, arteries appeared empty, so ancient anatomists assumed that the purpose of arteries was to transport air.

It was only in the 2nd century AD that the Greek physician, Galen, was able to determine the function of blood vessels and distinguish between venous (dark red) and arterial (brighter and thinner) blood. However, Galen believed that the arterial blood was created by venous blood passing from the left ventricle to the right through "pores" in the interventricular septum while air passed from the lungs via the pulmonary artery to the left side of the heart. As the arterial blood was cre-

Advances in Cardiovascular Pharmacology, edited by Philippe R. Housmans, MD, PhD and Gregory A. Nuttall, M.D.

ated, "sooty" vapors were created and passed to the lungs via the pulmonary artery to be exhaled.

In 1242, the Arab physician Ibn al-Nafis became the first person to accurately describe the process of blood circulation in the human body, including pulmonary circulation. He writes in his *Commentary on Anatomy in Avicenna's Canon*: "... the blood from the right chamber of the heart must arrive at the left chamber but there is no direct pathway between them. The thick septum of the heart is not perforated and does not have visible pores as some people thought or invisible pores as Galen thought. The blood from the right chamber must flow through the vena arteriosa (pulmonary artery) to the lungs, spread through its substances, be mingled there with air, pass through the arteria venosa (pulmonary vein) to reach the left chamber of the heart and there form the vital spirit ..."

Finally in 1628, William Harvey, an English physician, announced the discovery of the human circulatory system as his own and published an influential book *Exercitatio Anatomica de Motu Cordis et Sanguinis in Animalibus* (*An Anatomical Exercise on the Motion of the Heart and Blood in Animals*). While this book contributed significantly to our understanding of the mechanisms of circulation, Harvey was not able to identify the capillary system connecting arteries and veins; these were later described by Marcello Malpighi.

Arteries and veins, to a degree, can regulate their inner diameter by contraction of the muscular layer, thus changing the blood flow to downstream organs. This is mediated by the autonomic nervous system and modulated at a local level by many mediators released primarily by the endothelium. Vasoconstriction is regulated by vasoconstrictors such as paracrine factors (e.g., prostaglandins), a number of hormones (e.g., vasopressin and angiotensin) and neurotransmitters (e.g., epinephrine) from the nervous system. Vasodilation is a similar process mediated by antagonistically acting mediators, the most prominent of which is nitric oxide, which is termed endothelium-derived relaxing factor for this reason.

PHYSIOLOGICAL MODULATION OF VASCULAR SMOOTH MUSCLE TONE

Myogenic Tone

In the same manner that the Starling relationship (or length-dependent activation) is the fundamental mechanism regulating myocardial performance, so it is that myogenic tone is a fundamental mechanism underlying pressure-flow autoregulation. As anesthesiologists, we are very familiar with the autoregulatory curves. These curves define the blood pressure range over which flow is maintained constant, independent of blood pressure. On the other hand, below this threshold

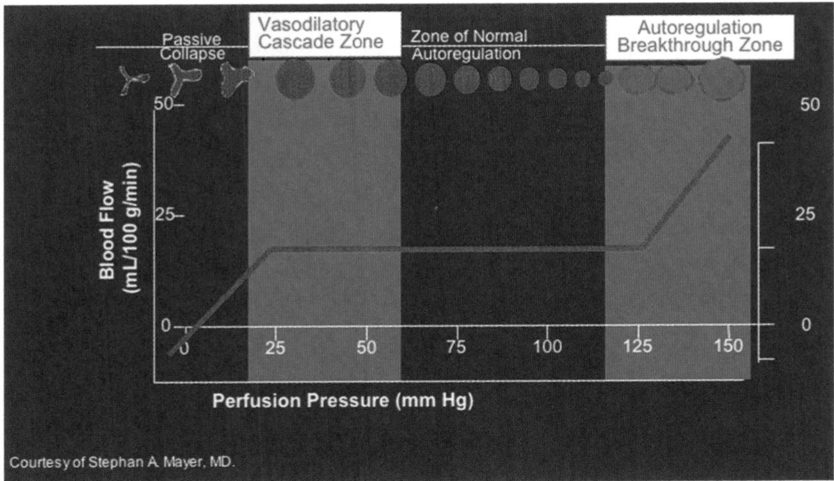

FIGURE 4–1. A normal pressure flow autoregulatory curve. When flow is independent of pressure, autoregulation is present and is mediated by active myogenic constriction of the arterioles. Below the autoregulatory threshold, flow becomes pressure-dependent.

blood flow remains pressure-dependent (Figure 4–1). The fundamental mechanisms underlying this phenomenon remains poorly understood (1, 2). The phenomenon of an increase in arteriolar constriction as a result of an increase in intraluminal pressure (myogenic tone) dates back to 1902 when Bayliss observed an increase in blood flow with a reduction in descending pressure acting on the vessel wall (3). Currently, it is well recognized that as intravascular pressure increases there is a development of tone as the vessel decreases its diameter (active smooth muscle contraction). Furthermore, it is well understood that the phenomenon of myogenic tone is Ca^{2+}-dependent; removal of Ca^{2+} leads to an increase in diameter with an increase in pressure (passive vessels dilation). It is thought that an increase in smooth muscle membrane tension leads to membrane depolarization and an opening of voltage gate Ca^{2+} channels. This led to activation of the contractile machinery and vasoconstriction. Furthermore, a sensitization of the contractile machinery to prevailing Ca^{2+} (as in the Frank-Starling mechanism) has been proposed (Figure 4–2). Finally, cytoskeletal arrangements have also been proposed to contribute to the mechanism (1, 2) (Figure 4–2). Recent sophisticated studies in vivo have implicated pressure-dependent increases in reactive oxygen species as proximate signaling molecules that mediate the responses. While 50 μM vessels from WT mice demonstrate a robust myogenic response (changing intravascular pressure from 10 to 90 mm Hg), mice deficient in one of the impor-

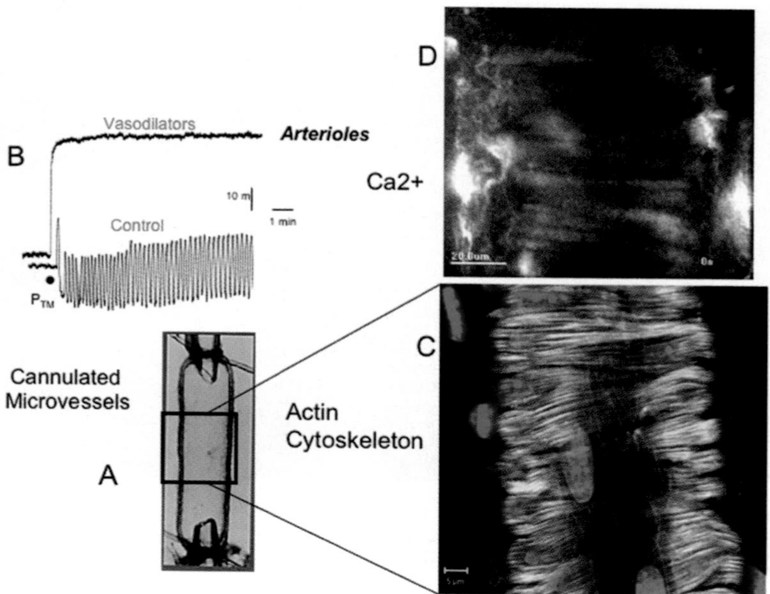

FIGURE 4–2. Myogenic tone is dependent on Ca^{2+} signaling as well as active re-arrangement of the cytoskeleton. The mechanism of myogenic tone can be studies in isolated pressurized arterioles (A). In the presence of vasodilators or absence of Ca^{2+}, an increase in pressure in the vessel led to a marked dilation of the arteriole. On the other hand, in the presence of Ca^{2+} the vessels develop an increase in tone such that with increase in pressure the diameter does not change or decreases (B). Staining of the actin cytoskeleton (silver) which is important in maintaining myogenic tone, is directed circumferentially with the nuclei (red) around the vessel. Active pressure development of tension is associated with Ca^{2+} sparks inside the vessel (D). Reactive oxygen species generation is critical for the development of myogenic tone. Increase in arteriolar pressure with resultant induction of myogenic tone (E), results in a production of reactive oxygen species as indicated by an increase in vascular green fluorescence using the ROS-sensitive dye DCF (F). Vessels from mice deficient in a component of the ROS-producing enzyme NADPH oxidase, p47 phox, do not develop myogenic tone when intravascular pressure is increased, suggesting that rROS play an important signaling role in myogenic tone (G). Adapted from Flavahan NA, et al.: Am J Physiol Heart Circ Physiol 2005;288:H660–9.; Nowicki PT, et al.: Circ Res 2001;89:114–6; and Miriel VA, et al.: J Physiol 1999;518:815–24.

tant subunits of the reactive oxygen species (ROS)-generating enzyme NADPH oxidase show no response, rapidly dilating (4) (Figure 4–2). Thus, while the exact nature of the myogenic response is not fully understood, vascular studies in animals and humans are allowing a more sophisticated understanding of the pathways involved in this important physiologic phenomenon.

Sympathetic Nervous System and the Neuroeffector Junction

It is well accepted that the α_1-adrenergic receptors are the most important mediators of noradrenergic vasoconstriction in vascular smooth muscle of arterioles. In addition to norepinephrine, the co-release of NPY and ATP is important in the synergistic augmentation of vasoconstriction (5, 6) (Figure 4–3A and 4–3B). The cloning and characterization of the different α-AR subtypes has led to a more sophisticated understanding of the subtypes that might be involved in mediating vasoconstriction at the neuroeffector junction. Recent in vivo and in vitro vascular biology studies support the idea that the α_{1B}-AR is the critical receptor mediating the noradrenergic response at the neuroeffector junction (7). This is in contrast to the α_{1A} and α_{1D} which might be important in mediating responses extra junctionally to circulating catecholamines (Figure 4–3C). This might in one sense explain the difference in response observed between endogenous sympathoactivation (pain and sympathetic stimulation) versus the response to exogenously administered catecholamines.

While the α_1-AR are critical in the regulation of visceral vasoconstriction, emerging evidence supports the idea that the α_2-AR are the

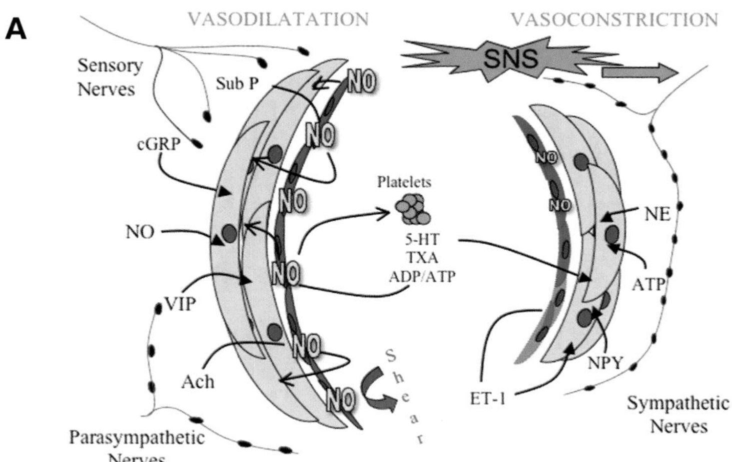

FIGURE 4–3. Schematic of the sympathetic neuroeffector junction. Efferent noradrenergic nerves release NE (and other mediators such as NPY and ATP) which activate α_1-adrenergic receptors on the vascular smooth muscle. Parasympathetic nerves also release neurotransmitters that mediate vasodilation. The endothelium modulates vascular smooth muscle tone by releasing paracrine molecules such as vasodilator NO, a vasoconstrictor endothelin (ET-1). Platelets can also contribute to vasoreactivity through the release of vasoactive molecules such as thromboxane (TXA) and serotonin (5-HT). Specific α_1-AR receptor subtypes appear to be important in mediating vasoconstriction at the neuroeffector

(figure continued next page)

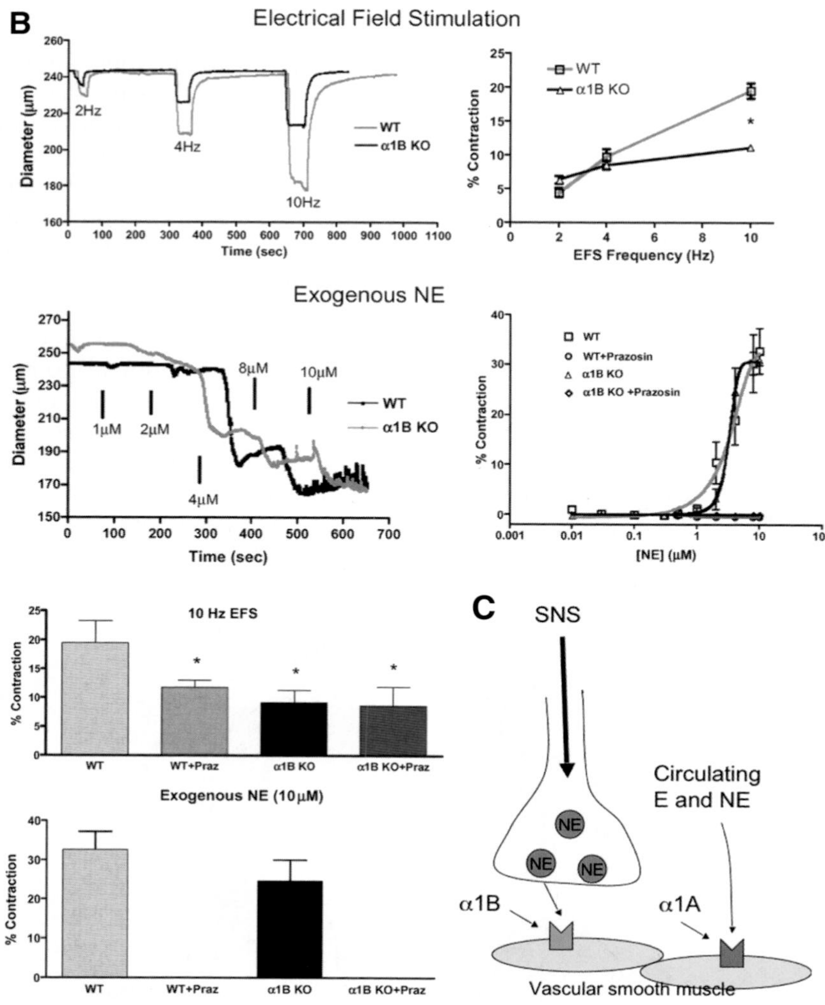

(FIG 4–3 CONT.) junction. Vasoconstriction mediated by endogenous release of NE induced by electrical stimulation (dose-dependent responses over 2, 4 and 10 Hz) are markedly attenuated in α_{1B}-AR KO mice as compared to WT. On the other hand, response to exogenous NE (added to the vessel bath) is no different in the 2 mouse strains (B). A schematic summarizing the model suggested by the above receptor subtype-specific findings (C). α_{2C} are thermosensitive receptors and mediate the vasoconstrictive effects of cold. As compared to the α_{2A}-receptor subtypes, the α_{2C} is not present on the cell membrane at 37°C and thus, cannot mediate the vasoconstrictive effect of agonists. On the other hand, at 28°C the receptors become expressed on the surface of the plasma membrane (D). This is

(figure continued next page)

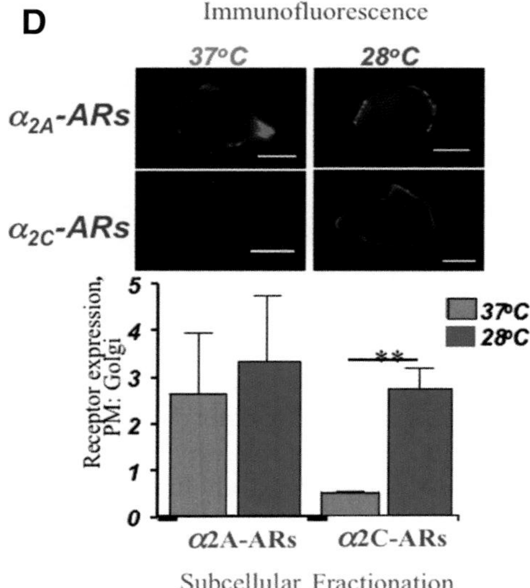

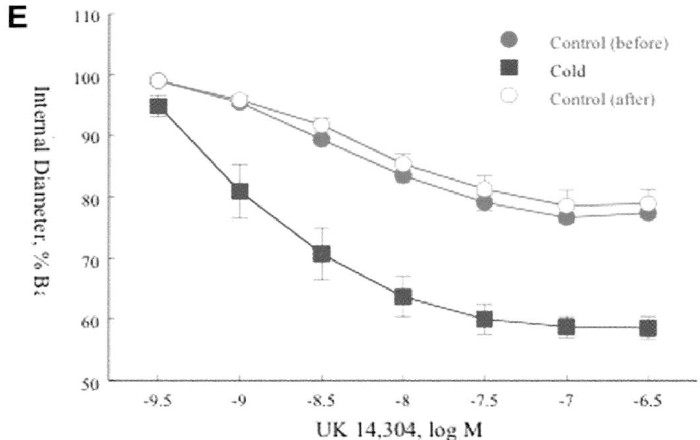

(FIG 4–3 CONT.) reflected functionally as an increase in vasoconstrictor responses to the α_2 specific agonist UK14,304 at 28 vs 37°C (E). Flavahan NA, et al.: Rheum Dis Clin North Am 2003; 29:275–91; Jeyaraj SC, et al.: Mol Pharmacol 2001;60:1195–200; and Chotani MA, et al.: Am J Physiol Heart Circ Physiol 2000; 278:H1075–83.

most important in mediating cutaneous vasoconstriction and hence one of the efferent arms of the thermoregulatory circuit. For example, the α_{2C}-AR was recently demonstrated to be thermosensitive. It is not expressed on the surface of cutaneous blood vessels at 37°C, however at 27°C the receptors are transported to the surface of the cell where they are expressed and respond to catecholamines (Figures 4–3D and 4–3E).

The thermosensitivity is thought to involve the Rho kinase pathway with the production of reactive oxygen species which are the proximate signaling molecules involved in the initiation of this process (8–10).

The Endothelium

The discovery that the endothelium is a critical organ system with a multitude of autocrine, paracrine, and endocrine functions, including mechanotransduction and modulator of inflammation rather than an inert lining of the blood vessels is probably the most important advance in vascular biology made during the past 30 years. In 1980, Furchgott and Zawadski demonstrated that blood vessels in which the intimal surface (endothelium) was physically denuded no longer demonstrated a vasodilatory effect to acetylcholine (in a vascular bioassay in organ chambers) (11). The mediator of this effect was labeled endothelium derived relaxing (EDRF). This was later identified by Ignarro, Murad, Palmer, and Moncado as the neurotransmitter gas nitric oxide (NO). A review of the multitude of mediators and signaling pathways that are involved in endothelium function are well beyond this chapter. Endothelial nitric oxide synthase, the enzyme responsible for the conversion of L-arginine to NO is regulated in a complex manner at a transcriptional, translational, and by post-translational level through modifications including phosphorylation and nitrosylation. In addition, the activity of the enzyme is regulated by co-factors (tetrahydrobiopterin, [BH4]) (12) and substrate L-arginine availability. Many of the pathways involved in the activation of nitric oxide synthase (NOS) are mechanosensitive. Laminar shear stress activates the enzyme (most likely the mechanism by which exercise improves endothelial function) (13) while oscillatory shear stress does not (a mechanism by which turbulence might contribute to endothelial dysfunction). An emerging idea with regard to dysfunction of the endothelium and dysregulation of NOS biology is referred to as "NOS uncoupling"(14) (Figure 4–4). In this process, a deficiency of BH_4, or substrate, leads to the inability of the enzyme to transfer electrons in the terminal process of NO synthesis. This leads to the enzyme acting as a NADPH oxidase-producing ROS superoxide. This process has been shown to contribute to the endothelial dysfunction associated with diabetes, atherosclerotic vascular disease, and erectile dysfunction. Ongoing work in our laboratory has determined that upregulation and activation of arginase, an enzyme that competes for L-arginine substrate in the endothelial cell, contributes to increased vascular oxidative stress in both aging and atherosclerotic vessels. Furthermore, the inhibition of arginase improves endothelial function in aging and attenuates the development of atherosclerosis in atherogenic mice. Thus, the coupling of NOS has important implications for the treatment of vascular diseases in which this nitroso-redox balance is disrupted.

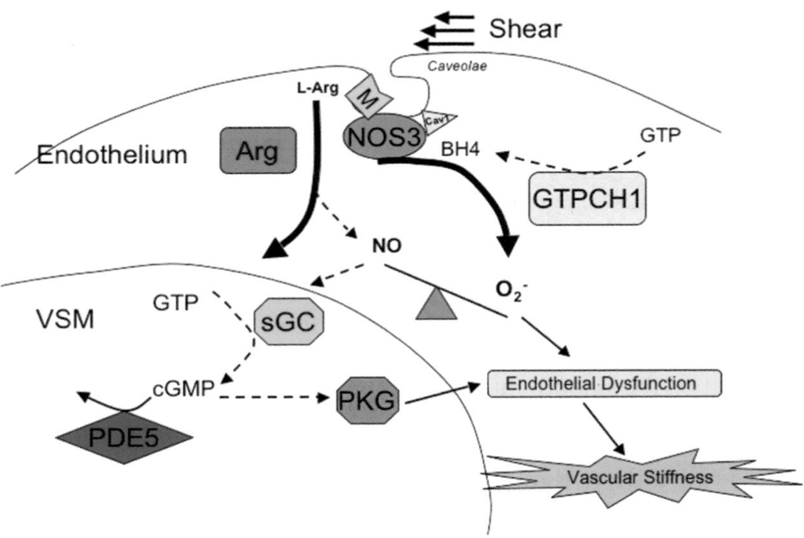

FIGURE 4–4. Both agonist (through the muscarinic receptor M) and shear stress-dependent activation of NOS leads to NO production and downstream signalling through soluble guanylyl cyclase (sGC) and protein kinase G (PKG) with resultant vasorelaxation. NOS uncoupling result from a depletion of substrate L-arginine (as might occur with an activation of the enzyme arginase (Arg) or with co-factor depletion or oxidation (tetrahydroibiopternin, BH4) leading to ROS generation by eNOS. GTP-cyclohydrolase 1 (GTPCH 1) is the critical rate-limiting enzyme in the synthesis of BH4. NOS uncoupling leads to endothelial dysfunction and impaired vascular health contributing to vascular stiffness and accelerated atherosclerosis.

PHARMACOLOGICAL MODULATION OF VASCULAR SMOOTH MUSCLE TONE

Vasopressin and Vasoplegic Syndromes

Vasoplegic syndrome (VS) is defined as an arterial pressure $<$50 mm Hg, cardiac index $>$2.5 L min^{-1} m^{-2}, right atrial pressure $<$5 mm Hg, left atrial pressure $<$10 mm Hg, and low SVR ($<$800 dyne s^{-1} cm^{-5}) during intravenous norepinephrine infusion ($\geq$0.5 μg kg^{-1} min^{-1}) (15). Vasoplegia is commonly associated with septic shock, the use of long-term angiotensin-converting enzyme inhibitors, as well as cardiac surgery, especially in patients undergoing LVAD implantation and heart transplantation. Vasoplegic syndrome responds poorly to norepinephrine therapy and leads to higher postoperative morbidity and mortality (16–18).

Vasopressin is an exogenous, parenteral form of antidiuretic hormone (ADH). Endogenous ADH is a hormone secreted by the hypothalamus and stored in the posterior pituitary gland. Vasopressin acts primarily as an antidiuretic hormone with little effect on arterial pressure at physiologic levels, resulting in avid free water retention. However, during hypotension, vasopressin levels increase to maintain blood pressure by vasoconstriction (19, 20). Commercial preparations of vasopressin exert the same pharmacologic effects as endogenous vasopressin. Vasopressin causes significant increases in mean arterial pressure and systemic vascular resistance, and results in a marked reduction in norepinephrine doses, with no appreciable change in cardiac index (21). Vasopressin stimulates vascular smooth muscle contraction in coronary, splanchnic, GI, pancreatic, skin, and muscular vascular beds. This effect is most prominent in the capillaries, small arterioles, and venules with less effect on the smooth musculature of large veins. Neither adrenergic agents nor vascular denervation has been shown to prevent this direct effect of vasopressin on smooth muscle contractile elements.

The precise mechanism of action of vasopressin is unclear. Whereas both catecholamines and vasopressin produce vasoconstriction by increasing intracellular calcium levels in vascular smooth muscle through activation of voltage-gated calcium channels, vasopressin inhibits the production of cyclic guanosine monophosphate and the adenosine triphosphate-activated potassium channels of vascular smooth muscle to produce vasoconstriction by activating the V1 receptors of vascular smooth muscles (22). Vasopressin also binds to oxytocin receptors to mediate a calcium-dependent vasodilatory response by stimulating the nitric oxide pathway in endothelial cells of pulmonary, coronary, and cerebral arteries.

While the vasopressin at high doses is thought to act through the V1 receptor to increase intracellular Ca^{2+}, recent data suggest that nanomolar (very low) concentrations might act synergistically with α_1-adrenergic receptors to enhance vasoconstriction (23). This occurs at concentrations of vasopressin (0.1 and 1 nM) that on their own have no intrinsic vasoconstrictor effect (Figures 4–5A and 4–5B). The mechanism of this "sensitization" might involve ATP-sensitive potassium channels (24–26). Blocking of these hyperpolarizing channels will make the membrane potential less negative, opening the voltage-sensitive Ca^{2+} channels and enhancing catecholamine mediated vasoconstriction (Figures 4–5C and 4–5D). So what is the potential pathophysiologic mechanism underlying the vasoplegic syndromes? It is now well established that the use of ACE inhibitors contributes to vasopressin-responsive vasoplegic syndromes (17, 27). ACE inhibitors prevent the activation of Ang II from Ang I. Another important role of ACE inhibitors is to prevent the breakdown of bradykinin. It is also well established that bradykinin is an important activator of the endothelium (BK-receptor dependent) leading to the release of NO and endothelium-derived hyperpolarizing factor (EDHF).

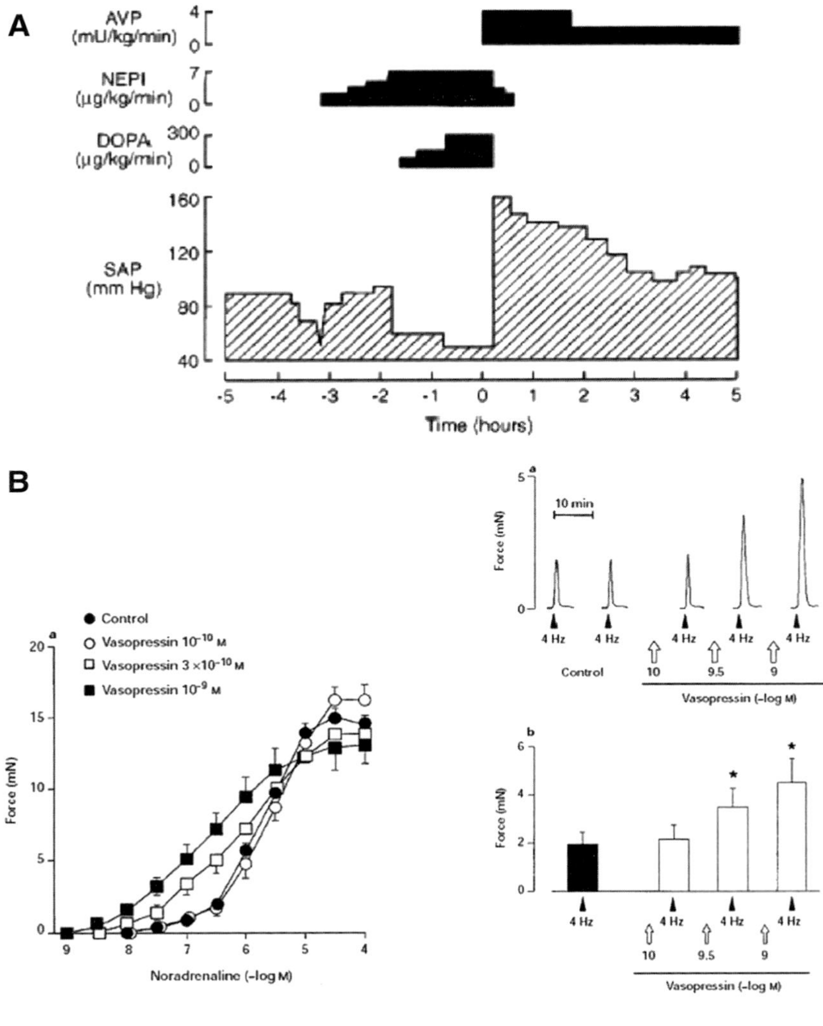

FIGURE 4–5. Vasopressin restores responsiveness to NE in septic shock and other vasoplegic syndromes (A). This is thought to be mediated by a mechanism that involves synergistic interaction between NE and vasopressin since vasopressin enhances responses to NE at doses that are not intrinsically vasoactive (0.1–1 nM) (B). This effect is thought to be mediated by the ability of vasopressin to block hyperpolarizing K_{ATP} channels. The open state probability of the channel is significantly reduced in patches from vascular smooth muscle upon exposure to vasopressin (C). Blocking of K_{ATP} channels results in a loss of hyperpolarization such that the membrane potential is less negative. This results in an

(figure continued next page)

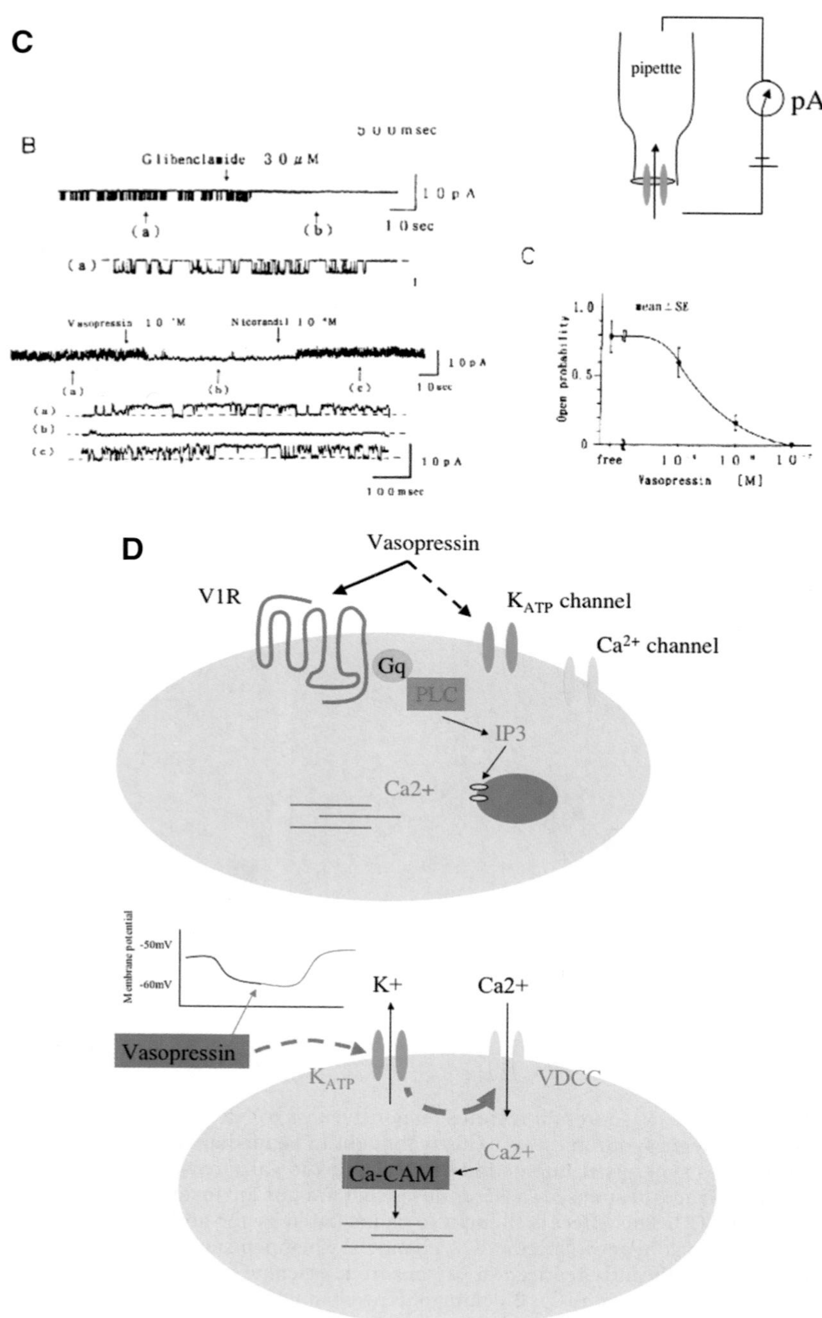

(FIG 4–5 CONT.) *(figure continued next page)*

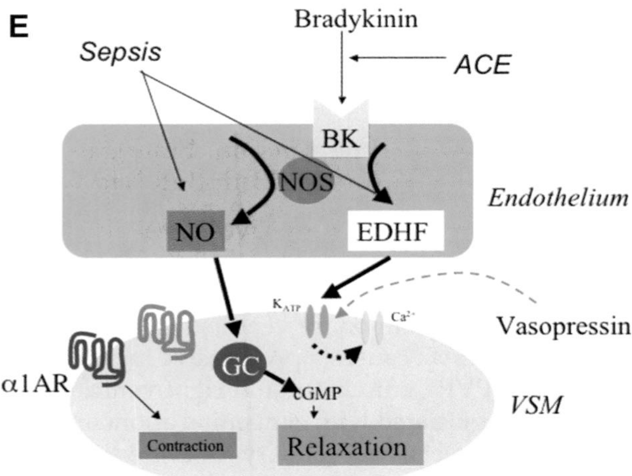

(FIG 4–5 CONT.) **opening of the voltage gated Ca^{2+} channels and ultimately a restoration of the vessel responsiveness to vasoconstrictor agonists (D). Mechanisms underlying potential vasoplegia in patients undergoing cardiac surgery, specifically those who have been treated with ACE inhibitors (E).**

This has important therapeutic implications in heart failure (increased NO leads to vasodilatation and prevention and remodelling). Following CPB, this may contribute to vasoplegia for the following reasons. CPB-mediated systemic inflammation leads to the activation of the kinin system with an increase in bradykinin production. The presence of ACE, as well as hypothermia, prevents the normal breakdown of BK with resultant increase. This in turn leads to a hyperpolarization of the membrane (EDHF release from the endothelium is mediated by the action of BK on the endothelial BK receptors) and a lack of responsiveness to vasoconstrictors. The addition of low-dose vasopressin alters the membrane potential, thus restoring catecholamine responsiveness (Figure 4–5E).

Numerous human trials of low-dose ($\leq$0.1 units/min) vasopressin have been conducted in vasodilatory shock to evaluate the hemodynamic effects of vasopressin. Of note, there are three randomized, controlled trials in patients with septic shock (28), vasodilatory shock after implantation of a left ventricular assist device (29), and vasodilatory shock (30). While the first two trials used normal saline as the control, Dunser et al. randomized patients to vasopressin plus norepinephrine vs. norepinephrine alone (30). All three trials show that vasopressin infusion increased mean arterial pressure and decreased the dose of catecholamine infusion. Preserved gastrointestinal perfusion was achieved with vasopressin plus norepinephrine in one trial (30) while vasopressin infusion increased urine output in two trials (31, 32). Low plasma vasopressin levels were found in five trials, including patients who had septic shock (31, 32) and postbypass vasodilatory shock (21, 29) and organ donors who had vasodilatory shock (33).

Therapy for Pulmonary Hypertension: Emerging Role of Phosphodiesterase Inhibitors and Inhaled Nitric Oxide

Over the past decade, many advances have been made in the therapy of pulmonary arterial hypertension (PAH), a condition characterized by an abnormal elevation of mean pulmonary arterial pressure (>25 mm Hg at rest) in the absence of pulmonary venous hypertension, respiratory, or embolic disorders. PAH causes a progressive increase in pulmonary vascular resistance (PVR), culminating in right ventricular failure and death. PAH may be associated with congenital anomalies (such as atrial or ventricular septal defects) or secondary to severe airway disease, such as hypoxemia from chronic obstructive pulmonary disease, late-stage pulmonary fibrosis, or adult respiratory distress syndrome. The familial form of PAH is an autosomal dominant disease with incomplete penetrance and is associated with mutations in the bone morphogenetic protein receptor II.

The Food and Drug Administration (FDA)-approved therapies for PAH, such as infused prostacyclins and an endothelin receptor antagonist, are associated with partial response. The disease is associated with high mortality so new and more effective therapies are needed.

The predominant PDE isoenzymes in pulmonary arteries are PDE5 (a specific cGMP inactivator) and PDE3 (a specific inactivator of cAMP, which is also inhibited by cGMP) (34). Animal data demonstrates that PDE5 is abundant in the normal lung and increases in the vessels of hypertensive lungs. This suggests that PDE5 limits vasodilation in hypertensive lungs and that inhibition of PDE5 could improve PAH.

Phosphodiesterase-5 (PDE5) inhibitors and other agents that modulate intracellular cGMP are now emerging as promising therapeutic options for PAH. PDE5 inhibitors slow the breakdown of cGMP and cAMP, and are potent acute pulmonary vasodilators in experimental models to partially reverse established pulmonary arterial hypertension and blunt chronic pulmonary hypertension (Figures 4–6A , 4–6B and 4–6C).

Sildenafil is a PDE5-inhibitor that slows the metabolism of cGMP (35). It is a potent vasodilator in its own right and can potentiate the effects of other vasodilators. Given its oral administration and favorable side-effect profile, sildenafil is particularly promising for the long-term therapy of PAH. Early nonrandomized studies of PAH patients given long-term sildenafil (25–100 mg PO three times daily for 5–20 months) showed reduced pulmonary artery systolic pressure on echocardiography compared with baseline as well as significant improvements in

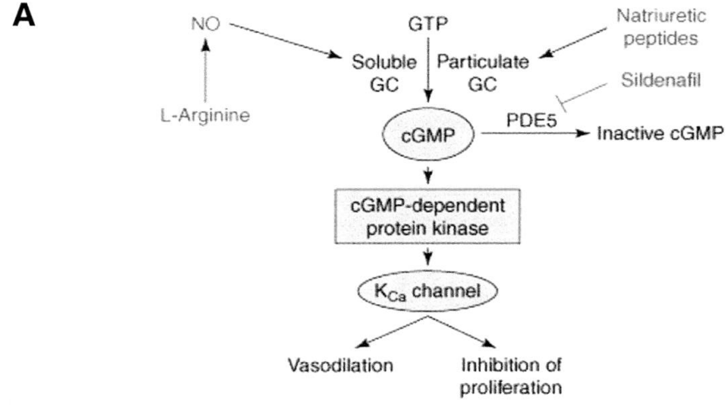

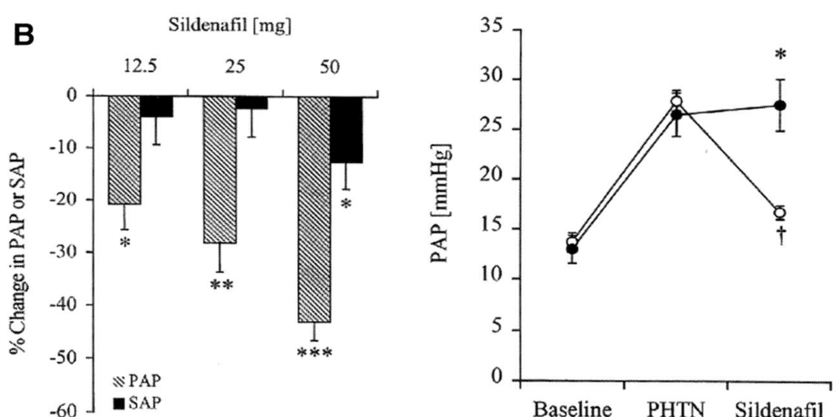

FIGURE 4–6. Schematic representation of the cGMP pathway that mediates vasodilation and inhibition of cellular proliferation (A). NO and natriuretic peptides stimulate soluble and particulate guanylate cyclase, respectively, to produce cGMP. Inhibition of PDE5 using sildenafil inhibits the breakdown of cGMP, augmenting pulmonary vasodilation and inhibiting cellular proliferation. GC, guanylyl cyclase; K_{Ca}, calcium channel (35). Sildenafil selectively and significantly reduces pulmonary pressures as compare to systemic blood pressure in an acute sheep model of PHTN (B). Interaction of iNO and sildenafil

(figure continued next page)

NYHA functional status and 6 minute walk distance (36, 37). Two placebo-controlled crossover trials have demonstrated the functional benefit of sildenafil. In the longer trial, 22 PAH patients received placebo or sildenafil (25–100 mg three times daily). The sildenafil group showed improved exercise tolerance, cardiac index, and quality of life scores after 6 weeks although there was no significant change in systolic pulmonary

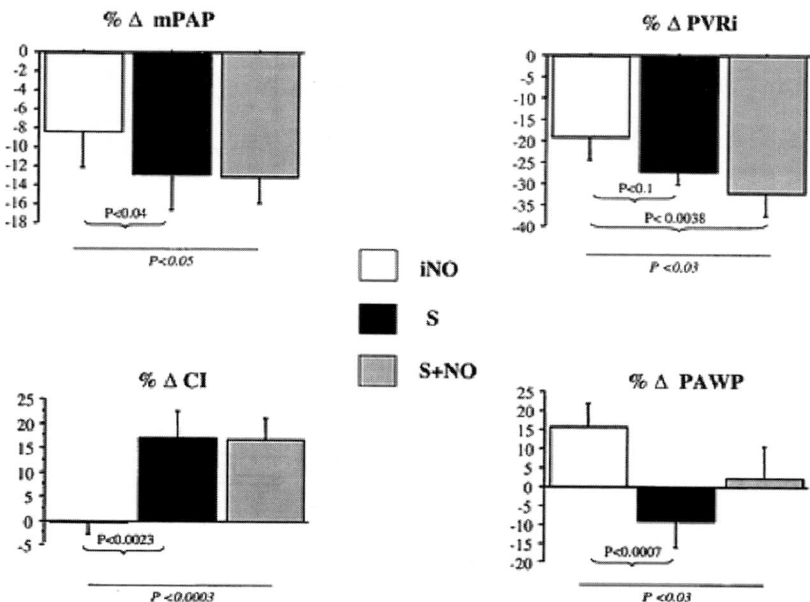

(FIG 4–6 CONT.) with regard to lowering pulmonary pressure and increasing cardiac output in patients with severe pulmonary hypertension (C). From Weimann, J, et al.: Anesthesiology 2000; 92:1702–12 and Michelakis E, et al.: Circulation 2002; 105:2398–403.

arterial pressure estimated by echocardiography (38). However, other PDE5 inhibitors such as longer-acting tadalafil or vardenafil have not been found to have similar effects on pulmonary circulation and oxygenation compared to sildenafil (39).

Inhaled nitric oxide (NO) is a potent and selective pulmonary vasodilator that improves oxygenation. As it is delivered directly to pulmonary resistance vessels and immediately inactivated by hemoglobin, inhaled NO is virtually devoid of systemic effects (40). Studies of acute right heart failure from open heart surgery, massive pulmonary embolism, lung transplantation. and acute respiratory distress syndrome demonstrate that while inhaled NO rapidly improves pulmonary hemodynamics and oxygenation, long-term results remain disappointing with high mortality rates despite therapy (41, 42). In addition, abrupt cessation of inhaled NO can lead to hemodynamic collapse. The difficulties and expense of administration of inhaled NO also limit its use in PAH therapy.

The combination of PDE5 inhibitors and agents that increase cGMP or cAMP can yield additive beneficial effects on pulmonary hemodynamics in patients with PAH. Sildenafil can potentiate and prolong the effects of inhaled NO (Figure 4–6C) and, when combined, the two agents produced a synergistic reduction in wedge pressure and PVR and an increased cardiac index more than when either agent was used alone (36). In a study by Kuhn et al. on PAH patients on long-term epoprostenol, 50 mg of sildenafil produced an additional 10% decrease in mean pulmonary arterial pressure, an 8% increase in cardiac output, and a 24% decrease in PVR compared with only a 13% decrease in PVR after inhaled NO (43). Such combination studies suggest that sildenafil can improve pulmonary hemodynamics in patients already on prostacyclins, though it is not yet known whether PDE5 inhibition potentiates the actions of endothelin receptor antagonists. The results from a large randomized trial currently underway that combines sildenafil with intravenous epoprostenol are eagerly awaited.

Hydralazine and Reversal of Nitrate Tolerance

Organic nitrates such as nitro-glycerine (NTG) have been one of the most widely used drugs for ischemic heart disease and chronic congestive heart failure (44, 45). However, prolonged systemic therapy with organic nitrates induces tolerance and endothelial dysfunction in patients with coronary artery disease and congestive heart failure, and even in healthy controls (46, 47). This phenomenon is known as nitrate tolerance and is due to a nitrate-induced stimulation of vascular (mitochondrial) superoxide and/or peroxynitrite production with the ensuing inhibition of ALDH2 leading to impaired NTG biotransformation (48).

The demonstration of increased endothelial superoxide formation in NTG tolerance suggests that treatment with antioxidants may prevent this phenomenon.

Hydralazine has also been shown to prevent the development of nitrate tolerance in both experimental models and patients with congestive heart failure (49, 50). It is a potent arteriolar dilator that stimulates reflex increases in vasoconstrictor stimuli in the form of circulating catecholamines and plasma rennin with associated increased circulating angiotensin II levels. While this may instinctively suggest a worsening of nitrate tolerance by enhancing the neurohormonal counter regulatory adjustments to nitrate, the fact that this does not occur indicates that hydralazine may have antioxidant properties.

The mechanisms whereby hydralazine exerts its antioxidant effects may include cyclic adenosine monophosphate- or hyperpolarization-induced inhibition of the expression and activity of the NADPH oxidase or direct ROS free radical scavenging effects. The scavenging of peroxynitrite may be of utmost importance, because peroxynitrite has been identified to cause NOS III uncoupling, tyrosine nitration of the PGI_2-S, and inhibition of activity of the NO target sGC (51) (Figures 4–7A and 4–7B).

The Veterans Heart Failure Trials (V-HeFT) demonstrated favorable interactions between hydralazine and ISDN, allowing improved left ven-

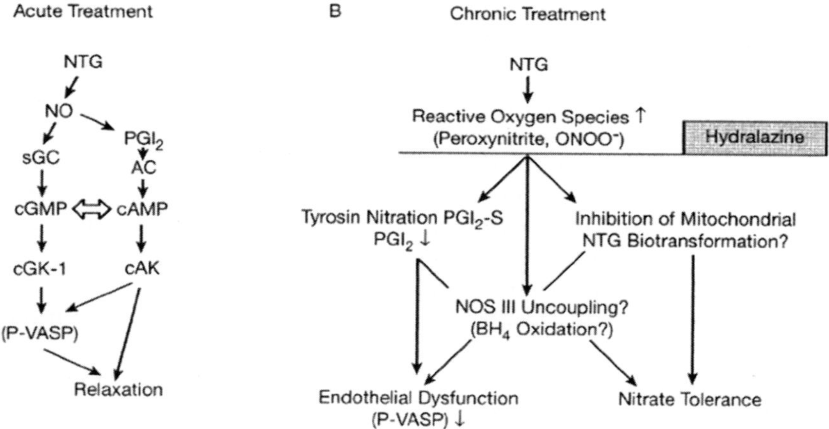

FIGURE 4–7. Schematic diagram depicting mechanisms underlying nitroglycerin (NTG)-induced vasodilation (A) and the vascular consequences of NTG-induced peroxynitrite formation (B). (A) Short-term NTG treatment causes vasorelaxation by releasing nitric oxide (NO) or an NO-related vasoactive metabolite, which in turn stimulates the soluble guanylyl cyclase (sGC) and release of prostacyclin (PGI_2). Activation of sGC and adenylyl cyclase (AC) increases the formation of second messengers such as cyclic guanosine monophosphate (cGMP) and cyclic adenosine monophosphate (cAMP). Signaling pathways activated by cAMP and cGMP may interact at different levels. Subsequent activation of the cGMP- and cAMP-dependent kinase (cGK-I and cAK) will induce vasorelaxation. Activation of the cGK-I, and to some extent cAK, will cause phosphorylation of the phosphorylated vasodilator-stimulated phosphoprotein (P-VASP). (B) Long-term NTG treatment stimulates the production of reactive oxygen species such as peroxynitrite ($ONOO^-$), which may in turn induce tolerance via inhibiting the activity of the NTG-metabolizing enzyme. $ONOO^-$ may also cause endothelial dysfunction by oxidizing the NO synthase (NOS) III cofactor tetrahydrobiopterin (BH_4) to dihydrobiopterin (BH_2) and by tyrosine nitration of the prostacyclin synthase (PGI_2-S) associated with a decrease in the cGK-I activity (decrease in P-VASP) (51).

tricular function, exercise capacity, and survival in a large patient population with severe heart failure (52). The recent African American Heart Failure Trial (A-HeFT) also showed that a fixed-dose combination of ISDN/hydralazine can decrease mortality, reduce the incidence of first hospitalization for heart failure, and improve quality of life (53).

Pleotropic Effects of Statins

Given the role of the vascular endothelium in the regulation of vascular wall homeostasis, impaired endothelial function has been attributed as the cause of various diseases such as hypertension, atherosclerosis, and heart failure. Hypercholesterolemia is associated with endothelial dys-

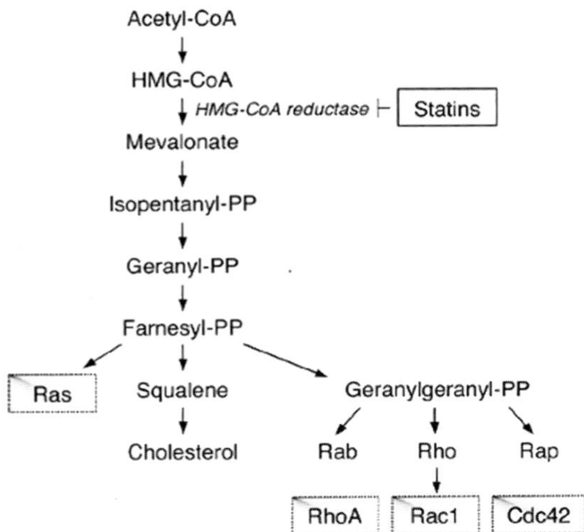

FIGURE 4–8. **Cholesterol biosynthesis pathway and the effects of statins. Inhibition of HMG-CoA reductase by statins decreases isoprenoid intermediates such as farnesyl-PP and geranylgeranyl-PP, which leads to an inhibition of isoprenylation of small GTPases such as Ras, Rho, Rab, and Rap. Among the Rho GTPases are RhoA, Rac1, and Cdc42. CoA indicates coenzyme A; PP, pyrophosphate (61).**

function and the impaired function of endothelial-derived NO and increases the risk for vascular disease (54, 55).

The lipid-lowering drugs, 3-hydroxy-3-methylglutaryl-coenzyme A (HMG-CoA) reductase inhibitors or statins, are used in the treatment of hypercholesterolemia and in the prevention of cardiovascular diseases (56, 57). Experimental and clinical studies suggest that statins exert their vascular protective effects by improving endothelial function via cholesterol-dependent and independent mechanisms.

It is thought that most, if not all, the beneficial effects of statins on endothelial function are attributable to cholesterol reduction. This is achieved by the inhibition of HMG-CoA reductase by statins, an enzyme in the liver that catalyzes the conversion of HMG-CoA to mevalonate. This conversion is the rate-limiting step in the hepatic synthesis of cholesterol biosynthesis (58) (Figure 4–8).

However, improvement in endothelial function from statin treatment has been found to occur before significant reduction in serum cholesterol levels (59). Thus, it is possible that the beneficial effects of statins on endothelial function extend beyond cholesterol reduction.

A hallmark of endothelial dysfunction is reduced bioavailability of NO, which could be caused by reduced expression of eNOS, impairment of eNOS activation, and increased inactivation of NO by oxidative stress. The cholesterol-independent or "pleiotropic" effects of statins include the up regulation and activation of endothelial NO synthase (eNOS). Because statins inhibit an early step in the cholesterol biosynthetic pathway, they also inhibit the synthesis of isoprenoids such as farnesylpyrophosphate and geranylgeranylpyrophosphate, which are important posttranslational lipid attachments for intracellular signalling molecules such as the Rho GTPases. Indeed, decrease in Rho GTPase responses as a consequence of statin treatment increases the production and bioavailability of endothelium-derived NO. The mechanism involves, in part, Rho/Rho-kinase (ROCK)-mediated changes in the actin cytoskeleton, which leads to decreases in eNOS mRNA stability. The regulation of eNOS by Rho GTPases, therefore, may be an important mechanism underlying the cardiovascular protective effect of statins (60).

CONCLUSION

The significant investment in cardiovascular research during the past 4 decades has paid off as we continue to develop an understanding of normal cellular and cardiovascular disease-related dysregulation of signalling pathways. This has led to the identification of key enzymes, channels, and receptors that can be modulated by small molecules, and form the basis of our current and future drug array. As cardiac anesthesiologists, we share the benefit of these advances as we increase the selection of drugs that allow us to treat tough pathophysiologic phenomena such as vasoplegic syndromes, pulmonary hypertension, ischemia, and heart failure. Furthermore these new agent allow us to optimize the patients' vascular health preoperatively and in so doing improve perioperative cardiovascular outcomes.

References

1. Hill MA, Davis MJ, Meninger GA, et al.: Arteriolar myogenic signalling mechanisms: implications for local vascular function. Clin Hemorheol Microcirc 2006; 34:67–79
2. Hill MA, Sun Z, Martinez-Lemus L, et al.: New technologies for dissecting the arteriolar myogenic response. Trends Pharmacol Sci 2007; 28:308–15
3. Bayliss WM: On the local reactions of the arterial wall to changes of internal pressure. J Physiol 1902; 28:220–31
4. Nowicki PT, Flavahan S, Hassanian H, et al.: Redox signaling of the arteriolar myogenic response. Circ Res 2001; 89:114–16

5. Yang XP, Chiba S: Interaction between neuropeptide YY1 receptors and alpha$_{1B}$-adrenoceptors in the neurovascular junction of canine splenic arteries. Eur J Pharmacol 2003; 466:311–15
6. Yang XP, Chiba S: Separate modulation of neuropeptide Y1 receptor on purinergic and on adrenergic neuroeffector transmission in canine splenic artery. J Cardiovasc Pharmacol 2001; 38:S17–S20
7. Townsend SA, Jung AS, Hoe YS, et al.: Critical role for the alpha-1B adrenergic receptor at the sympathetic neuroeffector junction. Hypertension 2004; 44:776–82
8. Bailey SR, Mitra S, Flavahan S, et al.: Reactive oxygen species from smooth muscle mitochondria initiate cold-induced construction of cutaneous arteries. Am J Physiol Heart Circ Physiol 2005; 289:H243–H250
9. Chotani MA, Flavahan S, Mitra S, et al.: Silent alpha 2C-adrenergic receptors enable cold-induced vasoconstriction in cutaneous arteries. Am J Physiol Heart Circ Physiol 2000; 278:H1075—H1083
10. Jeyaraj SC, Chotani MA, Mitra S, et al.: Cooling evokes redistribution of alpha$_{2C}$-adrenoceptors from Golgi to plasma membrane in transfected human embryonic kidney 293 cells. Mol Pharmacol 2001; 60:1195–1200
11. Furchgott R, Zawadzki J: The obligatory role of endothelial cells in the relaxation of arterial smooth muscle. Nature 1980; 288:373–6
12. Alp NJ, McAteer MA, Khoo JC, et al.: Increased endothelial tetrahydrobiopterin synthesis by targeted transgenic GTP-cyclohydrolase I overexpression reduces endothelial dysfunction and atherosclerosis in ApoE-knockout mice. Arterioscl Thromb Vasc Biol 2004; 24:445–50
13. Hambrecht R, Adams V, Erbs S, et al.: Regular physical activity improves endothelial function in patients with coronary artery disease by increasing phosphorylation of endothelial nitric oxide synthase. Circulation 2003; 107:3152–8
14. Forstermann U, Munzel T: Endothelial nitric oxide synthase in vascular disease: from marvel to menace. Circulation 2006; 113:1708–14
15. Ozal E, Kuralay E, Yildirim V, et al.: Preoperative methylene blue administration in patients at high risk for vasoplegic syndrome during cardiac surgery. Ann Thorac Surg 2005; 79:1615–19
16. Mekontso-Dessap A, Houel R, Soustelle C, et al.: Risk factors for post-cardiopulmonary bypass vasoplegia in patients with preserved left ventricular function. Ann Thorac Surg 2001; 71:1428–32
17. Carrel T, Englberger L, Mohacsi P, et al.: Low systemic vascular resistance after cardiopulmonary bypass: incidence, etiology, and clinical importance. J Card Surg 2000; 15:347–53
18. Gomes WJ, Carvalho AC, Palma JH, et al.: Vasoplegic syndrome after open heart surgery. J Cardiovasc Surg. 1998; 39:619–23

19. Minaker KL, Meneilly GS, Youn GJB, et al.: Blood pressure, pulse, and neurohumoral responses to nitroprusside-induced hypotension in normotensive aging men. J Gerontol 1991; 46:M151–M154
20. Cowley AWJ, Monos E, Guyton AC: Interaction of vasopressin and the baroreceptor reflex system in the regulation of arterial blood pressure in the dog. Circ Res 1974; 34:505–14
21. Argenziano M, Chen JM, Choudhri AF, et al.: Management of vasodilatory shock after cardiac surgery: identification of predisposing factors and use of a novel pressor agent. J Thorac Cardiovasc Surg 1998; 116:937–80
22. Gold JA, Cullinane S, Chen J, et al.: Vasopressin as an alternative to norepinephrine in the treatment of milrinone-induced hypotension. Crit Care Med 2000; 28:249–52
23. Noguera I, Medina P, Segarra G, et al.: Potentiation by vasopressin of adrenergic vasoconstriction in the rat isolated mesenteric artery. Br J Pharmacol 1997; 122:431–8
24. Kawano T, Tanaka K, Nazari H, et al.: The effects of extracellular pH on vasopressin inhibition of ATP-sensitive K+ channels in vascular smooth muscle cells. Anesth Analg 2007; 105:1714–19
25. Shi W, Cui N, Shi Y, et al.: Arginine vasopressin inhibits Kir6.1/SUR2B channel and constricts the mesenteric artery via V1a receptor and protein kinase C. Am J Physiol Regul Integr Comp Physiol 2007; 293:R191–R199
26. Wakatsuki T, Nakaya Y, Inoue I: Vasopressin modulates K^+-channel activities of cultured smooth muscle cells from porcine coronary artery. Am J Physio 1999; 263:H491–H496
27. Byrne JG, Leacche M, Paul S, et al.: Risk factors and outcomes for "vasoplegia syndrome" following cardiac transplantation. Eur J Cardiothorac Surg 2004; 25:327–32
28. Malay MB, Ashton RCJ, Landry DW, et al.: Low-dose vasopressin in the treatment of vasodilatory septic shock. . J Trauma 1999; 47:699–703
29. Argenziano M, Choudhri AF, Oz MC, et al.: A prospective randomized trial of arginine vasopressin in the treatment of vasodilatory shock after left ventricular assist device placement. Circulation 1997; 96:II286–II290
30. Dünser MW, Mayr AJ, Ulmer H, et al.: Arginine vasopressin in advanced vasodilatory shock: a prospective randomized, controlled study. Circulation 2003; 107:2313–19
31. Landry DW, Levin HR, Gallant EM, et al.: Vasopressin deficiency contributes to the vasodilation of septic shock. Circulation 1997; 95:1122–5
32. Patel BM, Chittock DR, Russell JA, et al.: Beneficial effects of short-term vasopressin infusion during severe septic shock. Anesthesiology 2002; 96:576–82

33. Briegel J, Forst H, Haller M, et al.: Stress doses of hydrocortisone reverse hyperdynamic septic shock: a prospective, randomized, double-blind, single-center study. Crit Care Med 1999; 27:723–32
34. Rabe KF, Tenor H, Dent G, et al.: Identification of PDE isozymes in human pulmonary artery and effect of selective PDE inhibitors. Am J Physio 1994; 266:L536-L543
35. Steiner MK, Preston IR, Klinger JR, et al.: Pulmonary hypertension: inhaled nitric oxide, sildenafil and natriuretic peptides. Curr Opin Pharmacol 2005; 5:245–50
36. Michelakis E, Tymchak W, Lien D, et al.: Oral sildenafil is an effective and specific pulmonary vasodilator in patients with pulmonary arterial hypertension: comparison with inhaled nitric oxide. Circulation 2002; 105:2398–403
37. Sastry BK, Narasimhan C, Reddy NKA, B, et al.: A study of clinical efficacy of sildenafil in patients with primary pulmonary hypertension. Indian Heart J 2002; 54:410–14
38. Sastry BK, Narasimhan C, Reddy NK, et al.: Clinical efficacy of sildenafil in primary pulmonary hypertension: a randomized, placebo-controlled, double-blind, crossover study. J Am Coll Card 2004; 43:1149–53
39. Ghofrani HA, Voswinckel R, Reichenberger F, et al.: Differences in hemodynamic and oxygenation responses to three different phosphodiesterase-5 inhibitors in patients with pulmonary arterial hypertension: a randomized prospective study. J Am Coll Card 2004; 44: 1488–96
40. Pepke-Zaba J, Higenbottam TW, Dinh-Xuan AT, et al.: Inhaled nitric oxide as a cause of selective pulmonary vasodilatation in pulmonary hypertension. Lancet 1991; 338:1173–74
41. Zapol WM, Falke KJ, Hurford WE, et al.: Inhaling nitric oxide: a selective pulmonary vasodilator and bronchodilator. Chest 1994; 105:87S-91S
42. Taylor RW, Zimmerman JL, Dellinger RP, et al.: Low-dose inhaled nitric oxide in patients with acute lung injury: a randomized controlled trial. JAMA 2004; 291:1603–09
43. Kuhn KP, Wickersham NE, Robbins IM, et al.: Acute effects of sildenafil in patients with primary pulmonary hypertension receiving epoprostenol. Exp Lung Res 2004; 30:135–45
44. Abrams J: Use of nitrates in ischemic heart disease. Curr Probl Cardiol 1992; 17:481–542
45. Elkayam U, Johnson JV, Shotan A, et al.: Double-blind, placebo-controlled study to evaluate the effect of organic nitrates in patients with chronic heart failure treated with angiotensin-converting enzyme inhibition. Circulation 1999; 99:2652–57

46. Caramori PR, Adelman AG, Azevedo ER, et al.: Therapy with nitroglycerin increases coronary vasoconstriction in response to acetylcholine. J Am Coll Card 1998; 32:1969–74
47. Gori T, Mak SS, Kelly S, et al.: Evidence supporting abnormalities in nitric oxide synthase function induced by nitroglycerin in humans. J Am Coll Card 2001; 38:1096–1101
48. Daiber A, Mülsch A, Hink U, et al.: The oxidative stress concept of nitrate tolerance and the antioxidant properties of hydralazine. Am J Cardiol 2005; 96:25i–36i
49. Münzel T, Kurz S, Rajagopalan S, et al.: Hydralazine prevents nitroglycerin tolerance by inhibiting activation of a membrane-bound NADH oxidase. A new action for an old drug. J Clin Invest 1996; 98:1465–70
50. Gogia H, Mehra A, Parikh S, et al.: Prevention of tolerance to hemodynamic effects of nitrates with concomitant use of hydralazine in patients with chronic heart failure. J Am Coll Card 1995; 26:1575–80
51. Hink U, Oelze M, Kolb P, et al.: Role for peroxynitrite in the inhibition of prostacyclin synthase in nitrate tolerance. J Am Coll Card 2003; 42:1826–34
52. Cohn JN: Role of nitrates in congestive heart failure. Am J Cardiol 1987; 60:39H-43H
53. Taylor AL, Ziesche S, Yancy C, et al.: Combination of isosorbide dinitrate and hydralazine in blacks with heart failure. N Eng J Med 2004; 351:2049–57
54. Sytkowski PA, Kannel WB, D'Agostino RB: Changes in risk factors and the decline in mortality from cardiovascular disease. The Framingham Heart Study. N Eng J Med 1990; 322:1635–41
55. Gordan T, Kannel WB: Premature mortality from coronary heart disease. The Framingham Study. JAMA 1971; 215:1617–25
56. (4S) TSSSS. Randomised trial of cholesterol lowing in 4444 patients with coronary heart disease. Lancet 1994; 344:1383–9
57. Study MBHP. Cholesterol lowing with simvastain in 20,536 high-risk individuals: a randomised placebo-controlled trial. Lancet 2002; 360:7–22
58. Rikitake Y, Liao JK: Rho GTPases, statins, and nitric oxide. Circ Res 2005; 97:1232–5
59. O'Driscoll G, Green D, Taylor RR: Simvastatin, an HMG-coenzyme A reductase inhibitor, improves endothelial function within 1 month. Circulation 1997; 95:1126–31
60. Hall A: Rho GTPases and the actin cytoskeleton. Science 1998; 279:509–14
61. Rikitake Y, Liao JK: Rho GTPases, statins, and nitric oxide. Circ Res 2005; 97:1332–5

Jacob Raphael, MD

5 Physiology and Pharmacology of Myocardial Preconditioning

Myocardial preconditioning (PC) has been the subject of intense laboratory and clinical research and is definitely one of the most important developments in the field of ischemic biology in the past 20 years. The implications of PC transcend the field of cardiovascular perioperative medicine and are of interest to anesthesiologists as well as cardiologists, surgeons, and many other physicians. This review chapter will focus particularly on the physiology and pharmacology of myocardial preconditioning and will discuss the aspects of volatile anesthetics and cardioprotection. It also will focus on several other drugs and biological agents that may have cardioprotective properties.

First, it is important to establish the definition of preconditioning and distinguish it from cardioprotection. Ischemic preconditioning (IPC) is the phenomenon whereby brief episodes of sublethal ischemia render the heart more resistant to subsequent prolonged ischemic injury. Here, the protection persists after the therapeutic intervention has dissipated, implying the existence of a cardiac "memory" (i.e., the heart "remembers" that it has been exposed to a PC stimulus and maintains a preconditioned phenotype even after the stimulus has been withdrawn). In contrast, with direct cardioprotection the enhanced resistance to ischemia-reperfusion injury occurs only while the therapeutic intervention is being applied; when the intervention is withdrawn, the protection disappears.

The phenomenon of PC was described initially in 1986 by Murry et al. (1). In this study, the authors made what at that time appeared to

Advances in Cardiovascular Pharmacology, edited by Philippe R. Housmans, MD, PhD and Gregory A. Nuttall, M.D.
Lippincott Williams & Wilkins, Baltimore © 2008.

be a paradoxical observation. They exposed a group of open-chest dogs to a sequence of four brief ischemic episodes (5-minute coronary occlusions interspersed with 5-minute reperfusion periods) and then subjected them to a prolonged, more severe ischemic insult (a 40-minute coronary occlusion followed by 4 days of reperfusion). Theoretically, one would have expected that the dogs that received the four brief coronary occlusions would exhibit greater infarct size because they had been exposed to an additional 20 minutes of ischemia. Surprisingly, it was found that infarct size was much smaller in the dogs that were exposed to the short periods of ischemia than in the controls, and that this effect was independent of differences in coronary collateral blood flow (Figure 5–1). These investigators coined the term "ischemic preconditioning" to describe this phenomenon, opening the gates for what has become one of the major themes of research in cardiovascular medicine in the past 2 decades. Following the fundamental publication of Murry et al., the number of studies dealing with PC has increased dramatically, such that in the past 10 years, for example, more than 5,000 publications were published in the English medical literature on this subject (Figure 5–2). Initially almost all studies were experimental; however, clinical studies

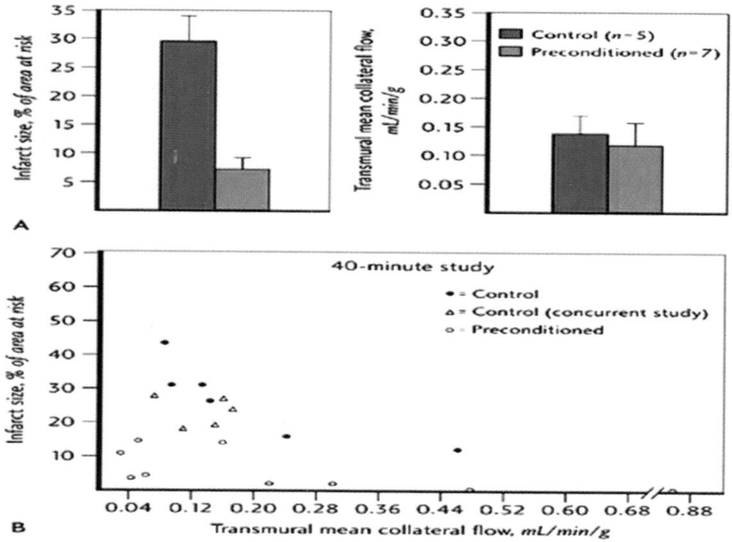

FIGURE 5–1. Bar graphs (A) and normogram (B) of infarct size as percentage of the area at risk and transmural collateral coronary blood flow in preconditioned and non-preconditioned dogs after 40 minutes of coronary occlusion and 4 days of reperfusion. Adapted with modifications with permission from Murry, et al. (1).

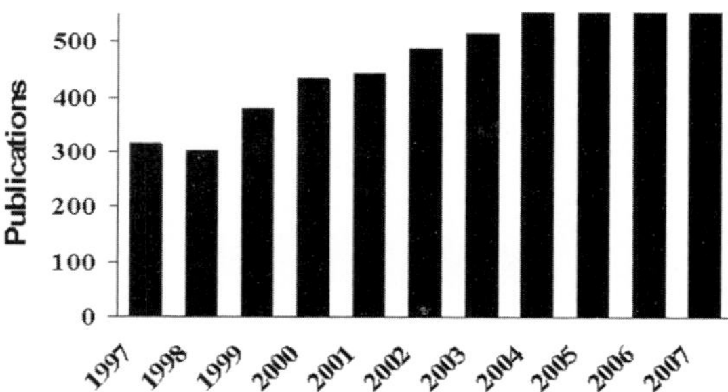

FIGURE 5–2. **Bar graph representing number of publications per year in the English scientific literature in the topic of myocardial preconditioning in the years 1997–2007.**

soon appeared and continued to increase—proof of the growing level of interest among clinicians in this phenomenon.

During the past 35 years, many cardioprotective therapies have been claimed to reduce myocardial infarct size in experimental animal models. However, few of these results have been reproducible, and none has been translated into clinical practice. As a result, after investing an enormous amount of time, money, and resources into the search for cardioprotective therapies, we still do not have a drug that has been specifically approved for the reduction of infarct size in patients with acute myocardial infarction. After many years of frustration with the failure to identify a single therapy to decrease myocardial infarct size, ischemic PC was discovered. It quickly became very clear that PC was an extremely powerful cardioprotective phenomenon. In many experimental models, IPC can reduce infarct size by as much as 80–90%—a degree of infarct size limitation that is rarely, if ever, observed with any other cardioprotective intervention. Furthermore, IPC was found to be remarkably reproducible. Ischemic PC exerts robust and highly reproducible protection, and appears to be a ubiquitous endogenous protective mechanism at the cellular level that has been observed in the heart of every species tested. This protection is also seen in other organs such as the liver, kidney, gut, and brain (2). The reduction in infarct size mediated by ischemic preconditioning disappears if the interval between the preconditioning protocol and the index ischemic period is longer than 3 or 4 hours (2). This loss of effect suggests that there is an associated "memory effect" and that protection is transient.

After the initial description of PC in 1986, the next major discovery came in 1993, when it was found that PC consists of two distinct phases: an *early phase*, which develops very quickly (within a few minutes from the exposure to the stimulus) but is rather short, lasting 2–4 hours, and

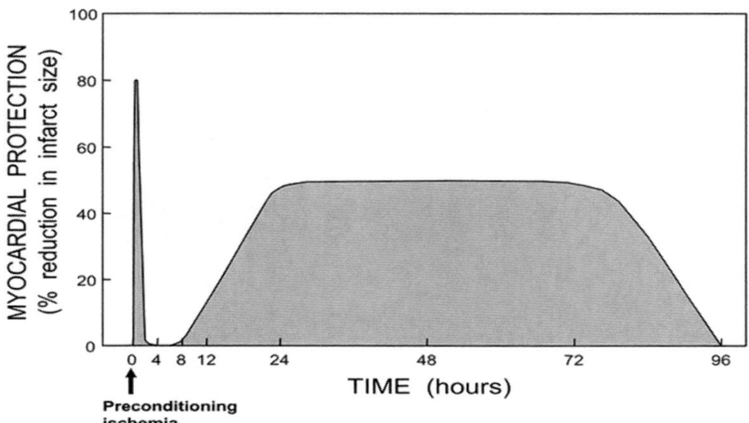

FIGURE 5–3. A diagram illustrating the two phases of protection. The early phase develops very quickly but is rather short, lasting up to 2–4 hours. The late phase develops more slowly (over a period of 12–24 hours) but lasts much longer (3–4 days). Adapted with modifications with permission from Marber, et al. (3).

a *late phase*, which develops more slowly (requiring 12–24 hours) but lasts much longer (3–4 days) (3) (Figure 5–3). The mechanisms for these two phases are completely different. The early phase is caused by rapid post-translational modification of preexisting proteins, whereas the late phase is caused by the synthesis of new cardioprotective proteins (which explains the time course of this phenomenon).

The range of protection also is different. The early phase is very effective in limiting lethal ischemia-reperfusion injury (i.e., infarction) but does not protect against reversible postischemic contractile dysfunction (myocardial "stunning"). The late phase protects against both infarction and stunning, although it is less powerful than the early phase in limiting infarct size.

MECHANISMS OF CARDIOPROTECTION BY ISCHEMIC PRECONDITIONING

The current paradigm suggests that the short ischemic episodes of preconditioning lead to the release of substances such as adenosine, bradykinin, endothelin, and endorphins. These substances bind to their G protein-coupled receptors on the surface of myocytes and activate several signal transduction cascades, which include phosphatidylinositol-3-kinase (PI3K)-Akt (4), extracellular signal-regulated kinase (Erk1/2) (2) and transcription factors such as the Hypoxia Inducible Factor (HIF) 1 (5) and nuclear factor κB (6, 7). Activation of these pro-survival mediators converges on the mitochondria, resulting in the opening of the ATP-dependent mitochondrial potassium channel (8, 9). Reactive oxygen species are then released (10), further signaling kinases are activated, such as protein kinase C, which is responsible for conveying the "memory effect" of ischemic preconditioning (2). It must be appreciated, however, that alternative protective mechanisms of IPC might exist that are independent of signal transduction pathways, such as those mediated by antioxidant and anti-inflammatory mechanisms.

During the second window of protection, signaling kinases mediate the transcription of distal mediators and effectors, such as inducible nitric oxide synthase (iNOS), manganese superoxide dismutase, heat-stress proteins, and cyclo-oxygenase 2 (COX-2), 24–72 hours after infarction, which manifest the late protection (2). How these signaling transduction pathways mediate protection and ultimately reduce infarct size is currently unknown. Suggested mechanisms include maintenance of mitochondrial ATP generation, reduced mitochondrial calcium accumulation, reduced generation of oxidative stress, inhibition of apoptosis, and prevention of mitochondrial permeability transition-pore (mPTP) opening (2, 11).

PHARMACOLOGICAL-INDUCED CARDIAC PROTECTION

Although PC was initially described as a response of the myocardium to ischemia, it soon became apparent that a similar phenotype can be elicited by a large number of stimuli, some of which are clinically relevant. For example, a number of pharmacological agents, including agonists of G protein-coupled receptors (GPCRs) (adenosine A_1 or A_3, bradykinin B_2, α_1-adrenergic, muscarinic M_2, angiotensin AT_1, endothelin, δ_1-opioid, etc.), nitric oxide (NO) donors, phosphodiesterase inhibitors, and various noxious stimuli (such as endotoxin and endotoxin derivatives, various cytokines, and reactive oxygen species) have all been found to elicit a PC-like phenotype (2, 12). The importance of these findings is the conclusion that ischemia is not the only stimulus capable of inducing a cardioprotected phenotype; stimuli that are less harmful or unpleasant (and thus more clinically relevant) also can do this.

A rapidly growing body of evidence indicates that volatile anesthetics protect myocardium against ischemic injury. Initially, several studies have suggested that isoflurane and other volatile agents may actually cause myocardial ischemia through "coronary steal" (13, 14). Later, the implication that isoflurane might produce myocardial ischemia through such a steal mechanism was dispelled by investigations conducted in animal models (15) as well as in humans with coronary artery disease (16, 17). Many laboratory and clinical investigations conducted since the resolution of the coronary steal controversy have shown convincingly that volatile anesthetics protect the heart against ischemia and reperfusion injury (18). Isoflurane, for instance, reduced myocardial infarct size in dogs, and this beneficial action was found to persist despite discontinuation of the volatile anesthetic before coronary artery occlusion (19). This phenomenon was termed anesthetic-induced preconditioning (APC) and was characterized by a short-term memory phase similar to that observed during ischemic preconditioning.

Anesthetic-induced preconditioning also has been described in other animal species, including rats (20) and rabbits (21). The efficacy of APC conferred by isoflurane to reduce infarct size has been shown to be dose dependent in rats (20), an animal model with minimal coronary collateral flow (22). Similarly, isoflurane and sevoflurane dose-dependently preserved the viability of isolated cardiac myocytes during ischemia (23).

Interestingly, recent findings show that isoflurane reduced myocardial damage when administered 24 hours before coronary artery occlusion and reperfusion in rabbit hearts in vivo (24). Pretreatment with isoflurane also preserved endothelial and vascular smooth muscle cell viability 12–48 hours after cytokine-induced injury (25). Therefore, volatile anesthetics also produce a late phase (i.e., a second window) of myocardial protection similar to IPC. In addition, sevoflurane reduced the duration of a brief ischemic episode required to protect against infarction during IPC (26). Sevoflurane also enhanced cardioprotection when administered 24 hours after an initial IPC stimulus (27). These findings show that administration of a volatile anesthetic combined with a brief ischemic event synergistically protects myocardium against subsequent damage as well.

Volatile anesthetics have been shown to produce coronary vasodilation by activating K_{ATP} channels (28) or by favorably affecting intracellular Ca^{2+} homeostasis in vascular smooth muscle. Sevoflurane increased collateral blood flow to ischemic myocardium when perfusion pressure was maintained (29). Sevoflurane also improved the functional recovery of coronary vascular reactivity and nitric oxide release in isolated hearts after global ischemia (30). Volatile anesthetics attenuated neutrophil and platelet aggregation (31) and also inhibited cytokine-induced cell death (25, 32) after ischemia-reperfusion injury in vitro. Finally, studies also show that volatile anesthetics attenuate apoptosis as well as necrosis after ischemia and reperfusion and shift the myocardium into an "anti-apoptotic" state by modulation of proteins of the BCL-2 family (33, 34)

The signal transduction pathways involved in APC are very similar to those responsible for IPC (35) (Figure 5–4). It is hypothesized that volatile anesthetics stimulate a trigger that initiates a cascade of events leading to activation of an end-effector that is responsible for resistance to injury. To date, adenosine type 1 (A_1) receptors (36, 37) protein kinase

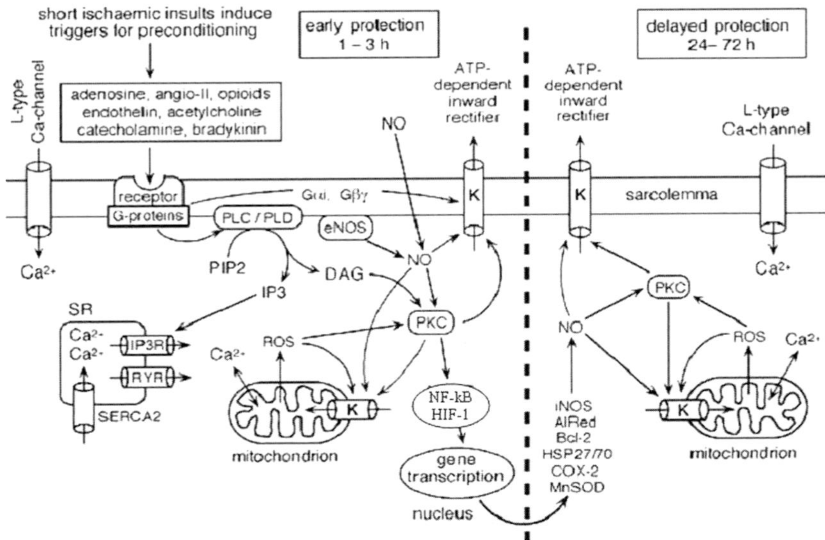

FIGURE 5–4. A schematic illustration of the signaling mechanisms involved in anesthetic preconditioning. Adapted with modifications with permission from Zaugg, et al. (35).

C (PKC) (38), inhibitory guanine nucleotide binding (G_i) proteins (39), reactive oxygen species (40, 41), and mitochondrial and sarcolemmal K_{ATP} channels (19, 42) have been shown to mediate APC. Recently several investigations also have demonstrated important roles for pro-survival kinases such as PI3K/Akt (43) and transcription factors such as HIF-1 (5) and nuclear factor κB (7).

THE CLINICAL POTENTIAL OF ISCHEMIC AND PHARMACOLOGICAL PRECONDITIONING

In vitro studies (44) suggest that the human myocardium can be preconditioned. The existence of this phenomenon in vivo has been suggested by several surrogate models of preconditioning in humans. In preinfarction angina, for example, antecedent angina improves clinical outcome after myocardial infarction (45). Repeated balloon-induced coronary occlusions during coronary catheterization were reported to decrease chest pain and attenuate ECG-related ischemic changes (46) and also to decrease subsequent ischemic events over a period of 1 year (47). Finally, intermittent aortic cross-clamping during cardiac surgery before the sustained period of global ischemia required for cardiopulmonary bypass also seems to provide cardioprotection (48).

Several preconditioning mimetic agents have been investigated in clinical studies of myocardial ischemia reperfusion, but with limited results. Only nicorandil has been investigated as a true preconditioning agent. This drug is believed to open ATP-dependent mitochondrial potassium channels and cause coronary vasodilatation. The Impact Of Nicorandil on Angina (IONA) study (49) examined nicorandil in patients with chronic stable coronary artery disease and demonstrated a small but significant reduction in major coronary events. Nicorandil also has cardioprotective effects when given as adjunctive therapy at the time of reperfusion after myocardial ischemia by primary percutaneous coronary intervention (PCI) (50). Other agents, such as adenosine and sodium-hydrogen exchanger inhibitors, have been investigated when given as adjuncts to reperfusion, as opposed to being investigated as true preconditioning mimetics, which necessitates giving the agent before the index ischemic period. Preclinical studies demonstrated that pharmacologic inhibition of the sodium-hydrogen exchanger before myocardial ischemia could reduce infarct size, through a reduction in myocardial calcium accumulation, to a level comparable to ischemic preconditioning (51). Unfortunately, the findings from subsequent clinical studies were not so clear and had conflicting results.

Many other drugs and pharmacological agents are under research for their preconditioning mimetic effects. Among those are found opioid receptor agonists (morphine, remifentanil) (20, 52, 53) that were determined to provide cardioprotection by themselves or enhance the protection achieved by ischemic or anesthetic preconditioning; the phosphodiesterase-5 inhibitor sildenafil (Viagra) (54, 55); and statins (56, 57). However, large randomized controlled clinical trials are yet to be done.

Several studies have shown a preconditioning effect for volatile anesthetics in cardiac surgery when administered prior to aortic cross clamping (58–60), however they consisted of small experimental groups and had to focus on surrogate outcome markers such as post-ischemic ventricular dysfunction and markers of cellular myocardial injury (troponin). In 2002, De Hert and colleagues (61) published a different protective approach. They administered sevoflurane throughout the entire operation (thus combining preconditioning and postconditioning), comparing it to propofol-based intravenous anesthesia. Although only 20 patients were enrolled in this study, there was a clear difference between the study groups: the patients in the sevoflurane group had a better LV function post CPB and lower levels of troponin (i.e., reduced myocardial injury) for 26 hours following surgery. Similar results were also confirmed in older patients with poor ventricular function (62). A recent study investigated different administration modalities of sevoflurane before (preconditioning), during, and after (postconditioning) cardiopulmonary bypass (63). The results indicated that only the administration of sevoflurane throughout the entire operation resulted in a decrease in troponin I release as well as decreased duration of in-hospital stay. Similar results were also found in a recent randomized controlled multicenter study comparing desflurane anesthesia to propofol-based intravenous anesthesia in off-pump coronary bypass (64). The patients in the desflurane group demonstrated decreased postoperative myocardial damage, resulting in a decreased need for inotropic support, eventually leading to a significant reduction in hospital stay. Taken together, there is data supporting a cardioprotective effect for volatile anesthetics administered during coronary surgery. However, the optimal dosing and timing for administration have not been determined. It seems that for maximal protection, administration of volatile agents is required for the entire duration of surgery. Larger randomized controlled trials are required for better understanding of the mechanisms of volatile anesthetics-induced protection in the clinical arena.

PRECONDITIONING OF THE AGED AND DISEASED HEART

Most experimental studies have evaluated the phenomenon of preconditioning in young and healthy hearts. Very few studies have evaluated ischemic or pharmacological PC in senescence or in the presence of underlying disease states that may affect the heart (e.g., diabetes, hypertension, and hypercholesterolemia). This approach, however, is far from clinical reality where older patients and those with concomitant comorbidities such as diabetes or hypertension would benefit most from these cardioprotective strategies.

The Aged Heart

Tolerance to stress in older animals is generally lower than that in younger animals, and most cardiac morbidity in humans occurs later in life. Because preconditioning of the aged myocardium is an important issue that may differ considerably from preconditioning of myocardium in the younger person, cardioprotection may need to be tailored to the aged population. Some investigators have found that age does not influence the myocardial tolerance to ischemia or the protective effect of ischemic preconditioning (65, 66); other studies question the ability of aged myocardium to be susceptible to preconditioning at all (67, 68). Schulman et al., for example, reported that aged rat hearts could not be preconditioned by ischemic or pharmacological means and that middle-aged rat hearts had only a blunted response to preconditioning compared with young adult hearts (69). They suggested defects within the signaling cascade of preconditioning in the aged heart. Evidence from an isolated heart model points in the same direction for anesthetic preconditioning, suggesting that the benefits of anesthetic preconditioning may indeed be reduced with advanced age (70). Nevertheless, as reported earlier, several clinical studies in elderly patients did demonstrate a protective effect with ischemic and anesthetic preconditioning (62, 65, 66), thus, the role of ischemic and pharmacological preconditioning in aged hearts needs to be further investigated before any conclusion can be drawn as to its applicability in the clinical situation.

Diabetes Mellitus and Preconditioning

Hyperglycemia (both acute and chronic) increases the risk for cardiac ischemic injury. Furthermore, endogenous protective signaling pathways are impaired and coronary blood flow to the ischemic myocardium is reduced during hyperglycemia. Several clinical trials have demonstrated strong correlation between perioperative hyperglycemia and an increased risk for postoperative morbidity and mortality after cardiac surgery (71–73). In a recent prospective study that included 200 diabetic patients who underwent coronary bypass surgery, Ouattara and colleagues (74) demonstrated a significant association between intraoperative hyperglycemia (blood glucose levels >200 mg/dL) and worse postoperative outcome in comparison to patients whose their intraoperative blood sugar level was well controlled (Figure 5–5). Adequacy of control of blood glucose concentration also will affect anesthetic preconditioning. High blood glucose concentrations have been shown to antag-

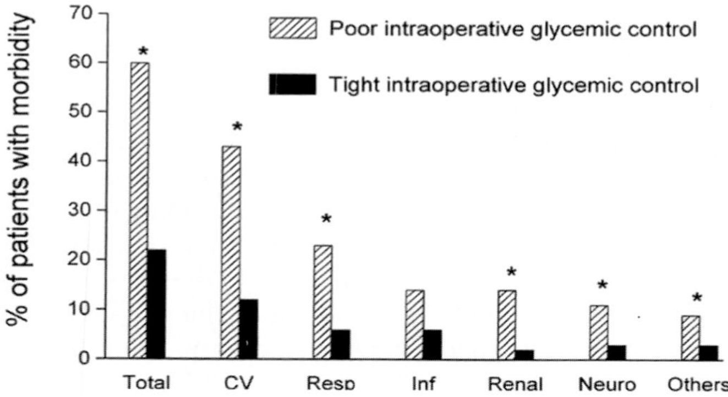

FIGURE 5–5. Incidence of in hospital morbidity in patients with good intraoperative glucose control compared to patients with poor intraoperative glycemic control. CV = cardiovascular morbidity; Inf = infectious morbidity; Neuro = neurological morbidity; Resp = respiratory morbidity. * $p < 0.05$ versus tight control. Adapted with modifications with permission from Outtara, et al. (74).

onize ischemic and anesthetic preconditioning in the presence and absence of diabetes in different animal models (75–78). Diabetic patients who are treated with sulfonylurea oral hypoglycemic drugs such as glibenclamide will most likely not benefit from any form of preconditioning. The target of sulfonylurea drugs is the K_{ATP} channel in the pancreatic β cells: closure of the K_{ATP} channel causes insulin release. K_{ATP} channels are also present in sarcolemmal and mitochondrial membranes of cardiac myocytes (79). Their activation has been implicated as both a trigger and effector of myocardial preconditioning, and both ischemic and anesthetic preconditioning are abolished by sulfonylurea drugs. Oral hypoglycemic agents should therefore be discontinued 24–48 hours before elective surgery. Instead, insulin should be used to maintain normoglycemia. Insulin has the added benefit of activating cell survival pathways, including the phosphatidylinositol 3′-kinase/Akt-dependent pathway to decrease infarct size and apoptotic myocyte death (80).

Preconditioning in Hypercholesterolemia

There has been controversy in the literature regarding the issue of whether hypercholesteremic animals can be preconditioned (81). Ueda et al. observed that in a rabbit model of myocardial infarction, a high cholesterol diet abolished ischemic preconditioning; however, the statin agent, pravastatin, at a dose that did not normalize serum cholesterol, restored IPC (82). In humans, it is well known that repetitive angioplasty balloon inflations can induce ischemic preconditioning. Kyriakides et al. studied 33 patients undergoing a minimum of three balloon inflations as part of a coronary angioplasty procedure (83). Thirteen patients had a total cholesterol level of <200 mg/dL and 20 had total cholesterol levels of >200 mg/dL. While in the normal cholesterol group, mean ST segment elevation on surface ECGs decreased from 0.21 mV during the first balloon inflation to 0.11 mV, during a third inflation ($P < 0.05$), in those patients with cholesterol levels of >200 mg/dL, the decrease was from 0.18 to 0.14 MV (P = nonsignificant). Thus, in this study, hypercholesterolemia prevented the normal decrease in myocardial ischemia associated with angioplasty-induced preconditioning. Ungi and colleagues also observed that hypercholesterolemia attenuated the beneficial effects of preconditioning during coronary angioplasty (84). In a recent meta-analysis Hindler et al. evaluated the efficacy of statin therapy to improve outcomes after cardiac, vascular, or noncardiac surgery (85). Statin therapy was associated with a 44% reduction in early postoperative mortality, irrespective of the type of surgical procedure involved. In a case-control study of 2,816 patients undergoing major vascular surgery, perioperative mortality in patients receiving statins was reduced 4.5-fold as compared with that in patients who did not take this medication (86). Statins have been shown to modulate vascular function by increasing expression of nitric oxide synthase and enhancing nitric oxide production. Increases in nitric oxide reduce endothelial dysfunction, attenuate leukocyte-endothelium interactions, and decrease platelet aggregation. Statins also have been demonstrated to scavenge reactive oxygen species, decrease endothelial cell apoptosis, and produce antithrombotic effects. Statins exert antiinflammatory effects that contribute to atherosclerotic plaque stability. In addition, statins reduce vascular smooth muscle proliferation in response to injury and may contribute to a decrease in the incidence of restenosis after percutaneous coronary intervention (87). Despite recent studies advocating the benefit of perioperative statin therapy, the American Heart Association Clinical Advisory on the Use and Safety of Statins concluded that it may be prudent to withhold statins during hospitalization for major surgery (88). Despite the American Heart Association Clinical Advisory, acute withdrawal of statin therapy may pose a significant risk to patients with cardiovascular disease. Cardiac event rate was investigated in 1,616 patients admitted with an acute coronary syndrome (89). Statin treatment was associated with a 3-fold reduction in 30-day mortality as compared with patients who did not receive these drugs. In contrast, mortality rates were dramatically increased by nearly 7-fold in patients in whom statin therapy was withdrawn during or after admission to the hospital (Figure 5–6). The mechanism for this deleterious effect remains unclear, but experimental evidence suggests that acute statin withdrawal enhances oxidative stress and produces endothelial dysfunction (90). Taken together, the data suggest that peri-

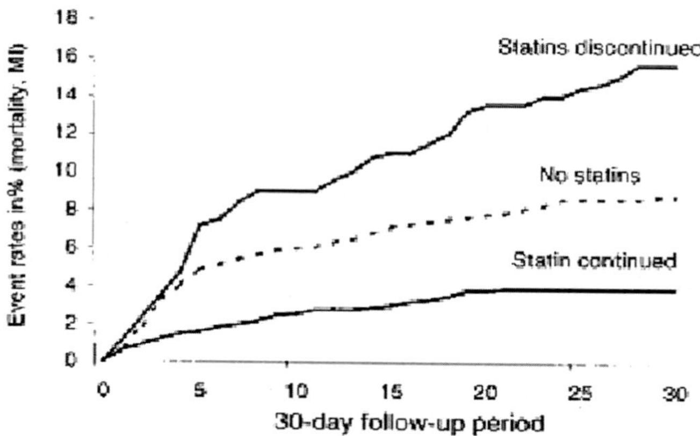

FIGURE 5–6. Event rate curves (death, non-fatal MI) during 30-day follow up period for patients with continued statin therapy, withdrawn statin therapy and without statin therapy. Adapted with modifications with permission from Heeschen, et al. (89).

operative statin therapy may decrease cardiovascular morbidity and reduce mortality after cardiac and noncardiac surgery in high-risk patients; however, the timing for initiation and the optimal duration of therapy to minimize side effects are still unclear and further studies are needed to answer these questions.

MYOCARDIAL POSTCONDITIONING

To harness the cardioprotective potential of preconditioning, the intervention needs to be implemented before the onset of myocardial ischemia. In the settings of an acute myocardial infarction, this timing is difficult to achieve. The approach might be possible, however, during elective coronary catheterization and cardiac surgery, in which the onset of myocardial ischemia is predictable. Given the prerequisite for a preconditioning agent to be present before the onset of myocardial ischemia, attention in the field of cardioprotection has focused on modifying events occurring at the time of myocardial reperfusion (i.e., postconditioning).

Postconditioning describes the reduction in infarct size induced by the application of alternating episodes of myocardial ischemia and reperfusion or cardioprotective pharmacological agents at the end of the index ischemic period. This concept was first introduced in 2003 by Zhao et al. (91). They demonstrated that the in vivo application of three 30-second episodes of alternating left anterior descending artery reocclusion and reperfusion, immediately following a 1-hour period of sustained occlusion, produced a significant reduction in infarct size. This effect is comparable to that of ischemic preconditioning. Since its introduction, ischemic postconditioning has been demonstrated in vivo in several different species, as well as ex vivo in the rat heart and rat myocytes. In addition to ischemia and similarly to preconditioning, volatile anesthetics also have been found to be cardioprotective when administered at the end of the index ischemia and early reperfusion (i.e., anesthetic postconditioning) (92).

MECHANISMS OF CARDIOPROTECTION BY ISCHEMIC POSTCONDITIONING

As with ischemic preconditioning, the exact mechanism by which ischemic postconditioning reduces infarct size is unknown. Study findings suggest that protection is dependent on adenosine-receptor stimulation, activation of the survival kinases (PI3K-Akt) (93), Erk1/2 (94), and inhibition of mPTP opening (95) (Figure 5–7). Ischemic postconditioning also is accompanied by a reduction in factors known to mediate myocardial reperfusion injury, such as oxidative stress, apoptotic factors, and neutrophil accumulation (91). Interestingly, although both pre-

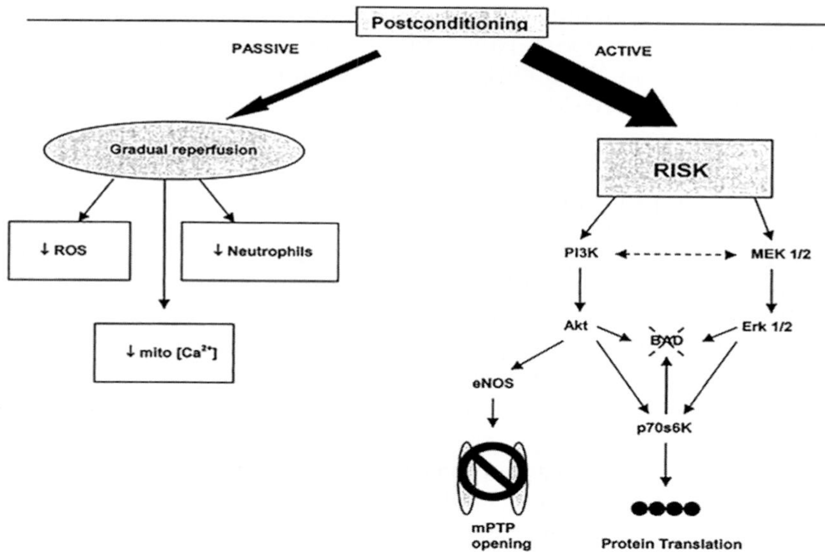

FIGURE 5–7. A schematic illustration of the signaling mechanisms involved in anesthetic preconditioning. Adapted with modifications with permission from Tsang, et al. (93).

conditioning and postconditioning activate very similar protective mechanisms in the heart, a recent study by Lucchinetti et al. showed evidence of opposing genomic responses in cardioprotection by pre- and postconditioning (96).

THE CLINICAL POTENTIAL OF MYOCARDIAL POSTCONDITIONING

Dependent on the clinical scenario of myocardial ischemia and reperfusion, the application of intermittent myocardial ischemia and reperfusion might be difficult to implement and justify. For example, the use of ischemic postconditioning would not be possible in an AMI patient referred for thrombolysis, in cases of unstable angina, in patients presenting with non-ST-segment elevation myocardial infarction, or in the event of a cardiac arrest. Such a protocol might be possible to apply in a patient with myocardial infarction referred for PCI, elective PCI, or at the time of cardiac surgery. Justification for applying intermittent episodes of balloon inflation or cross-clamping of the aorta at the time of myocardial reperfusion might, however, be difficult.

Taken together and considering the fact that the survival kinases (PI3K-Akt, ERK 1, and ERK 2) mediate the protection induced by ischemic postconditioning, a more practical approach would be to pharmacologically activate these kinases at the time of reperfusion to harness the powerful cardioprotective potential of ischemic postconditioning. Importantly, this approach can be readily applied to all clinical scenarios of myocardial ischemia and reperfusion (97).

As with preconditioning, volatile anesthetic agents have been found to protect the heart against ischemia and reperfusion also when administered during reperfusion. Several animal studies have demonstrated this cardioprotective effect and suggested that it is mediated by similar mechanisms that are activated in ischemic postconditioning (92, 98–100). Several studies in coronary bypass patients suggest that it may also have clinical implications (63).

CONCLUSIONS

The field of myocardial protection has had several major implications in cardiovascular and perioperative medicine. First, it has revealed that the heart possesses a remarkable phenotypic plasticity that enables it to overcome ischemia-reperfusion induced injury. Second, myocardial protection can be achieved not only by ischemia, but also by using cardioprotective agents such as volatile anesthetics, opioids, and statins.

Although the cardioprotective potential of preconditioning is hindered by the requirement to intervene before onset of ischemia—which is unpredictable in the setting of an acute myocardial infarction—postconditioning might allow a clinical intervention at the time of myocardial reperfusion to reduce infarct size after infarction. The recruitment of a common signaling pathway at the time of myocardial reperfusion in preconditioning and postconditioning provides a potential target for cardioprotection through the use of pharmacologic agents to activate survival kinases (PI3K-AKT, ERK 1, and ERK 2), directly inhibit mPTP opening or both. Future trials will be required to validate this novel approach to cardioprotection in clinical practice and identify the most effective pharmacologic agents.

References

1. Murry CE, Jennings RB, Reimer KA: Preconditioning with ischemia: a delay of lethal cell injury in ischemic myocardium. Circulation 1986; 74:1124–36
2. Yellon DM, Downey JM: Preconditioning the myocardium: from cellular physiology to clinical cardiology. Physiol Rev 2003; 83:1113–51
3. Marber MS, Latchman DS, Walker JM, Yellon DM: Cardiac stress protein elevation 24 hours after brief ischemia or heat stress is asso-

ciated with resistance to myocardial infarction. Circulation 1993; 88:1264–72
4. Hausenloy DJ, Tsang A, Mocanu MM, Yellon DM: Ischemic preconditioning protects by activating prosurvival kinases at reperfusion. Am J Physiol Heart Circ Physiol 2005; 288:H971–6
5. Cai Z, Manalo DJ, Wei G, et al.: Hearts from rodents exposed to intermittent hypoxia or erythropoietin are protected against ischemia-reperfusion injury. Circulation 2003; 108:79–85
6. Valen G: Signal transduction through nuclear factor κB in ischemia-reperfusion and heart failure. Basic Res Cardiol 2004; 99:1–7
7. Zhong C, Zhou Y, Liu H: Nuclear factor κB and anesthetic preconditioning during myocardial ischemia-reperfusion. Anesthesiology 2004; 100:540–6
8. Garlid KD, Paucek P, Yarov-Yarovoy V, et al.: Cardioprotective effect of diazoxide and its interaction with mitochondrial ATP-sensitive K^+ channels. Possible mechanism of cardioprotection. Circ Res 1997; 81:1072–82
9. Raphael J, Drenger B, Rivo J, Berenshtein E, Chevion M, Gozal Y: Ischemic preconditioning decreases the reperfusion-related formation of hydroxyl radicals in a rabbit model of regional myocardial ischemia and reperfusion: the role of K_{ATP} channels. Free Radic Res 2005; 39:747–54
10. Vanden Hoek TL, Becker LB, Shao Z, Li C, Schumacker PT: Reactive oxygen species released from mitochondria during brief hypoxia induce preconditioning in cardiomyocytes. J Biol Chem 1998; 273:18092–8
11. Hausenloy DJ, Maddock HL, Baxter GF, Yellon DM: Inhibiting mitochondrial permeability transition pore opening: a new paradigm for myocardial preconditioning? Cardiovasc Res 2002; 55:534–43
12. Bolli R: The late phase of preconditioning. Circ Res 2000; 87:972–83
13. Reiz S, Balfors E, Sorensen MB, Ariola S, Jr., Friedman A, Truedsson H: Isoflurane—a powerful coronary vasodilator in patients with coronary artery disease. Anesthesiology 1983; 59:91–7
14. Becker LC: Is isoflurane dangerous for the patient with coronary artery disease? Anesthesiology 1987; 66:259–61
15. Moore PG, Kien ND, Reitan JA, White DA, Safwat AM: No evidence for blood flow redistribution with isoflurane or halothane during acute coronary artery occlusion in fentanyl-anesthetized dogs. Anesthesiology 1991; 75:854–65
16. Pulley DD, Kirvassilis GV, Kelermenos N, et al.: Regional and global myocardial circulatory and metabolic effects of isoflurane and halothane in patients with steal-prone coronary anatomy. Anesthesiology 1991; 75:756–66

17. Diana P, Tullock WC, Gorcsan J, 3rd, Ferson PF, Arvan S: Myocardial ischemia: a comparison between isoflurane and enflurane in coronary artery bypass patients. Anesth Analg 1993; 77:221–6
18. Tanaka K, Ludwig LM, Kersten JR, Pagel PS, Warltier DC: Mechanisms of cardioprotection by volatile anesthetics. Anesthesiology 2004; 100:707–21
19. Kersten JR, Schmeling TJ, Pagel PS, Gross GJ, Warltier DC: Isoflurane mimics ischemic preconditioning via activation of K_{ATP} channels: reduction of myocardial infarct size with an acute memory phase. Anesthesiology 1997; 87:361–70
20. Ludwig LM, Patel HH, Gross GJ, Kersten JR, Pagel PS, Warltier DC: Morphine enhances pharmacological preconditioning by isoflurane: role of mitochondrial K_{ATP} channels and opioid receptors. Anesthesiology 2003; 98:705–11
21. Cason BA, Gamperl AK, Slocum RE, Hickey RF: Anesthetic-induced preconditioning: previous administration of isoflurane decreases myocardial infarct size in rabbits. Anesthesiology 1997; 87:1182–90
22. Maxwell MP, Hearse DJ, Yellon DM: Species variation in the coronary collateral circulation during regional myocardial ischaemia: a critical determinant of the rate of evolution and extent of myocardial infarction. Cardiovasc Res 1987; 21:737–46
23. Zaugg M, Lucchinetti E, Spahn DR, Pasch T, Schaub MC: Volatile anesthetics mimic cardiac preconditioning by priming the activation of mitochondrial K_{ATP} channels via multiple signaling pathways. Anesthesiology 2002; 97:4–14
24. Tanaka K, Ludwig LM, Krolikowski JG, et al.: Isoflurane produces delayed preconditioning against myocardial ischemia and reperfusion injury: role of cyclooxygenase-2. Anesthesiology 2004; 100:525–31
25. de Klaver MJ, Buckingham MG, Rich GF: Isoflurane pretreatment has immediate and delayed protective effects against cytokine-induced injury in endothelial and vascular smooth muscle cells. Anesthesiology 2003; 99:896–903
26. Toller WG, Kersten JR, Pagel PS, Hettrick DA, Warltier DC: Sevoflurane reduces myocardial infarct size and decreases the time threshold for ischemic preconditioning in dogs. Anesthesiology 1999; 91:1437–46
27. Mullenheim J, Ebel D, Bauer M, et al.: Sevoflurane confers additional cardioprotection after ischemic late preconditioning in rabbits. Anesthesiology 2003; 99:624–31
28. Cason BA, Shubayev I, Hickey RF: Blockade of adenosine triphosphate-sensitive potassium channels eliminates isoflurane-induced coronary artery vasodilation. Anesthesiology 1994; 81:1245–55

29. Kersten JR, Schmeling T, Tessmer J, Hettrick DA, Pagel PS, Warltier DC: Sevoflurane selectively increases coronary collateral blood flow independent of K_{ATP} channels in vivo. Anesthesiology 1999; 90:246–56
30. Novalija E, Fujita S, Kampine JP, Stowe DF: Sevoflurane mimics ischemic preconditioning effects on coronary flow and nitric oxide release in isolated hearts. Anesthesiology 1999; 91:701–12
31. Kowalski C, Zahler S, Becker BF, et al.: Halothane, isoflurane, and sevoflurane reduce postischemic adhesion of neutrophils in the coronary system. Anesthesiology 1997; 86:188–95
32. de Klaver MJ, Manning L, Palmer LA, Rich GF: Isoflurane pretreatment inhibits cytokine-induced cell death in cultured rat smooth muscle cells and human endothelial cells. Anesthesiology 2002; 97:24–32
33. Raphael J, Abedat S, Rivo J, et al.: Volatile anesthetic preconditioning attenuates myocardial apoptosis in rabbits after regional ischemia and reperfusion via Akt signaling and modulation of Bcl-2 family proteins. J Pharmacol Exp Ther 2006; 318:186–94
34. Jamnicki-Abegg M, Weihrauch D, Pagel PS, et al.: Isoflurane inhibits cardiac myocyte apoptosis during oxidative and inflammatory stress by activating Akt and enhancing Bcl-2 expression. Anesthesiology 2005; 103:1006–14
35. Zaugg M, Lucchinetti E, Uecker M, Pasch T, Schaub MC: Anaesthetics and cardiac preconditioning. Part I. Signalling and cytoprotective mechanisms. Br J Anaesth 2003; 91:551–65
36. Kersten JR, Orth KG, Pagel PS, Mei DA, Gross GJ, Warltier DC: Role of adenosine in isoflurane-induced cardioprotection. Anesthesiology 1997; 86:1128–39
37. Roscoe AK, Christensen JD, Lynch C, 3rd: Isoflurane, but not halothane, induces protection of human myocardium via adenosine A1 receptors and adenosine triphosphate-sensitive potassium channels. Anesthesiology 2000; 92:1692–701
38. Cope DK, Impastato WK, Cohen MV, Downey JM: Volatile anesthetics protect the ischemic rabbit myocardium from infarction. Anesthesiology 1997; 86:699–709
39. Toller WG, Kersten JR, Gross ER, Pagel PS, Warltier DC: Isoflurane preconditions myocardium against infarction via activation of inhibitory guanine nucleotide binding proteins. Anesthesiology 2000; 92:1400–7
40. Mullenheim J, Ebel D, Frassdorf J, Preckel B, Thamer V, Schlack W: Isoflurane preconditions myocardium against infarction via release of free radicals. Anesthesiology 2002; 96:934–40

41. Tanaka K, Weihrauch D, Kehl F, et al.: Mechanism of preconditioning by isoflurane in rabbits: a direct role for reactive oxygen species. Anesthesiology 2002; 97:1485–90
42. Ismaeil MS, Tkachenko I, Gamperl AK, Hickey RF, Cason BA: Mechanisms of isoflurane-induced myocardial preconditioning in rabbits. Anesthesiology 1999; 90:812–21
43. Raphael J, Rivo J, Gozal Y: Isoflurane-induced myocardial preconditioning is dependent on phosphatidylinositol-3-kinase/Akt signalling. Br J Anaesth 2005; 95:756–63
44. Walker DM, Walker JM, Pugsley WB, Pattison CW, Yellon DM: Preconditioning in isolated superfused human muscle. J Mol Cell Cardiol 1995; 27:1349–57
45. Rezkalla SH, Kloner RA: Ischemic preconditioning and preinfarction angina in the clinical arena. Nat Clin Pract Cardiovasc Med 2004; 1:96–102
46. Tomai F, Crea F, Gaspardone A, et al.: Ischemic preconditioning during coronary angioplasty is prevented by glibenclamide, a selective ATP-sensitive K^+ channel blocker. Circulation 1994; 90:700–5
47. Laskey WK, Beach D: Frequency and clinical significance of ischemic preconditioning during percutaneous coronary intervention. J Am Coll Cardiol 2003; 42:998–1003
48. Jenkins DP, Steare SE, Yellon DM: Preconditioning the human myocardium: recent advances and aspirations for the development of a new means of cardioprotection in clinical practice. Cardiovasc Drugs Ther 1995; 9:739–47
49. Effect of nicorandil on coronary events in patients with stable angina: the Impact Of Nicorandil in Angina (IONA) randomised trial. Lancet 2002; 359:1269–75
50. Ono H, Osanai T, Ishizaka H, et al.: Nicorandil improves cardiac function and clinical outcome in patients with acute myocardial infarction undergoing primary percutaneous coronary intervention: role of inhibitory effect on reactive oxygen species formation. Am Heart J 2004; 148:E15
51. Bolli R: The role of sodium-hydrogen ion exchange in patients undergoing coronary artery bypass grafting. J Card Surg 2003; 18 Suppl 1:21–6
52. Schultz JE, Hsu AK, Gross GJ: Morphine mimics the cardioprotective effect of ischemic preconditioning via a glibenclamide-sensitive mechanism in the rat heart. Circ Res 1996; 78:1100–4
53. Zhang Y, Irwin MG, Wong TM: Remifentanil preconditioning protects against ischemic injury in the intact rat heart. Anesthesiology 2004; 101:918–23

54. Kukreja RC, Ockaili R, Salloum F, Xi L: Sildenafil-induced cardioprotection in rabbits. Cardiovasc Res 2003; 60:700–1; author reply 702–3
55. Kukreja RC, Salloum F, Das A, et al.: Pharmacological preconditioning with sildenafil: Basic mechanisms and clinical implications. Vascul Pharmacol 2005; 42:219–32
56. Kersten JR, Fleisher LA: Statins: The next advance in cardioprotection? Anesthesiology 2006; 105:1079–80
57. Elrod JW, Lefer DJ: The effects of statins on endothelium, inflammation and cardioprotection. Timely Top Med Cardiovasc Dis 2005; 9:E20
58. Tomai F, De Paulis R, Penta de Peppo A, et al.: Beneficial impact of isoflurane during coronary bypass surgery on troponin I release. G Ital Cardiol 1999; 29:1007–14
59. Belhomme D, Peynet J, Louzy M, Launay JM, Kitakaze M, Menasche P: Evidence for preconditioning by isoflurane in coronary artery bypass graft surgery. Circulation 1999; 100:II340–4
60. Julier K, da Silva R, Garcia C, et al.: Preconditioning by sevoflurane decreases biochemical markers for myocardial and renal dysfunction in coronary artery bypass graft surgery: a double-blinded, placebo-controlled, multicenter study. Anesthesiology 2003; 98:1315–27
61. De Hert SG, ten Broecke PW, Mertens E, et al.: Sevoflurane but not propofol preserves myocardial function in coronary surgery patients. Anesthesiology 2002; 97:42–9
62. De Hert SG, Cromheecke S, ten Broecke PW, et al.: Effects of propofol, desflurane, and sevoflurane on recovery of myocardial function after coronary surgery in elderly high-risk patients. Anesthesiology 2003; 99:314–23
63. De Hert SG, Van der Linden PJ, Cromheecke S, et al.: Cardioprotective properties of sevoflurane in patients undergoing coronary surgery with cardiopulmonary bypass are related to the modalities of its administration. Anesthesiology 2004; 101:299–310
64. Guarracino F, Landoni G, Tritapepe L, et al.: Myocardial damage prevented by volatile anesthetics: a multicenter randomized controlled study. J Cardiothorac Vasc Anesth 2006; 20:477–83
65. Loubani M, Ghosh S, Galinanes M: The aging human myocardium: tolerance to ischemia and responsiveness to ischemic preconditioning. J Thorac Cardiovasc Surg 2003; 126:143–7
66. Kloner RA, Przyklenk K, Shook T, Cannon CP: Protection Conferred by Preinfarct Angina is Manifest in the Aged Heart: Evidence from the TIMI 4 Trial. J Thromb Thrombolysis 1998; 6:89–92

67. Riess ML, Camara AK, Rhodes SS, McCormick J, Jiang MT, Stowe DF: Increasing heart size and age attenuate anesthetic preconditioning in guinea pig isolated hearts. Anesth Analg 2005; 101:1572–6
68. Abete P, Ferrara N, Cacciatore F, et al.: Angina-induced protection against myocardial infarction in adult and elderly patients: a loss of preconditioning mechanism in the aging heart? J Am Coll Cardiol 1997; 30:947–54
69. Schulman D, Latchman DS, Yellon DM: Effect of aging on the ability of preconditioning to protect rat hearts from ischemia-reperfusion injury. Am J Physiol Heart Circ Physiol 2001; 281:H1630–6
70. Sniecinski R, Liu H: Reduced efficacy of volatile anesthetic preconditioning with advanced age in isolated rat myocardium. Anesthesiology 2004; 100:589–97
71. Lazar HL, Chipkin SR, Fitzgerald CA, Bao Y, Cabral H, Apstein CS: Tight glycemic control in diabetic coronary artery bypass graft patients improves perioperative outcomes and decreases recurrent ischemic events. Circulation 2004; 109:1497–502
72. Puskas F, Grocott HP, White WD, Mathew JP, Newman MF, Bar-Yosef S: Intraoperative hyperglycemia and cognitive decline after CABG. Ann Thorac Surg 2007; 84:1467–73
73. Doenst T, Wijeysundera D, Karkouti K, et al.: Hyperglycemia during cardiopulmonary bypass is an independent risk factor for mortality in patients undergoing cardiac surgery. J Thorac Cardiovasc Surg 2005; 130:1144
74. Ouattara A, Lecomte P, Le Manach Y, et al.: Poor intraoperative blood glucose control is associated with a worsened hospital outcome after cardiac surgery in diabetic patients. Anesthesiology 2005; 103:687–94
75. Ebel D, Mullenheim J, Frassdorf J, et al.: Effect of acute hyperglycaemia and diabetes mellitus with and without short-term insulin treatment on myocardial ischaemic late preconditioning in the rabbit heart in vivo. Pflugers Arch 2003; 446:175–82
76. Kehl F, Krolikowski JG, Mraovic B, Pagel PS, Warltier DC, Kersten JR: Hyperglycemia prevents isoflurane-induced preconditioning against myocardial infarction. Anesthesiology 2002; 96:183–8
77. Kersten JR, Schmeling TJ, Orth KG, Pagel PS, Warltier DC: Acute hyperglycemia abolishes ischemic preconditioning in vivo. Am J Physiol 1998; 275:H721–5
78. Tanaka K, Kehl F, Gu W, Krolikowski JG, Pagel PS, Warltier DC, Kersten JR: Isoflurane-induced preconditioning is attenuated by diabetes. Am J Physiol Heart Circ Physiol 2002; 282:H2018–23
79. Grover GJ, Garlid KD: ATP-Sensitive potassium channels: a review of their cardioprotective pharmacology. J Mol Cell Cardiol 2000; 32:677–95

80. Gao F, Gao E, Yue TL, et al.: Nitric oxide mediates the antiapoptotic effect of insulin in myocardial ischemia-reperfusion: the roles of PI3-kinase, Akt, and endothelial nitric oxide synthase phosphorylation. Circulation 2002; 105:1497–502
81. Kremastinos DT: The phenomenon of preconditioning today. Hellenic J Cardiol 2005; 46:1–4
82. Ueda Y, Kitakaze M, Komamura K, et al.: Pravastatin restored the infarct size-limiting effect of ischemic preconditioning blunted by hypercholesterolemia in the rabbit model of myocardial infarction. J Am Coll Cardiol 1999; 34:2120–5
83. Kyriakides ZS, Psychari S, Iliodromitis EK, Kolettis TM, Sbarouni E, Kremastinos DT: Hyperlipidemia prevents the expected reduction of myocardial ischemia on repeated balloon inflations during angioplasty. Chest 2002; 121:1211–5
84. Ungi I, Ungi T, Ruzsa Z, et al.: Hypercholesterolemia attenuates the anti-ischemic effect of preconditioning during coronary angioplasty. Chest 2005; 128:1623–8
85. Hindler K, Shaw AD, Samuels J, Fulton S, Collard CD, Riedel B: Improved postoperative outcomes associated with preoperative statin therapy. Anesthesiology 2006; 105:1260–72; quiz 1289–90
86. Poldermans D, Bax JJ, Kertai MD, et al.: Statins are associated with a reduced incidence of perioperative mortality in patients undergoing major noncardiac vascular surgery. Circulation 2003; 107:1848–51
87. Davignon J, Laaksonen R: Low-density lipoprotein-independent effects of statins. Curr Opin Lipidol 1999; 10:543–59
88. Pasternak RC, Smith SC, Jr., Bairey-Merz CN, Grundy SM, Cleeman JI, Lenfant C: ACC/AHA/NHLBI Clinical Advisory on the Use and Safety of Statins. Stroke 2002; 33:2337–41
89. Heeschen C, Hamm CW, Laufs U, Snapinn S, Bohm M, White HD: Withdrawal of statins increases event rates in patients with acute coronary syndromes. Circulation 2002; 105:1446–52
90. Vecchione C, Brandes RP: Withdrawal of 3-hydroxy-3-methylglutaryl coenzyme A reductase inhibitors elicits oxidative stress and induces endothelial dysfunction in mice. Circ Res 2002; 91:173–9
91. Zhao ZQ, Corvera JS, Halkos ME, et al.: Inhibition of myocardial injury by ischemic postconditioning during reperfusion: comparison with ischemic preconditioning. Am J Physiol Heart Circ Physiol 2003; 285:H579–88
92. Chiari PC, Bienengraeber MW, Pagel PS, Krolikowski JG, Kersten JR, Warltier DC: Isoflurane protects against myocardial infarction during early reperfusion by activation of phosphatidylinositol-3-kinase signal transduction: evidence for anesthetic-induced postconditioning in rabbits. Anesthesiology 2005; 102:102–9

93. Tsang A, Hausenloy DJ, Mocanu MM, Yellon DM: Postconditioning: a form of "modified reperfusion" protects the myocardium by activating the phosphatidylinositol 3-kinase-Akt pathway. Circ Res 2004; 95:230–2
94. Yang XM, Proctor JB, Cui L, Krieg T, Downey JM, Cohen MV: Multiple, brief coronary occlusions during early reperfusion protect rabbit hearts by targeting cell signaling pathways. J Am Coll Cardiol 2004; 44:1103–10
95. Argaud L, Gateau-Roesch O, Raisky O, Loufouat J, Robert D, Ovize M: Postconditioning inhibits mitochondrial permeability transition. Circulation 2005; 111:194–7
96. Lucchinetti E, da Silva R, Pasch T, Schaub MC, Zaugg M: Anaesthetic preconditioning but not postconditioning prevents early activation of the deleterious cardiac remodelling programme: evidence of opposing genomic responses in cardioprotection by pre- and postconditioning. Br J Anaesth 2005; 95:140–52
97. Yellon DM, Hausenloy DJ: Realizing the clinical potential of ischemic preconditioning and postconditioning. Nat Clin Pract Cardiovasc Med 2005; 2:568–75
98. Krolikowski JG, Weihrauch D, Bienengraeber M, Kersten JR, Warltier DC, Pagel PS: Role of Erk1/2, p70s6K, and eNOS in isoflurane-induced cardioprotection during early reperfusion in vivo. Can J Anaesth 2006; 53:174–82
99. Krolikowski JG, Bienengraeber M, Weihrauch D, Warltier DC, Kersten JR, Pagel PS: Inhibition of mitochondrial permeability transition enhances isoflurane-induced cardioprotection during early reperfusion: the role of mitochondrial KATP channels. Anesth Analg 2005; 101:1590–6
100. Weihrauch D, Krolikowski JG, Bienengraeber M, Kersten JR, Warltier DC, Pagel PS: Morphine enhances isoflurane-induced postconditioning against myocardial infarction: the role of phosphatidylinositol-3-kinase and opioid receptors in rabbits. Anesth Analg 2005; 101:942–9

Antoine G. M. Aya, MD, PhD
Pierre-Géraud Claret, MD, MSc
Jean-Emmanuel de La Coussaye, MD, PhD

6 Cardiac Electrophysiology: Pharmacological Applications

Cardiac electrophysiology refers to all processes leading to the occurrence and the propagation of the cardiac electrical activity throughout the cardiac tissue, which is essential to initiate the cardiac muscle contraction and thus blood circulation. Knowledge about cardiac electrophysiology is the basis of the understanding of cardiac arrhythmia mechanisms and of the principles of their treatments. At the cellular level, the generation and conduction of the cardiac impulse is due to ionic currents flowing across cell membranes, through specialized membrane structures referred to as ion channels. Thereafter, at a more macroscopic scale, the impulse is transmitted from cell to cell, throughout the heart via conduction pathways. This electrical activity is highly regulated, mainly by the autonomic nervous system. Ion channels, conduction mechanisms and pathways, and regulation processes are different targets of antiarrhythmic agents.

CARDIAC ELECTROPHYSIOLOGY AT THE SUBCELLULAR AND CELLULAR LEVELS: ION CHANNELS AND ACTION POTENTIALS

The Cell Membrane and Cardiac Ion Channels

In cardiac cells, as in any cell, the cell membrane is composed of two hydrophilic layers made up of phospholipids and cholesterol lining a hydrophobic core. The molecules of the phospholipid bilayer interact

Advances in Cardiovascular Pharmacology, edited by Philippe R. Housmans, MD, PhD and Gregory A. Nuttall, M.D.
Lippincott Williams & Wilkins, Baltimore © 2008.

with the intra- and extracellular media, while the central core accounts for the relative impermeability of the cell membrane to charged ions. Therefore, several specialized protein structures (receptors, coupling proteins, enzymes, pumps, ion channels) embedded in the membrane are required to allow the transfer of ions and various molecules across the cell membrane. Ion channels are transmembrane proteins through which ions cross the hydrophobic core of the plasma membrane. They control the cell electrical excitability and determine conduction properties. Their production is genetically determined and their defect or dysfunction lead to diseases called channelopathies (1, 2). Ion channels are distributed over the whole cell membrane, but with a higher density at the gap junctions that are specialized structures implicated in cell to cell communication. Ion channels are classified into two groups: ligand-gated ion channels which are activated by the binding of substances such as acetylcholine or ATP, and voltage-gated ion channels which are activated by changes in the membrane potential. Ligand-gated ion channels are involved in the adaptation of the cardiac tissue to pathologic changes of its environment, while voltage-gated ion channels determine the electrophysiologic properties of normal cells. Four types of voltage-gated ion channels are responsible for the impulse generation and propagation in the cardiac cells. They are called sodium, calcium, potassium, and chloride channels according to the ion to which they are most selectively permeable. Sodium and calcium currents are depolarizing currents while potassium currents repolarize the cell membrane. Some types of channels have several subtypes with various effects. This is especially the case for calcium (I_{CaL} and I_{CaT}) (3) and potassium (I_{to}, I_{Kur} I_{Kr}, I_{Ks}, I_{K1}, I_{KACh}, I_{KATP}, I_{Kp}) channels (4, 5). Main currents involved in action potentials and their main functional roles are summarized in Table 6-1.

With regard to the structure, ion channels are large glycoproteins spanning the cell membrane. A channel is composed of several subunits, the most important of which is the pore-forming α-subunit. The α-subunit is generally made up of 4 domains designated I, II, III, and IV, linked by short covalent linking segments in sodium and calcium channels, and by noncovalent segments in most potassium channels (6). Each domain is composed of 6 α-helical transmembrane segments named S1–S6 (Figure 6–1). However, some potassium channels such as Kir channels contain only 1 or 2 segments. S5 and S6 and the S5–S6 linker line the pore of the channel. The S4 segments of each of the 4 homologous domains contain positively charged arginine and lysine residues that detect changes in the transmembrane field, and thus are the voltage sensors of the channel. A shift in the position of the S4 segments induced by membrane depolarization opens the channel pore, allowing the selective and passive flux of a single ion species down its concentration gradient

TABLE 6–1. Main ionic currents involved in action potentials

Ionic current	Functional role
Sodium currents	
I_{Na}: fast inward voltage-gated sodium current	Responsible for the depolarization (phase 0) and conduction in fast-response cells
I_{bNa}: baseline sodium current	Contributes to the generation of slow diastolic spontaneous depolarization of automatic cells (phase 4)
Calcium currents	
I_{CaL}: voltage-gated slow (L-Type) calcium current	Responsible for the depolarization (phase 0) of slow-response cells
I_{CaT}: voltage-gated transient (T-Type) calcium current	Role in the initiation of the depolarization (phase 0) of slow-response cells
I_f: pacemaker funny current	Responsible for the generation and control of slow diastolic spontaneous depolarization of automatic cells (phase 4)
Potassium currents	
I_{to}: transient outward current	Activated immediately after depolarization, contributes to early repolarization (phase 1)
I_{Kur}: ultra-rapid component of the delayed rectifier current I_K	Major role in late repolarization (phase 3) in atrial cells
I_{Kr}: rapid component of the delayed rectifier current I_K	Contributes to late repolarization (phase 3) in atrial and ventricular cells
I_{Ks}: slow component of the delayed rectifier current I_K	Contributes to late repolarization (phase 3) in atrial and ventricular cells
I_{K1} (I_{Kir}): inward rectifier current	Maintains resting potential in non-automatic cells (phase 4), role in plateau phase (phase 2)
I_{KACh}: acetylcholine-induced rectifier current	Hyperpolarization of cardiac cells, slowing of sinus pacemaker, shortening of atrial action potential duration
I_{KATP}: ATP-dependent rectifier current	Myocardial protection in ischemia

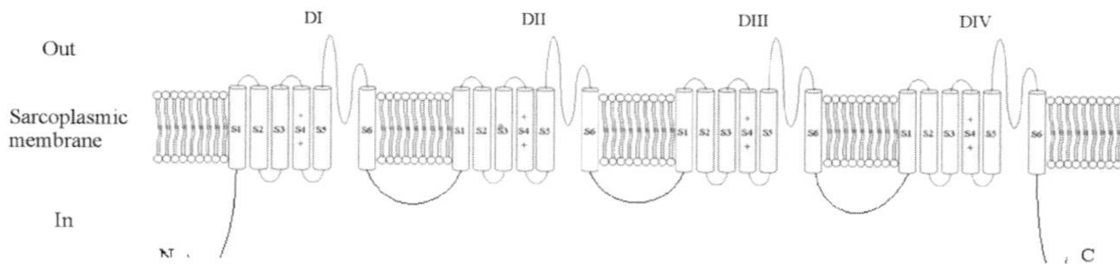

FIGURE 6–1. **The α-subunit of the voltage-gated sodium channel. Four transmembrane domains (DI to DIV). Each domain is made of six transmembrane segments (S1 to S6). The S4 segment of each domain is a voltage sensor.**

between the intra- and extracellular media. The III-IV linker is implicated in the channel fast inactivation.

Membrane ion channels can show 3 different states: the rested state during which the channel pore is closed, the activated state characterized by the opening of the channel allowing the occurrence of an ionic flux, and the inactivated state during which the inner pore is occluded, interrupting the ionic flow (7). The shift of a rested channel to the activated state can be induced by ligand binding or by changes in membrane potential. Almost simultaneously, fast inactivation is initiated. However, rested channels can reach inactivated state without previous activation. An inactivated channel is refractory to any stimulus, and moves to the rested state before being available for a new activation process.

The Membrane Action Potential

Like any cell, cardiac cells are polarized as a result of concentration gradients in ions between intra- and extracellular media, mainly sodium and potassium. This gradient is maintained by pumps (Na^+-K^+ ATPase) regulating the extracellular and intracellular concentrations of Na^+ and K^+ ions, respectively. As a result, the extracellular sodium concentration is 10-fold its intracellular concentration (142 vs. 14 mmol/L), and the intracellular potassium concentration is 30-fold its extracellular concentration (140 vs. 4 mmol/L). At a given moment, the membrane potential is the result of several ionic currents flowing throughout the membrane. In resting fast conducting cells, most potassium channels are open, allowing a transmembrane K^+ diffusion following its concentration gradient. As a result, the resting potential of these cells (-85 to -70 mV) is close to the K^+ electrochemical equilibrium potential (-98 mV). Because Na^+ and K^+ flows are equilibrated, the resting potential is stable during diastole. Therefore, an exogenous stimulus is required to depolarize these cells. In nodal and His-Purkinje cells, there is a net inward current during diastole, so that these cells show a maximum diastolic rather than a resting potential, from which the membrane spontaneously depolarizes, and develops an action potential when the membrane potential reaches the threshold potential.

Action potential (AP) is a sequence of changes in electrical transmembrane potential over time, due to coordinated activation and inactivation of several ionic currents. As 2 types of conducting cells are described, 2 types of AP can be distinguished: the fast and slow APs (Figure 6–2). Both have a depolarization phase due to inward currents and characterized by the reversal of the intracellular electronegativity, and a repolarization phase due to outward currents and during which the membrane resting potential is restored. The fast AP shows 5 phases. The inward current responsible for the depolarization phase (phase 0) is

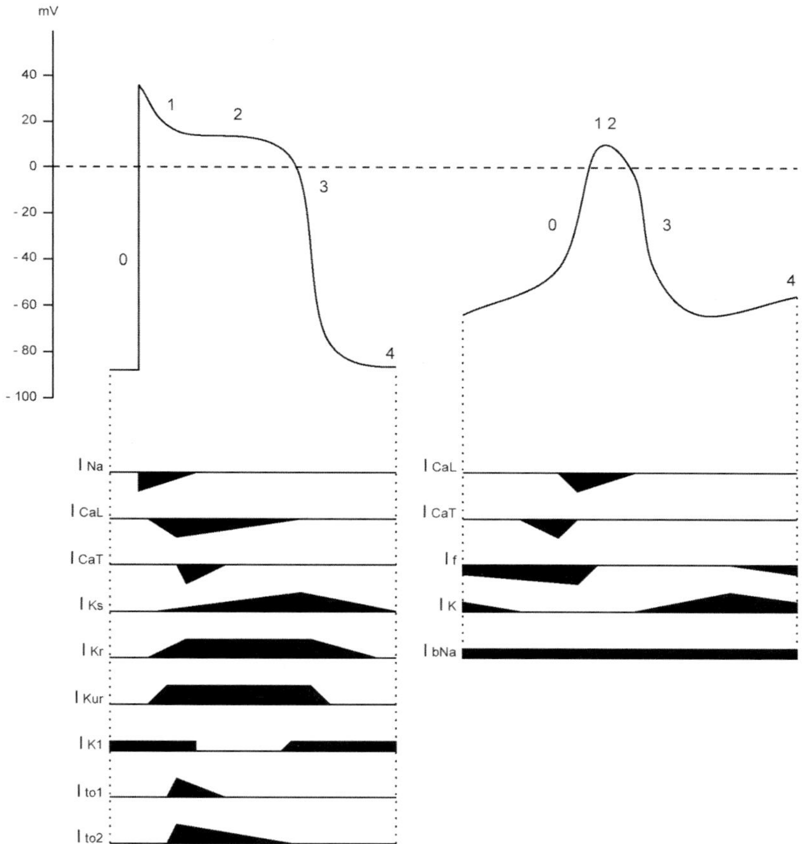

FIGURE 6–2. Schematic representation of normal fast (left) and slow (right) action potentials, and of the kinetic of various currents contributing to different phases

a Na^+ current (I_{Na}) which brings the membrane potential from the resting to a positive value which maximum is called overshoot (+30 m$\mathring{V}$). The maximal upstroke velocity of this phase ($\dot{V}_{max}$) is considered as an accurate estimate of the membrane conduction velocity (8). $\dot{V}_{max}$ is correlated with the depth of the resting membrane electronegativity. Therefore, $\dot{V}_{max}$ is decreased and conduction velocity is slowed by any factor that induces a partial membrane depolarization, such as ischemia, hypoxia, or acidosis. After the overshoot, the membrane potential decreases slowly, showing 4 additional phases due to the inactivation of I_{Na} and the activation of several calcium and potassium currents. Phase 1, also called fast repolarization, is triggered by the activation of I_{to}. This current is mainly observed in Purkinje and epicardial cells. This contributes to the epicardial versus endocardial differences in electrophysiologic properties and to different pharmacologic effects on these cell types (9–11). Phase 2 is a plateau phase (also called slow repolarization) due to the activation of I_{CaT} and I_{CaL} which offset the electrical effects of I_{to}. The inactivation of these calcium currents and the activation of several potassium currents allow the membrane potential to return to the resting value during phase 3, also referred to as final repolarization. Phase 4 is a resting phase, except in Purkinje fibers, which depolarize slowly.

Some differences are observed between the slow and the fast AP. The depolarization phase is triggered by inward calcium currents (I_{CaT} and I_{CaL}) which are activated by the spontaneous diastolic slow depolarization of these cell membranes. The plateau phase is almost absent. During phase 4, inward sodium (I_{bNa}) and calcium (I_f) currents are activated and induce a spontaneous diastolic slow depolarization, defining automaticity.

The heart is made of several cell types. Cardiomyocytes account for 75% of the cell volume, but only 30–40% of cell numbers. Most nonmuscle cells are fibroblasts, since endothelial cells and vascular smooth muscle cells represent small populations (12). Although recent data suggest that fibroblasts may play a role in cardiac conduction in both normal and pathologic cardiac conditions (13–15), structurally, it is usually accepted that 3 myocardial cell types are involved in the generation and the propagation of cardiac impulse throughout the whole heart: nodal cells, cardiomyocytes, and the His-Purkinje tracts. Nodal cells are small fascicular cells constituting sinoatrial (SA) and atrioventricular (AV) nodes. These cells are characterized by their ability to depolarize spontaneously and generate cardiac impulse, the SA node having the highest frequency of depolarization. Another characteristic is that the conduction velocity of nodal cells is slow. Cardiomyocytes (i.e., atrial and ventricular wall cells) are long fascicular cells responsible for the muscle function. These cells are unable to depolarize spontaneously, and show fast conduction veloc-

TABLE 6–2. Values of electrophysiologic parameters with reference to the cell type

Electrophysiologic parameter	SA node	AV node	Purkinje fibers	Myocytes*
Resting potential (mV)	–50 to –60	–60 to –70	–90 to –95	–80 to –90
Action potential				
Amplitude (mV)	60 to 70	70 to 80	120	110 to 120
Maximum potential (mV)	0 to 10	5 to 15	30	30
Duration (ms)	100 to 300	100 to 300	300 to 500	100 to 300#
Vmax (V/s)	1 to 10	5 to 15	500 to 700	100 to 200
Conduction velocity (m/s)	<0.05	0.1	2 to 3	0.3 to 0.4

*Atrial and ventricular myocytes
200 to 300 ms for ventricular myocytes

ity. Cells from the His-Purkinje system are morphologically close to cardiomyocytes, show fast conduction velocity, but depolarize spontaneously. However, the frequency of this automatic activity is lower than that of SA and AV nodes.

From an electrophysiologic point of view, cardiac cells are divided into 2 groups according to the conduction velocity: slow-conducting or slow-response (nodal cells) and fast-conducting or fast-response cells (cardiomyocytes and specialized conducting cells). The characteristics of their action potentials and conduction velocities are shown in Table 6-2. In each group, subtypes of cells are distinguished based on their topography in the heart. The differences between subtypes are due to qualitative and quantitative differences in ion channel equipments, and account for different responses of these cell subtypes to various physiologic or pharmacologic stimuli. Thus, differences between atrial versus ventricular myocytes (16, 17) explain that ketamine decreases the atrial wavelength and therefore tend to have arrhythmogenic properties in atrial tissue (18), while it increases the ventricular wavelength and has ventricular antiarrhythmic properties (19). Similarly, it was shown that the ventricular wall contains at least 3 functionally different subtypes of ventricular myocytes: epicardial, midmyocardial (M-cells), and endocardial cells. M-cells are characterized by a longer duration of repolarization compared to the other cell subtypes (10, 20). With reference to responses to pharmacologic agents, it was shown, for example, that propranolol and tetrodotoxin induce a shortening of the action potential duration of endocardial cells while they lengthen it in epicardial cells (9).

CARDIAC ELECTROPHYSIOLOGY AT THE TISSUE AND ORGAN LEVELS: CARDIAC CONDUCTION

Conduction in Cardiac Tissue

The process of cell membrane conduction agrees with the cable theory (21). Membrane properties, especially the depth of the resting membrane potential and ionic conductance to sodium in fast-conducting cells and calcium in slow-conducting cells, are the main determinants of conduction. As a result, $\dot{V}_{max}$ is correlated to the amplitude of depolarizing currents, large I_{Na} or I_{Ca} producing high conduction velocities in fast- and slow-conducting cells, respectively. However, this relationship is not linear in fast-conducting cells, because the size of neighboring cells and amplitude of the depolarizing current also play a role (22–25). Nevertheless, any pharmacologic agent that inhibits I_{Na} decreases $\dot{V}_{max}$ and slows conduction velocity.

Tissue conduction depends on cell membrane properties as well as the tissue architecture, i.e., intracellular resistances (cytoplasm and gap junctions), extracellular resistances (extracellular medium and other and non-conducting cells), and other structural barriers such as blood vessels. However, an impulse spreads throughout the cardiac tissue by passing from a depolarized cell to a less depolarized neighbor via specialized low-resistance structures known as gap junctions. Therefore, gap junctional intercellular coupling is a main determinant of myocardial conduction (26, 27). Gap junctional channels connect intracellular spaces of adjacent cells, allowing the cell-to-cell transmission of electrical signals as well as biochemical substances. They are made up of proteins called connexins (Cx). Three isoforms of connexins are expressed in cardiac tissue: Cx43, Cx45, and Cx40 (28). Each isoform forms a channel distinguishable by its unitary conductance, voltage sensitivity, and permeability to ions and dye (29). However, Cx43 is the major connexion in cardiac tissue; its absence (homozygous mutation) leads to lethal cardiomyopathy (30), a 50% expression (heterozygous mutation) leading to QRS widening with slow ventricular conduction but normal atrial conduction, suggesting a greater functional importance of Cx43 in ventricular versus atrial tissue (31). The qualitative and quantitative isoform composition in connexins varies with age (32), and from one cardiac tissue to another (33), contributing to differences in conduction profiles between different tissues throughout the heart.

The density of gap junctions is the highest at the intercalated discs at the end of the rectangular shaped cardiac cells (34, 35). Therefore, conduction velocity is 2–3 times greater in the direction of the long axis of the cardiac fibers (longitudinal conduction-θ_L) than in the transverse direction (transverse conduction-θ_T), because the number of junctions through which the impulse must travel is less in the former than in the latter directions (36, 37). This directional dependence defines anisotropy of cardiac conduction, which can be quantified in cardiac tissue by an anisotropic ratio (θ_L/θ_T) (Figure 6–3). Anisotropy is determined by several structural (cell geometry, cell size, gap junction, and ion channel distribution) and functional (stimulation rate, gap junctional conductance) factors, and can be uniform such as in normal cardiac tissue, or nonuniform such as in diseased hearts (38). Nonuniformity can result from Cx redistribution, the presence of fatty and fibrous tissues interposed in between myocytes due to aging (39, 40), or to tissue healing after myocardial infarction (41, 42).

The transmission of an electric impulse from one cell to another depends on the ratio between the amount of charge generated by the depolarized membrane and the amount of charge required to depolarize the adjacent cell, with ratio referred to as the safety factor (36). Because of anisotropy and the discontinuous nature of impulse propagation through the cardiac tissue, the safety factor is different in the lon-

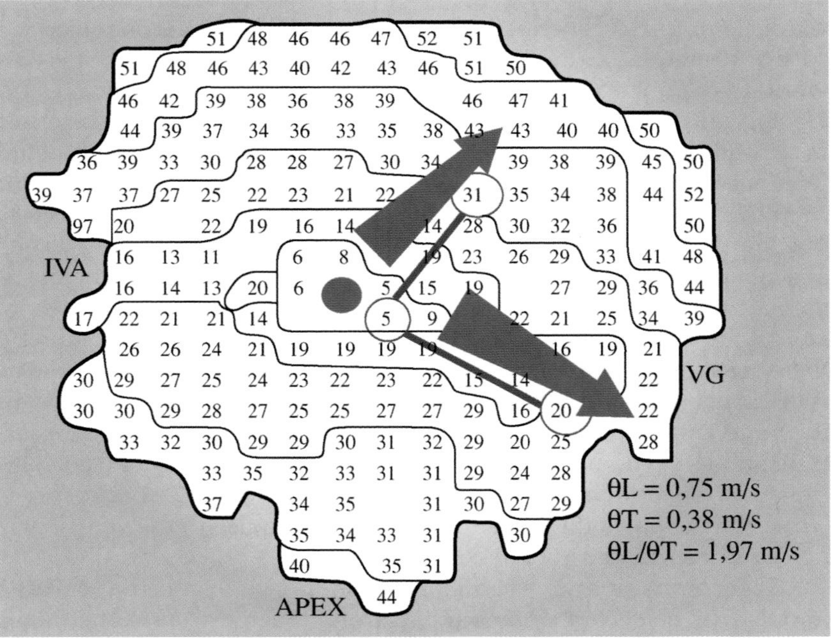

FIGURE 6–3. Mapping of epicardial conduction in an isolated rabbit heart. The green point represents the stimulating electrodes. Numbers are activation times. Drawing isochrones reveals longitudinal and transverse conduction axes. Conduction velocities are calculated between a pair of electrodes along these axes. IVA: left anterior descending artery. VG: left ventricle.

gitudinal versus transverse directions. It was demonstrated that the safety factor is higher in the transverse direction (36, 39, 43), but different results were observed in aged atria (40), sheep (44), and rabbit epicardial tissue (45). In addition, the mechanism of conduction alteration (decreased excitability or cellular uncoupling) may also be implicated. Decreased excitability leads to a decrease in the safety factor and to the rapid occurrence of a conduction block despite a relatively moderate slowing in conduction velocity. In contrast, the safety factor increases in case of cellular uncoupling, allowing the maintenance of conduction despite a marked slowing in conduction velocity. This could be due to the role played by I_{CaL} in conduction in cases of cellular uncoupling (46). In ventricular tissue, longitudinal conduction is correlated to $\dot{V}_{max}$ and I_{Na}, and reflects the role of membrane excitability while the transverse conduction reflects mainly the role of cellular coupling in ventricular conduction, and alteration of either of these parameters may preferably impacts the longitudinal or transverse conduction (45, 47, 48).

Cardiac Conduction

Cardiac impulse is generated by sinoatrial (SA) cells and conducted via special structures (atrioventricular node, His bundle, and Purkinje network) to the myocardial tissue. These structures are anatomically and cytologically well described (49). The SA node is made up of clusters of nodal cells surrounded by transitional cells which functions to ensure intercluster electrical connections to allow synchronized nodal electrical activity and to connect electrically the nodal cells with the atrial cells. The human SA node is richly innervated by branches of both the vagus and sympathetic systems. The structure of the AV node is close to that of the SA node, and it also has a rich vagal and sympathetic innervation. His bundle is the only electrical pathway for ventricular activation by the sinusal impulse. It is made up of an array of slender and insulated transitional cells, and its innervation is supplied by the vagus nerve. In the interventricular septum, the His bundle divides into two branches, right and left to both ventricles, the latter dividing further into an anterior and a posterior branch. His bundle is connected to the Purkinje network which allows the transmission of the impulse to the ventricular myocardium via transitional cells (50).

Electrophysiologic studies in humans suggested that cardiac impulse can be generated by the synchronous activity of several rather than a single anatomic pacemaker (51). Whatever the mechanism of its generation, the cardiac impulse travels throughout the atrial tissue via the atrial myocardium and interatrial conduction pathways such as Bachmann bundle (52, 53) and initiates atrial contraction. Thereafter, the impulse reaches the AV node; is transiently slowed before going through the His bundle, its branches, and the Purkinje network; and finally reaches the ventricular myocardium. The impulse propagation throughout the ventricular myocardium initiates the ventricular contraction. The symmetrical and synchronous activation of the ventricles accounts for narrow QRS complexes on surface ECG.

Cardiac Repolarization

At the cellular level, repolarization corresponds to phase 3 of the membrane AP and is characterized by the inactivation of inward currents while several outward currents, mainly potassium currents, are activated. This allows the transmembrane electrical gradient to be restored; the ionic gradient is restored later with the action of ionic pumps. Repolarization is a critical phase in ventricular cells, because its alteration leads to severe pathologic conditions responsible for life-threatening arrhythmias such as long QT or short QT syndromes. Ventricular cells show a fast-type AP, with a plateau phase (phase 2) contributing to the determination of the AP duration. In fact, the plateau phase is characterized by a high membrane resistance or a low current flow, so that any change—even a mild change of one inward or outward current—can lead to a significant lengthening or shortening of the AP duration. The initial part of repolarization, the so-called absolute refractory period, is characterized by the inability of the cell membrane to generate an AP, whatever the stimulus. This is because the transmembrane gradient of the depolarizing ion (Na^+ or Ca^{2+}) is not sufficient to generate an effective depolarizing current (I_{Na} or I_{Ca}). The final phase, before complete recovery of excitability, is called the relative refractory period. During this phase, the membrane is able to generate partial depolarizing currents, characterized by slow rates of rise of depolarization and therefore slow conduction with a low safety factor. When several partial AP are generated as a result of a high pacing rate or by using multiple extrastimuli, each AP is conducted slower than the preceding one because of a beat-to-beat slowing in the safety factor. This can lead to a functional conduction block facilitating the occurrence of reentry arrhythmias.

At the tissue level, repolarization is assessed using the duration of the monophasic AP or the duration of refractory period. Repolarization is shortened by high pacing rates, and in cases of increased temperature or decreased pH. Refractory period is a stable and homogenous parameter. This homogeneity is accounted for by the lack of increased spatial dispersion in the duration of refractory period throughout a given tissue. Increased spatial dispersion in repolarization is arrhythmogenic (54-56), and can be observed in pathologic conditions such as myocardial ischemia or with the use of some pharmacologic agents (57). The high velocity of the cardiac conduction also allows a temporal homogeneity in repolarization, i.e., there is no delay in the times of occurrence of repolarization phases between two separated areas of a same tissue. However, in case of major conduction slowing or conduction block, a temporal dispersion of repolarization can occur, facilitating functional conduction blocks and leading to reentrant circuits.

In humans, repolarization is evaluated by using the duration of the monophasic AP or the duration of refractory period during electrophysiologic studies. However, in daily practice, the duration of the QT interval is used to reflect the duration of the cellular action potential. As this parameter is influenced by heart rate, a correction is usually applied, most frequently using the Bazett's formula: $QTc = QT/(RR)^{1/2}$, with RR expressed in milliseconds. The normal value of the QTc is <430 msec in men, and <450 msec in women (58). Long QT is defined by an increase of these values by 20 msec, and subjects with long QTc are vulnerable for reentrant arrhythmias. The QTc value is homogenous from an ECG lead to another. The occurrence of an interlead dispersion of the QTc value (reflecting spatial dispersion of AP duration) is associated with an increased risk of reentrant arrhythmias (59).

REGULATION OF THE CARDIAC ELECTRICAL ACTIVITY BY THE AUTONOMIC NERVOUS SYSTEM

Sympathetic and parasympathetic nerves that supply the heart form a plexus located at the base: the cardiac plexus. Various staining and binding techniques (histochemical, immunohistochemical, scintigraphic, immunofluorescence) showed the presence of numerous small sympathetic and vagal nerves distributed along the conduction system. The density of these nerves decreases from the SA node in the following order: SA node, AV node, His bundle and branches, atrial and ventricular myocardium (60). Density also decreases with advancing age (61). Sympathetic nerves are uniformly distributed throughout the conduction system, although the norepinephrine concentration is 3-fold higher in the SA node, the AV node, and the atrial tissue compared with the ventricular myocardium. Therefore, sympathetic stimulation leads to tachycardia by increasing the SA node pulse rate and the AV nodal conduction. Vagal nerves are heterogeneously distributed since their density is higher in the SA and AV nodes than in the myocardium. As a result, parasympathetic stimulation leads to a slowing in heart rate by decreasing the SA pulse rate and the AV nodal conduction. The cardiac electrophysiologic activity is modulated by the autonomic nervous system mainly via norepinephrine and acetylcholine (62), mediators which act on β-adrenergic and muscarinic membrane receptors, respectively. The resulting modulation of the intracellular concentration of cAMP allows the regulation of ionic currents implicated in the AP. Then, acetyl-

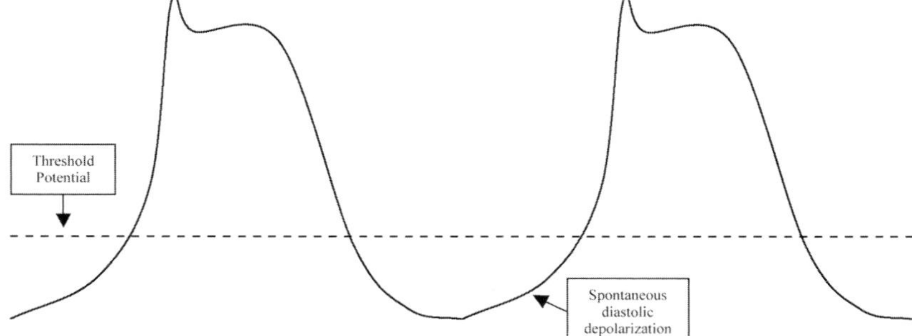

FIGURE 6–4. **Schematic representation of abnormal automaticity.**

choline decreases I_{CaL} and I_f in the SA node and induces bradycardia. In contrast, norepinephrine and epinephrine increase I_{CaL} and I_f and cause tachycardia. The comparison in density suggests that the parasympathetic system is dominant in the atrium while the sympathetic tone is dominant in the ventricles. In addition, cholinergic fibers represent almost two-thirds of the cardiac autonomic nerves, suggesting that the parasympathetic tone is predominant in the regulation of the cardiac electrophysiologic activity. Other nerves mainly located in the His-Purkinje system are peptidergic with sympathetic peptides or other mediators such as substance P. The local release of these mediators contributes to the regulation of the electrophysiologic activity of the His-Purkinje system.

MECHANISMS OF ARRHYTHMIAS

Two different types of mechanisms lead to cardiac arrhythmias: disorders of impulse formation and disorders of impulse conduction (63). However, mechanisms of both types can occur simultaneously, one inducing the arrhythmic event and the other sustaining it.

Disorders of impulse formation are divided into abnormal automaticity and triggered activity. Abnormal automaticity is the ability for a nonautomatic cardiac fiber to depolarize spontaneously in phase 4 of its AP (Figure 6–4). This abnormal spontaneous depolarization is facilitated by ischemia, anoxia, hyperkalemia, increased cardiac fiber tension, and catecholamines. As action potential may be conducted slowly in partially depolarized fibers, conduction blocks are likely to occur in the neighboring tissues of these abnormal automatic foci. Then, reentrant circuits can appear around these blocks and maintain the so-created arrhythmia.

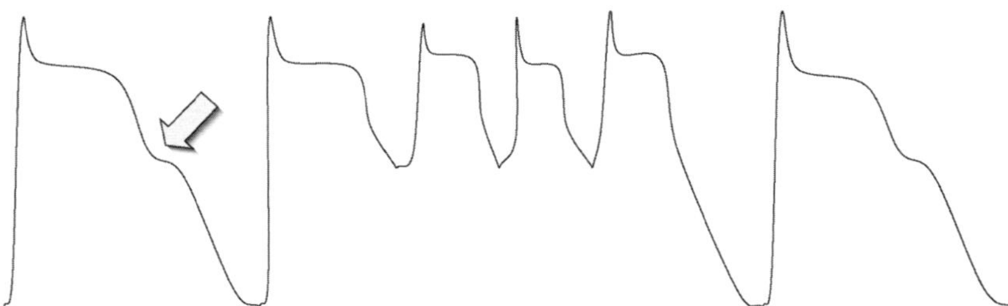

FIGURE 6–5. Schematic representation of triggered activity: a non-sustained tachycardia triggered by early afterdepolarization (arrow)

Triggered activity is defined as AP-induced by afterdepolarizations. As afterdepolarizations are oscillations of membrane potentials occurring after or during a normal action potential and reaching the threshold value (Figure 6–5), a triggered activity is a consequence of a preceding AP (64). Afterdepolarizations are either early or delayed. Early afterdepolarizations (EAD) occur during Phase 2 or 3 of the AP and are facilitated by ischemia, anoxia, bradycardia, hypokalemia, and all factors and agents that lengthen repolarization. Delayed afterdepolarizations (DAD) occur after complete repolarization and are facilitated by tachycardia, catecholamines, digitalis, and late myocardial infarction.

Disorders of impulse conduction can be described as conduction blocks and reentry. As stated earlier, conduction block can be facilitated by abnormal automaticity. More commonly, conduction block can occur during tachycardia as a result of incomplete recovery of refractoriness. In addition, blocks can occur on the myocardial tissue and/or on the specialized conduction pathways.

The occurrence of reentry requires an electrophysiologic circuit including an anatomic or functional unidirectional conduction block, the slowing of conduction and the ability of cell to cell conduction around this block, depending on the duration of the refractory periods. While anatomic blocks result from alterations of the myocardial structure, functional blocks occur in cases of slowing of conduction with increased anisotropy (45), use-dependent block (65, 66), or increased dispersion of refractoriness (55). An example of reentry is presented in Figure 6–6.

PHARMACOLOGY OF ANTIARRHYTHMIC DRUGS

Several agents such as digitalis, magnesium, and adenosine can suppress arrhythmias by correcting electrolytic or acid-base disorders and/or by improving cardiac failure or coronary artery disease.

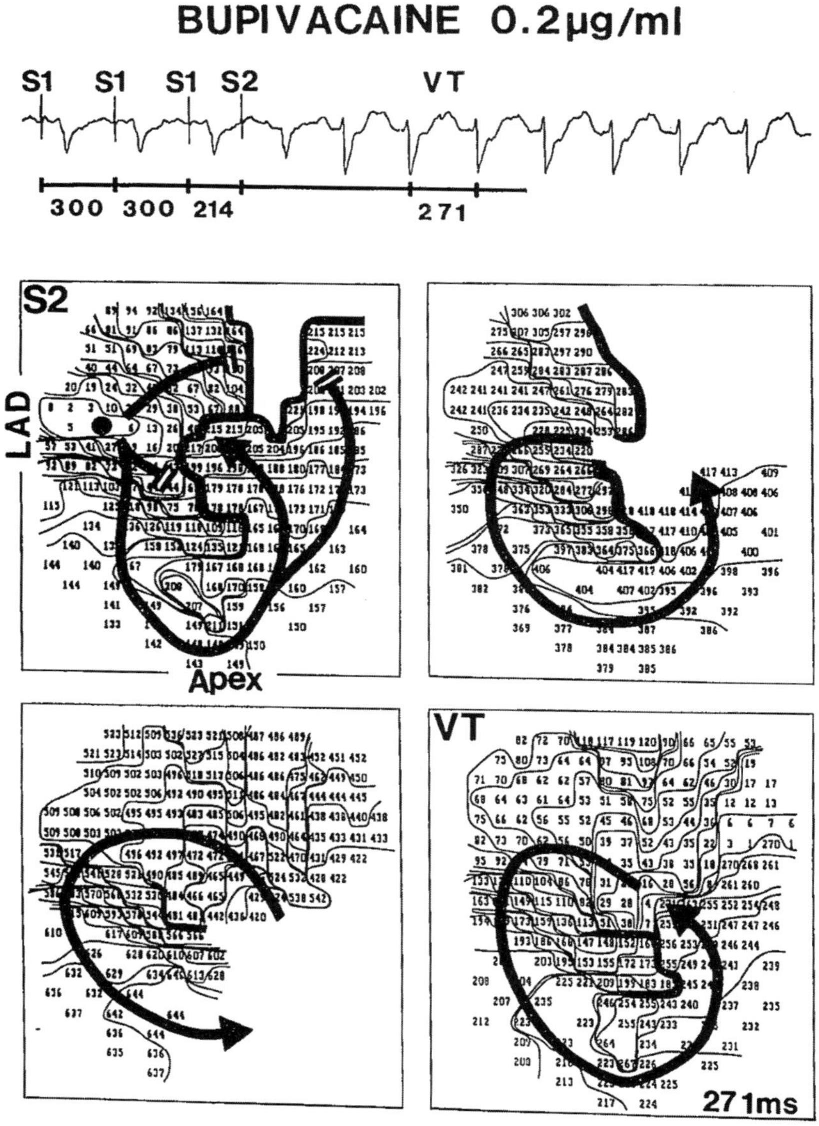

BUPIVACAINE 0.2μg/ml

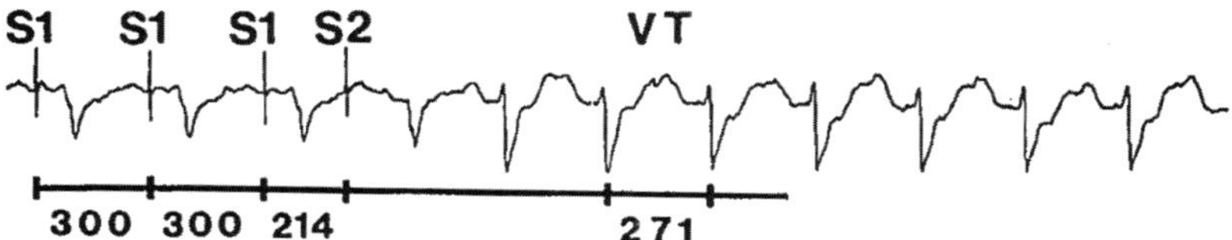

FIGURE 6–6. Mapping of the initiation and the development of a ventricular tachycardia on a rabbit epicardial preparation treated with bupivacaine. From de La Coussaye JE, Brugada J, Allessie MA: Electrophysiologic and arrhythmogenic effects of bupivacaine: a study with high resolution ventricular epicardial mapping in rabbit hearts. Anesthesiology 1992; 77:132–41

However, the "antiarrhythmic" term refers specifically to drugs that induce changes in ionic currents involved in the cardiac AP. Nevertheless, the in vivo antiarrhythmic property of an agent results from its concomitant effects on cardiac electrophysiology, on myocardial blood supply, and on the autonomic nervous system.

Several systems have been used to classify antiarrhythmic agents. Although debated, the Vaughan-Williams classification, based on 4 classes of antiarrhythmic action, remains in widespread clinical use (67). The debate comes from the fact that this system is based on cellular electrophysiologic effects only, and that a given drug can possess more than one class of action. Other classifications based on the electrophysiologic and/or clinical data have therefore been proposed. The working group on arrhythmias of the European Society of Cardiology proposed a new classification (The Sicilian Gambit) (68) including electrophysiologic effects, effects on the autonomic nervous system, and actions on arrhythmogenic mechanisms. However, because this classification system is far more complicated and because the Vaughan Williams classification is commonly used, it will be followed in this chapter (Tables 6-3 and 6-4). The list of antiarrhythmic drugs is not exhaustive because it is limited to agents currently recommended for the treatment of cardiac arrhythmias (69, 70). As indications for the use of antiarrhythmics for the treatment of patients with cardiac arrhythmias are provided in several guidelines from cardiac societies (69, 70), the current review is focused on the effects of antiarrhythmic agents (71, 72) on electrophysiologic parameters and their resulting antiarrhythmic properties, and possible implications for anesthesiologists.

Class I Antiarrhythmic Drugs

All class I antiarrhythmic agents inhibit the fast inward sodium current I_{Na} (73), thereby decreasing the $\dot{V}_{max}$ and slowing conduction velocities in fast-conducting cells. The effect on I_{Na} appears as a widening of QRS complexes. The characteristics of this effect and the nature of ancillary effects such as those on potassium currents lead to the distinction of 3 subgroups of class I agents, referred to as Ia, Ib, and Ic. The classification of class 1 agents and their effects are summarized in Table 6-3. With reference to sodium channels, the efficiency of class I antiarrhythmic drugs depends on the functional state of the channel and therefore on the heart rate. Quinidine and flecainide mainly act in the activated state of the cardiac sodium channel while lidocaine mainly interacts with activated and inactivated channels (74). Moreover, the kinetic of block and recovery is different in the subclasses. Another parameter determining efficacy is the in- out kinetic of class I agents on the sodium channel receptors (fast or slow block and recovery) (75). Class Ib antiarrhythmic

Table 6–3. Mechanisms of action and effects of class I antiarrhythmic agents

Class and drugs	Ionic mechanisms of action	Effects on AP	Clinical and ECG effets
Class Ia *Quinidine* *Procainamide* *Disopyramide*	Moderate to marked inhibition of I_{Na} Significant inhibition of I_{to}, I_{Kr} and I_{Kur}	Dose-dependent decrease in $\mathring{V}_{max}$ in fast-response cells Prolongation of APD at low concentration	Slowing in conduction velocities in fast-response cells (widening of QRS complexes) Lengthening of ERP QT and JT intervals lengthening
Class Ib *Lidocaine* *Mexiletine* *Diphenylhydantoine*	Mild to moderate inhibition of I_{Na} (mainly on abnormal cells) No or minor effect on potassium channels	Mild decrease in $\mathring{V}_{max}$ in fast-response cells No effect or shortening of APD	QRS unchanged QT interval unchanged
Class Ic *Flecainide* *Propafenone* *Cibenzoline*	Marked inhibition of I_{Na} No or minor effect on potassium channels	Marked dose- and use-dependent decrease in $\mathring{V}_{max}$ in fast-response cells No effect or slight prolongation APD	QRS widening Slight prolongation and dispersion of ERP JT interval unchanged

drugs have fast kinetics, class Ic have slow kinetics, and class 1a have intermediate kinetics (76). Thus, the faster the heart rate or the more depolarized the cardiac cells, the more inhibited the $\dot{V}_{max}$ because antiarrhythmic drugs induce greater receptor saturation. This effect is more potent with class Ic antiarrhythmic agents, which tend to be effective at all heart rates. Regarding potassium channels, the blocking effect of class Ia agents is more potent than that of class Ic agents, with a resulting larger prolongation of repolarization.

In addition to a dose-dependant blockade of I_{Na}, class 1a agents potently inhibit one or more of the potassium currents I_{to} (77), I_{Kr} (78), and I_{Kur} (79) at low concentrations—actions accounting for their most important electrophysiologic effects: prolongation of repolarization (80, 81). They also exhibit vagolytic effects that tend to facilitate atrioventricular nodal conduction. Finally, quinidine is more potent than procainamide and disopyramide (82, 83). Class Ia agents, mainly quinidine and disopyramide, can cause proarrhythmic complications (reentrant or Torsade de pointes tachycardias) both via conduction slowing and related to a dose-dependent effect, and via delayed repolarization by promoting afterdepolarization (80, 81).

TABLE 6–4. Mechanisms of action and effects of class II, III, and IV antiarrhythmic agents

Class and drugs	Ionic mechanisms of action	Effects on AP	Clinical and ECG effects
Class II			
Propranolol *Esmolol* *dl-Sotalol* *Atenolol* *Metoprolol*	Competitive blockade of β-adrenoceptors with indirect blockade of calcium currents and I_f Inhibition of I_{Na}, enhancement of I_{K1} (high concentrations propranolol) Inhibition of I_{Kr} and I_{to} (dl-sotalol)	Decrease in the slope of spontaneous depolarization (phase 0) of slow-response cells (SA and AV nodes), Enhanced repolarization of abnormal cells Prolongation of APD in fast-response cells	Slowing in heart rate, prolongation of PR interval, prolongation of AV node refractoriness Increased fibrillation threshold Prolongation of refractoriness in atrial and ventricular tissues
Class III			
Amiodarone *d-Sotalol* *Azimilide* *Ibutilide* *Dofetilide*	Block of potassium currents, mainly I_{Kr}(selective effect for dofetilide), but also I_{Ks} (azimilide), I_{K1}, I_{Na}, I_{CaL} (amiodarone, dronedarone)	Homogeneous prolongation of APD in fast-response cells Reduced automaticity (amiodarone, dronedarone)	Prolongation of QT interval and of atrial and ventricular effective refractory periods Slowing in heart rate and in AV node conduction
Class IV			
Verapamil *Diltiazem*	Direct inhibition of I_{CaL}	Decrease in the slope of spontaneous depolarization (phase 0) of slow-response cells (SA and AV nodes)	Shortening of the fast AP plateau Slowing in heart rate and atrio-ventricular conduction

Class Ib agents are less potent sodium channel blockers than class Ia and Ic agents, and have almost no significant effects on potassium channels. In fact, their inhibitory effect on I_{Na} is mainly observed in abnormal conditions such as hyperkalemia, acidosis, hypoxia, and ischemia (81, 84). Lidocaine is especially efficient to suppress ischemia/reperfusion-induced arrhythmias, by decreasing excitability of ischemic cells (85). Mexiletine can be given orally. Diphenylhydantoine has central sympatholytic effects, and its electrophysiologic effects depend on its plasma level, kalemia, pH, age, and cardiac fiber state.

Class Ic agents are the most potent class I agents with regard to I_{Na} inhibition. These agents induce PR lengthening and QRS widening without major alteration of ventricular repolarization. The sodium channel blockade is prolonged, so these agents exhibit a strong use-dependent effect, the conduction slowing/QRS widening being more important with increasing heart rate (86–88). However, as shown with flecainide, this use-dependency also can lead to conduction blocks and reentrant arrhythmias (47, 89, 90). Flecainide also has been shown to cause conduction defects at rest and at exercise (86, 91) and atrio-ventricular blocks. The other drugs of this sub-class show electrophysiologic effects characteristic of other sub-classes. Propafenone has slight class II and IV effects. Cibenzoline has slight class Ia and class IV effects in vitro and in vivo, and is slightly vagolytic.

Class II Antiarrhythmic Drugs

Class II is represented by β-adrenoceptor blockers, agents that have many other properties than that used for the treatment of arrhythmias. With reference to their antiarrhythmic effects, β-blockers act by phosphorylation of β_1-adrenoceptors, thereby blocking sympathetic activity of the heart. β-blockers also inhibit I_f current. As a result, these agents decrease the rate of spontaneous depolarization of pacemaker cells and slow the heart rate, mainly in the presence of a high adrenergic tone. They also induce a slowing of conduction in the AV node. Some β-blockers have intrinsic sympathomimetic activity and/or membrane-stabilizing actions. Some β-blockers such as esmolol are relatively cardioselective, whereas others such as propranolol act on β-adrenoceptors on other tissue types, potentially inducing extra-cardiac side effects. In addition, at high concentrations, propranolol inhibits I_{Na}, and therefore shows quinidine-like effects. This agent also enhances repolarization of abnormal cells, as do class Ib agents, probably by increasing I_{K1}. Esmolol is available for intravenous use, and its elimination half-life is so short that esmolol is an agent of choice for the short-term or emergency treatment of cardiac arrhythmias. Class II antiarrhythmic agents have demonstrated convincing interests in postmyocardial infarction and in the perioperative management of high-risk cardiovascular patients by clearly reducing their mortality rates (92, 93).

Sotalol is a potent noncardioselective β-blocker without intrinsic sympathomimetic activity and/or membrane-stabilizing effects. It also shows class III antiarrhythmic effects since it inhibits I_{Kr} and I_{to} (94, 95). Therefore, sotalol prolongs repolarization in a dose-dependent manner, an effect that is increased by hypothermia and bradycardia (96, 97). In fact, sotalol is marketed as a racemic mixture (de-sotalol), in which the blocking effect is due to the l-sotalol isomer, whereas the d-sotalol isomer only has class III effects. High blood levels of sotalol can promote Torsade de pointes tachycardia (98).

Class III Antiarrhythmic Drugs

Class III antiarrhythmic agents block potassium channels, delay repolarization, and prolong refractoriness. This group is composed of amiodarone, d-sotalol (see supra), and relatively new agents: dronedarone, azimilide, and dofetilide. Although the risk varies from one agent to another, all class III agents produce a propensity to Torsade de pointes tachycardia.

The electrophysiologic effects of amiodarone are complex and are different when it is given acutely by intravenous route, or chronically, where the effects are more pronounced (99). The class III effect is observed as a homogenous prolongation of myocardial refractoriness. It is due to the inhibition of several potassium currents, including I_K, I_{K1}, I_{KATP}, I_{KACh}, and I_{KNa}. Other effects of amiodarone are due to the blockade of I_{Na} and I_{CaL} (100). Acute administration of amiodarone does not or slightly prolongs the effective refractory period of atria, His-Purkinje system, and of ventricles, but markedly lengthens those of AV node and accessory pathways (101). Moreover, amiodarone slows SA spontaneous rate and conduction through AV nodes (102). During chronic administration, amiodarone prolongs refractory periods in most cardiac tissues. Furthermore, in addition to its class III actions, it shows use-dependent class IV (103, 104) and class I effects (105, 106). Amiodarone produces noncompetitive β-adrenergic blockade (107) and inhibits the conversion of T4 into T3. These effects increase with long-standing treatments. Finally, amiodarone inhibits the microsomal Na-K-ATPase activity (108).

Other class III agents have been developed more recently. Dronedarone, an analogue of amiodarone, has its electrical and pharmacological profiles of effects, without side effects related to the thyroid. Dronedarone inhibits I_{Kr}, I_{K1}, I_{KAch}, I_{Na}, and slows I_{CaL} in isolated cardiomyocytes (109, 110). Dronedarone also has antiadrenergic properties (111). It is poorly tolerated in patients with heart failure and ventricular dysfunction. Azimilide blocks I_{Na}, I_{Ca}, I_{Kr}, and I_{Ks} (112), thereby increasing the action potential duration and prolonging myocardial repolarization. QT interval and effective refractory period are also prolonged. Ibutilide induces a persistent sodium current sensitive to dihydropyridine calcium channel blockers and potently blocks I_{Kr}. These effects result in a prolongation of myocardial action potential duration (113). Dofetilide is a pure I_{Kr} blocker that induces a prolongation in action potential duration and effective refractory period of atrial and ventricular myocytes in a reverse-frequency-dependent manner. It can be given orally or by intravenous route. It is generally well tolerated.

Class IV Antiarrhythmic Drugs

Class IV antiarrhythmic drugs are represented by the nondihydropyridine calcium channel blockers. Two agents are usually used as antiarrhythmics: verapamil and diltiazem (114). Although diltiazem tends to be less potent than verapamil, both agents have qualitatively similar actions and block I_{CaL} channels mainly in their inactivated or activated state (115, 116). Therefore, they are more effective at high heart rates. Calcium channel blockers decrease the slope of spontaneous diastolic depolarization and the $\dot{V}_{max}$ of phase 0 of slow action potentials (117). As a result, they induce a frequency-dependent depression of the SA node automaticity and of AV node anterograde conduction (118). On the other cardiac tissues (atria, His, Purkinje, and ventricles), calcium channel blockers shorten the AP plateau phase (phase 2), giving a triangular aspect to the fast AP. However, conduction velocity is not altered. Therefore, calcium channel blockers do not exhibit antiarrhythmic actions on atria or ventricles, except in cases of partial depolarization and/or ischemia (119). Calcium channel blockers depress myocardial contractility, can be responsible for severe sinus bradycardia, atrioventricular conduction defects, and cardiac failure in cases of overdosage or preexisting cardiac failure.

ELECTROPHYSIOLOGIC EFFECTS OF ANESTHETIC AGENTS AND THEIR POSSIBLE INTERACTIONS WITH ANTIARRHYTHMIC DRUGS

Most anesthetic agents exhibit cardiac electrophysiologic effects. These effects need to be taken into account when choosing agents to be given to patients with diseased heart in order to avoid additive or synergic arrhythmogenic effects.

Volatile Anesthetics

Volatile anesthetics inhibit several ionic currents (Table 6-5), but their main target is I_{CaL} (120). As a result, these agents slow the spontaneous

Table 6–5. Cellular and clinical effects of volatile anesthetic agents and opiates

Anesthetic agents	Ionic mechanisms of action	Cellular effects	Clinical effects
Volatile anesthetics *Halothane* *Isoflurane* *Sevoflurane* *Desflurane*	Concentration- and voltage-dependant inhibition of I_{CaL} and I_{Na} Inhibition of I_K (desflurane) and I_{to} (halothane, sevoflurane), I_{Kr} (isoflurane), I_{Ks} (sevoflurane)	Concentration-dependent decrease in $\mathring{V}_{max}$ in slow and fast-response cells Prolongation of slow and fast APD Biphasic effect on fast-response APD (halothane, isoflurane)	Slowing in heart rate and AV nodal conduction Slowing in ventricular conduction velocity Increase in AV nodal ERP Increase of ventricular ERP Increase (low concentrations) and decrease in ventricular ERP (halothane, isoflurane)
Opiates *Morphine* *Fentanyl* *Sufentanil* *Alfentanil* *Remifentanil*	Inhibition of I_{Na}, increase in I_{CaL} and I_{K1} (morphine) Increase in I_{KATP} (fentanyl)	Hyperpolarization and prolongation of APD in fast- and slow-response cells	Slowing in heart rate and AV nodal conduction Increase in AV and in ventricular nodal ERP Role in preconditioning

rate of the SA node, decrease conduction, and lengthen ERP in the AV node (121). In addition to the block of I_{CaL}, volatile anesthetics induce a depression of the sarcoplasmic reticulum, contributing to a depressive effect on myocardial contractility (122, 123). These effects are more potent for halothane compared with newer volatile anesthetics. Volatile anesthetics also inhibit I_{Na}, decrease $\dot{V}_{max}$ of fast action potential, and slow conduction in fast-response cells, mainly by altering the cell-to-cell conduction (124–126). However, this effect seems to be more potent on atrial than on ventricular tissue. Furthermore, volatile anesthetics inhibit several potassium channels (127, 128): I_K (halothane, desflurane), I_{Kr} (isoflurane), I_{Ks} (sevoflurane), and I_{to} (halothane, sevoflurane). As a result, most volatile anesthetics have been shown to prolong action potential duration in fast-response cells (129), and the QTc interval in the clinical setting (130–132). However, at least for halothane and isoflurane, a biphasic effect was observed on effective refractory period and on action potential duration, respectively (133, 134). In ventricular cells and epicardium, low concentrations of halothane and isoflurane lead to a prolongation, whereas high concentrations shortened ventricular effective refractory periods and action potential duration. Clinically, volatile anesthetics induce concentration-dependent bradycardia with a lengthening of the PR interval, and the effects on ventricular conduction are probably of lower magnitude than those observed at a cellular level, at least in normal cardiac tissues.

Because of their effects on ion channels, volatile anesthetics have at least class I and IV antiarrhythmic properties. Therefore, a theoretical additive effect leading to severe bradycardia or AV nodal conduction block could be expected when these agents are given to patients treated with antiarrhythmics. While the risk is suggested by experimental studies (especially verapamil vs. diltiazem) (135, 136), associating volatile anesthetics with antiarrhythmics could be beneficial. For example, it was shown that in humans anesthetized with volatile anesthetics, intravenous diltiazem decreases the rate of ventricular premature contractions and slows the ventricular rate in atrial fibrillations (137). Both pro- and antiarrhythmic properties have been shown with volatile anesthetics. Briefly, the proarrhythmic effect of volatile anesthetics is observed in hyperadrenergic states, because these agents sensitize myocytes to the arrhythmogenic effects of epinephrine (138–140). On the other hand, several studies show that volatile anesthetics have antiarrhythmic effects in cases of regional or global cardiac ischemia (141–144).

Opiates

The clinical effects of opiates are complex because these agents act both directly via tissue-associated opioid receptors, and indirectly via receptors located in areas in the brain and nuclei that regulate the cardiovascular functions. Opioid receptors, especially κ, have been identified in the heart tissues, with a maximum density in the right atrium. The presence of μ-receptors and their distribution are debated. Experimental data show that, at high concentrations, morphine blocks I_{Na} but increases I_{CaL} and I_{K1}. The resulting effects are hyperpolarization and moderate prolongation of action potential duration in myocytes (145). Fentanyl and sufentanil also prolong the duration of action potential in fast-response cells (146,147). In addition, fentanyl was shown to increase I_{KATP} (148).

In vivo, opiates induce a dose-dependent bradycardia, a lengthening of the AV nodal conduction, and an increase in AV node and ventricular effective refractory periods (149). Romero et al. reported on isolated rat atria that the negative chronotropic effect of morphine is not modified by naloxone, by atropine, or after reserpine pretreatment (150). Because of their effects on repolarization, opiates may have class III-like antiarrhythmic properties. Indeed, Saini et al. demonstrated in anesthetized dogs with hemorrhagic shock that fentanyl increases the fibrillation threshold (151). Rabkin reported that morphine and dynorphine (an endogenous opiate) decrease the severity of arrhythmias induced by digoxin in guinea pigs (152). However, the autonomic nervous system might play a role in the antiarrhythmic effects of opiates, which are observed at very high concentrations (153). Finally, these effects could increase the effects of calcium channel blockers and of β-blockers (154, 155).

Intravenous Agents

Thiopental inhibits sodium and several potassium currents (156–158). This leads to a prolongation of the action potential duration and effective refractory periods in atrial and ventricular tissues, and to a slowing in AV nodal conduction (Table 6–6). However, the clinical relevance of these effects seems to be limited. Propofol inhibits I_{CaL}, slightly I_K, and at high concentration I_{to} (159–162). Its cardiac electrophysiologic effects are almost similar to those of thiopental (163). Ketamine potently inhibits I_{Na}, I_{CaL}, I_K, and I_{K1} (159, 164). As a result, this agent slows the SA spontaneous rate (19), although a sinus tachycardia is observed in vivo, which is related to sympathetic stimulation with catecholamine release. Ketamine also induces a slowing in conduction velocity in atrial and ventricular tissues, as well as in AV node (165, 166). With regard to repolarization, experimental data suggest that ketamine leads to a shortening of atrial effective refractory period (18), whereas this parameter is prolonged at the ventricular level (19). While ketamine could promote atrial reentrant arrhythmias, it has antiarrhythmic properties on the ventricular tissue, as it prolongs homogenously ventricular refractoriness. The effects of benzodiazepines and etomidate on cardiac ion channels are

TABLE 6–6. Cellular and clinical effects of intravenous and local anesthetic agents

Anesthetic agents	Ionic mechanisms of action	Cellular effects	Clinical effects
Intravenous anesthetics			
Thiopental *Propofol* *Ketamine*	Inhibition of I_{CaL}, I_K, I_{K1}, I_{to}, I_{Kr} Inhibition of I_{CaL}, I_K(mild), I_{to} (high con centration) Inhibition of I_{Na}, I_{CaL}, I_{K1}, I_K	Prolongation of APD in fast- and slow-response cells Prolongation of APD in fast- and slow-response cells Slows the rate of rise of phase 0 in both slow- and fast-response cells Prolongation of fast APD	Increase in atrial and ventricular ERP Slowing in heart rate and AV nodal conduction Slowing in heart rate and AV nodal conduction Slowing in heart rate and AV nodal conduction Slowing in atrial and ventricular conduction Shortening in atrial ERP Lengthening in ventricular ERP
Local anesthetics			
Lidocaine *Bupivacaine* *Ropivacaine* *Levobupivacaine*	Inhibition of I_{Na} Inhibition ofcalcium and potassium channels at high concentrations, as well as other cellular and intra- cellular targets	Concentration- and use-dependent decrease in $\mathring{V}_{max}$ in slow- and fast-response cells Moderate prolongation of fast APD Slight lengthening in ventricular ERP	Slowing in heart rate and AV nodal conduction Slowing in ventricular conduction

observed only at pharmacologic concentrations, so they do not exhibit a significant effect on electrophysiologic parameters in clinical practice.

Droperidol has quinidine-like effects. It increases anterograde and retrograde refractory periods in accessory pathways in patients having Wolff-Parkinson-White syndrome. However, as droperidol prolongs ventricular repolarization (167), large doses of droperidol can theoretically induce torsades de pointes, probably by creating triggered activity induced by early afterdepolarizations. Vecuronium bromide slightly increases heart rate and myocardial contractility in vitro. In vivo, combined with opiates, it can worsen opiate-induced bradycardia and/or facilitate the occurrence of junctional rhythm or atrioventricular block (168). This effect is increased by the administration of calcium channel or β-blockers (155). Physostigmine or edrophonium used to reverse muscle relaxant action classically facilitates bradycardia or atrioventricular block. These disorders are more frequent during anaesthesia using fentanyl and vecuronium bromide (169), and are reversed by large doses of atropine.

Local Anaesthetic Agents

Local anaesthetic drugs have direct action on conduction due to their class 1 antiarrhythmic property (Table 6–6). These effects on the infranodal conduction are clinically relevant only in the case of overdosage, especially with the most potent agents, bupivacaine and etidocaine. The magnitude of conduction slowing varies from one agent to another, and depends on the concentration (170, 171). Indeed, the sodium channel blockade and recovery kinetic depends on the agent and concentration. For example, the kinetic is fast with lidocaine (fast-in-fast-out), while it depends on concentration with bupivacaine: slow-in-slow-out at low concentration, fast-in-slow-out at high concentration (172). This is due to the fact that lidocaine blocks sodium channels in the activated and inactivated states and unbinds rapidly from the resting channels (154 ms), allowing a rapid recovery of membrane excitability. In contrast, bupivacaine blocks sodium channels preferentially in the inactivated state, dissociates slowly from rested channels (1.5 s), thereby inducing a block accumulation. As a result, bupivacaine shows a stronger use-dependent effect on cardiac conduction than lidocaine, ropivacaine, and levobupivacaine (65, 171, 173). At high concentrations, local anesthetics also inhibit potassium (174) and calcium currents (175), and alter other targets such as β-adrenergic receptors, mitochondria, and some enzyme functions (176). All these effects account for the arrhythmogenic risks associated with the use of potent local anesthetics. Therefore, lidocaine and mepivacaine should be preferred in patients taking antiarrhythmic drugs. Indeed, worsening of hemodynamic status and of conduction velocities was demonstrated in anesthetized dogs receiving bupivacaine combined with β-blockers (175), calcium channel inhibitors (177), and class 1 antiarrhythmic drugs (178). Finally, verapamil, more than diltiazem, potentiates ECG and hemodynamic effects of "anaesthetic" doses of bupivacaine versus lidocaine in awake dogs (179).

References

1. Tan HL, Bezzina CR, Smits JPP, Verkerk AO, Wilde AAM: Genetic control of sodium channel function. Cardiovasc Res 2003; 57:961–73
2. Marcus FI: Depolarization/repolarization, electrocardiographic abnormalities, and arrhythmias in cardiac channelopathies. J Electrocardiol 2005; 38:60–3
3. Hofmann F, Lacinova L, Klugbauer N: Voltage-dependent calcium channels: from structure to function. Rev Physiol Biochem Pharmacol 1999; 139:33–87
4. Li GR, Feng J, Yue L, Carrier M, Nattel S: Evidence for two components of delayed rectifier K^+ current in human ventricular myocytes. Circ Res 1996; 78:689–96.
5. Tamargo J, Caballero R, Gomez R, Valenzuela C, Delpon E: Pharmacology of cardiac potassium channels. Cardiovasc Res 2004; 62:9–33
6. Catterall WA, Cestèle S, Yarov-Yarovoy V, Yu FH, Konoki K, Scheuer T: Voltage-gated ion channels and gating modifier toxins. Toxicon 2007; 49:124–41
7. Mantegazza M, Yu FH, Catterall WA, Scheuer T: Role of the 5-terminal domain in inactivation of brain and cardiac sodium channels. Proc Natl Acad Sci 2001; 98:15348–53
8. Buchanan JW, Saito T, Gettes LS: The effects of antiarrhythmic drugs, stimulation frequency, and potassium-induced resting membrane potential changes on conduction velocity and dV/dt_{max} in guinea pig myocardium. Circ Res 1985; 56:696–703
9. Krishnan SC, Antzelevitch C: Sodium channel block produces opposite electrophysiological effects in canine ventricular epicardium and endocardium. Circ Res 1991; 69:277–91
10. Anyukhovsky EP, Sosunov EA, Rosen MR: Regional differences in electrophysiological properties of epicardium, midmyocardium, and epicardium. In vitro and in vivo correlations. Circulation 1996; 94:1981–8
11. Rithalia A, Gibson CN, Hopkins PM, Harrison SM: Halothane inhibits contraction and action potential duration to a greater extent in subendocardial than subepicardial myocytes from rat left ventricle. Anesthesiology 2001; 95:1213–9
12. Nag AC: Study of non-muscle cells of the adult mammalian heart: a fine structural analysis and distribution. Cytobios 1980; 28:41–61

13. Camelliti P, Green CR, LeGrice I, Kohl P: Fibroblast network in rabbit sinoatrial node: structural and functional identification of homogeneous and heterogeneous cell coupling. Circ Res 2004; 94:828–35
14. Kohl P, Camelliti P, Burton FL, Smith GL: Electrical coupling of fibroblasts and myocytes: relevance for cardiac propagation. J Electrocardiol 2005; 38:45–50
15. Miragoli M, Gaudesius G, Rohr S: Electrotonic modulation of cardiac impulse conduction by myofibroblasts. Circ Res 2006; 98:801–10
16. Giles WR, Imiazumi Y: Comparison of potassium currents in rabbit atrial and ventricular cells. J Physiol 1988; 405:123–45
17. Li GR, Lau CP, Shrier A: Heterogeneity of sodium currents in atrial vs epicardial ventricular myocytes of adult guinea pig hearts. J Mol Cell Cardiol 2002; 34:1185–94
18. Napolitano CA, Raatikainen MJP, Martens JR, Dennis DM: Effects of intravenous anesthetics on atrial wavelength and atrioventricular nodal conduction in guinea pig heart. Potential antidysrhythmic properties and clinical implications. Anesthesiology 1996; 85:393–402
19. Aya AGM, Robert E, Bruelle P, Lefrant JY, Juan JM, Peray P, Eledjam JJ, de La Coussaye JE: Effects of ketamine on ventricular conduction, refractoriness, and wavelength. Potential antiarrhythmic effects: A high-resolution epicardial mapping in rabbit hearts. Anesthesiology 1997; 87:1417–27
20. Liu DW, Gintant GA, Antzelevitch C: Ionic bases for electrophysiological distinctions among epicardial, midmyocardial, and endocardial myocytes from the free wall of the canine left ventricle. Circ Res 1993; 72:671–87
21. Weidmann S: The electrical constants of Purkinje fibers. J Physiol 1952; 118 :348–60
22. Strichartz GR, Cohen I: V_{max} as a measure of G_{Na} in nerve and cardiac membranes. Biophys J 1978; 23:153–6
23. Cohen CJ, Bean BP, Tsien RW: Maximum upstroke velocity (V_{max}) as an index of available sodium conductance: Comparison of V_{max} and voltage clamp measurements of I_{na} in rabbit Purkinje fibers. Circ Res 1984; 54:636–51
24. Sheets MF, Hanck DA, Fozzard HA: Nonlinear relation between V_{max} and I_{na} in canine cardiac Purkinje cells. Circ Res 1988; 63:386–8
25. Spach MS, Heidlage JF, Darken ER, Hofer E, Raines KH, Starmer CF: Cellular V_{max} reflects both membrane properties and the load presented by adjoining cells. Am J Physiol 1992; 263:H1855–H1863

26. Weingart R, Rüdisüli A, Maurer P: Cell to cell communication. In: Zipes DP, Jalif J, eds. Cardiac Electrophysiology—From Cell to Bedside. Philadelphia:WB. Saunders Company; 1990: 122-127
27. Severs NJ, Rothery S, Dupont E, et al.: Immunocytochemical analysis of connexin expression in the healthy and diseased cardiovascular system. Microsc Res Tech 2001; 52:301–22
28. Davis LM, Kanter HL, Beyer EC, Saffitz JE: Distinct gap junction protein phenotypes in cardiac tissues with disparate conduction properties. J Am Coll Cardiol 1994; 24:1124–32
29. Veenstra RD: Size and selectivity of gap junction channels formed from different connexins. J Bioenerg Biomembr 1996; 28:317–37
30. Guerrero PA, Schuessler RB, Davis LM, et al.: Slow ventricular conduction in mice heterozygous for a connexin43 null mutation. J Clin Invest 1997; 99:1991–8
31. Thomas SA, Schuessler RB, Berul CI, Beaedslee MA, Beyer EC, Mendelsohn ME, Saffitz JE: Disparate effects of deficient expression of connexin43 on atrial and ventricular conduction: evidence for chamber-specific molecular determinants of conduction. Circulation 1998; 24:686–91
32. Chen SC, Davis LM, Westphale EM, Beyer EC, Saffitz JE: Expression of multiple gap junction proteins in human fetal and infant hearts. Pediatr Res 1994; 36:561–6
33. Davis LM, Rodefeld ME, Green K, Beyer EC, Saffitz JE: Gap junction protein phenotypes of the human heart and conduction system. J Cardiovasc Electrophysiol 1995; 6:813–22
34. Hoyt RH, Cohen ML, Saffitz JE: Distribution and three-dimensional structure of intercellular junctions in canine myocardium. Circ Res 1989; 64:563–74
35. Saffitz JE, Kanter HL, Green KG, Tolley TK, Beyer EC: Tissue specific determinants of anisotropic conduction velocity in canine atrial and ventricular myocardium. Circ Res 1994; 74:1065–70
36. Spach MS, Miller WT Jr, Geselowitz DB, Barr RC, Kootsey JM, Johnson EA: The discontinuous nature of propagation in normal canine cardiac muscle: evidence for recurrent discontinuities of intracellular resistance that affect the membrane currents. Circ Res 1981; 48:39–54
37. Spach MS, Miller WT, Dolber PC, Kootsey JM, Sommer JR, Mosher CE: The functional role of structural complexities in the propagation of depolarization in the atrium of the dog: cardiac conduction disturbances due to discontinuities of effective axial resistivity. Circ Res 1982; 50:175–91

38. Valderrabano M: Influence of anisotropic conduction properties in the propagation of the cardiac action potential. Progress Biophys Mol Biol 2007; 94:144–68
39. Spach MS, Dolber PC: Relating extracellular potentials and their derivatives to anisotropic propagation at a microscopic level in human cardiac muscle. Evidence for electrical uncoupling of side-to-side fiber connections with increasing age. Circ Res 1986; 58:356–71
40. Koura T, Hara M, Takeuchi S, et al.: Anisotropic conduction properties in canine atria analyzed by high-resolution optical mapping: preferential direction of conduction block changes from longitudinal to transverse with increasing age. Circulation 2002; 105:2092–8
41. Ursell PC, Gardner PI, Albala A, Fenoglio JJ Jr, Wit AL: Structural and electrophysiological changes in the epicardial border zone of canine myocardial infarcts during infarctus healing. Circ Res 1985; 56:436–51
42. De Bakker JM, van Capelle FJ, Janse MJ, et al.: Slow conduction in the infarcted human heart. "Zigzag" course of activation. Circulation 1993; 88:915–26
43. Leon LJ, Roberge FA: Directional characteristics of action potential propagation in cardiac muscle: a model study. Circ Res 1991; 69:378–95
44. Delgado C, Steinhaus B, Delmar M, Chialvo DR, Jalife J. Directional differences in excitability and margin of safety for propagation in sheep ventricular epicardial muscle. Circ Res 1990; 67:97–110
45. Schalij MJ, Lammers WJEP, Rensma PL, Allessie MA: Anisotropic conduction and reentry in perfused epicardium of rabbit left ventricle. Am J Physiol 1992; 263:H1466–H1478
46. Shaw RM, Rudy Y: Ionic mechanisms of propagation in cardiac tissue. Roles of sodium and L-type calcium currents during reduced excitability and decreased gap junction coupling. Circ Res 1997; 81:727–41
47. Brugada J, Boersma L, Kirchhof CHJ, Allessie MA: Proarrhythmic effects of flecainide. Evidence for increased susceptibility to reentrant arrhythmias. Circulation 1991; 84:1808–18
48. Schalij MJ, Boersma L, Huijberts M, Allessie MA: Anisotropic reentry in a perfused 2-dimensional layer of rabbit ventricular myocardium. Circulation 2000; 102:2650–8
49. James TN: Structure and function of the sinus node, AV node and His Bundle of the human heart: Part I-Structure. Prog Cardiovasc Dis 2002; 45:235–67
50. Tranum-Jensen J, Wilde AMM, Vermeulen JT, Janse MJ: Morphology of electrophysiologically identified junctions between Purkinje

fibers and ventricular muscle in rabbit and pig hearts. Circ Res 1991; 69:429–37

51. Cosio FG, Martin-Penato A, Pastor A, Nunez A, Montero MA, Cantale CP, Schames S: Atrial activation mapping in sinus rhythm in the clinical electrophysiology laboratory: observations during Bachmann's bundle block. J Cardiovasc Electrophysiol 2004; 15:524–31
52. Ho SY, Sanchez-Quintana D, Cabrera JA, Anderson RH: Anatomy of the left atrium: implications for radiofrequency ablation of atrial fibrillation. J Cardiovasc Electrophysiol 1999; 10:1525–33
53. Roithinger FX, Cheng J, SippensGroenewengen A, et al.: Use of electroanatomic mapping to delineate transseptal atrial conduction in humans. Circulation 1999; 100:1791–7
54. Gough WB, Mehra R, Restivo M, Zeiler RH, El-Sherif N: Reentrant ventricular arrhythmias in the late myocardial infarction in the dog. 13. Correlation of activation and refractory maps. Circ Res 1985; 57:432–42
55. Robert E, Aya AGM, de La Coussaye JE, et al.: Dispersion-based reentry: mechanism of initiation of ventricular tachycardia in isolated rabbit hearts. Am J Physiol 1999; 276:H413–23
56. Boersma L, Zetelaki Z, Brugada J, Allessie M: Polymorphic reentrant ventricular tachycardia in the isolated rabbit heart studied by high-density mapping. Circulation 2002; 105:3053–61
57. Antzelevitch C: Ionic, molecular, and cellular bases of QT-interval prolongation and torsade de pointes. Europace 2007; 9 suppl 4:iv4–15
58. Stramba-Badiale M, Locati EH, Martinelli A, Courville J, Schwartz PJ: Gender and the relationship between ventricular repolarization and cardiac cycle length during 24-h Holter recordings. Eur Heart J 1997; 18:1000–6
59. Bode F, Karasik P, Katus HA, Franz MR: Upstream stimulation versus downstream stimulation. Arrhythmogenesis based on repolarization dispersion in the human heart. J Am Coll Cardiol 2002; 40:731–6
60. Crick SJ, Wharton J, Sheppard MN, et al.: Innervation of the human cardiac conduction system. A quantitative immunohistochemical and histochemical study. Circulation 1994; 89:1697–1708
61. Chow LT, Chow SS, Anderson RH, Gosling JA: Autonomic innervation of the human cardiac conduction system: changes from infancy to senility—an immunohistochemical and histochemical analysis. Ann Rec 2001; 264:169–82
62. Hedman AE, Thavanainen KU, Hartikainen JE, Hakumaki MO: Effect of sympathetic modulation and sympatho-vagal interaction

on the heart rate variability in anaesthetized dogs. Acta Physiol Scand 1995; 155:205–14

63. Zipes DP: Mechanisms of clinical arrhythmias. J Cardiovasc Electrophysiol 2003; 14:902–12
64. Cranefield PF: Action potentials, after potentials, and arrhythmias. Circ Res 1977; 41:415–23
65. de La Coussaye JE, Brugada J, Allessie MA: Electrophysiologic and arrhythmogenic effects of bupivacaine: a study with high resolution ventricular epicardial mapping in rabbit hearts. Anesthesiology 1992; 77:132–41
66. Robert E, Bruelle P, de La Coussaye JE, et al.: Electrophysiologic and proarrhythmogenic effects of therapeutic and toxic doses of imipramine. A study with high resolution ventricular epicardial mapping in rabbit hearts. J Pharmacol Exp Ther 1996; 278:170–8
67. Vaughan Williams EM: Classification of antiarrhythmic actions. In: Williams, EM, ed. Antiarrhythmic Drugs. Berlin: Springer-Verlag; 1989:45–68
68. Task Force of the Working Group on Arrhythmias of the European Society of Cardiology: The "Sicilian Gambit." A new approach to the classification of antiarrhythmic drugs based on their actions on arrhythmogenic mechanisms. Circulation 1991; 84:1831–51
69. Fuster V, Rydén LE, Cannom DS, et al.: ACC/AHA/ESC 2006 guidelines for the management of patients with atrial fibrillation. Executive summary: a report of the American College of Cardiology/American Heart Association Task Force on Practice Guidelines and the European Society of Cardiology Committee for Practice Guidelines (Writing Committee to revise the 2001 Guidelines for the management of patients with atrial fibrillation). Circulation 2006; 114:700–52
70. Zipes DM, Camm AJ, Borggrefe M, et al.: ACC/AHA/ESC 2006 guidelines for the management of patients with ventricular arrhythmias and the prevention of sudden cardiac death: a report of the American College of Cardiology/American Heart Association Task Force and the European Society of Cardiology Committee for Practice Guidelines (Writing Committee to develop the 2001 Guidelines for the management of patients with ventricular arrhythmias and the prevention of sudden cardiac death). Circulation 2006; 114:e385–484
71. Lafuente-Lafuente C, Mouly S, Longás-Tejero MA, Mahé I, Bergmann JF: Antiarrhythmic drugs for maintaining sinus rhythm after cardioversion of atrial fibrillation. Arch Intern Med 2006; 166:719–28

72. Lafuente-Lafuente C, Mouly S, Longás-Tejero MA, Bergmann JF: Antiarrhythmics for maintaining sinus rhythm after cardioversion of atrial fibrillation. Cochrane Database Syst Rev. 2007; (4):CD005049
73. Kohlhardt M, Fichtner H, Froebe U, Herzig JW: On the mechanism of drug-induced blockade of Na^+ currents: interaction of antiarrhythmic compounds with DPI-modified single cardiac Na^+ channels. Circ Res 1989; 64:867–81
74. Clarkson CW, Follmer CH, Ten Eick RE, Hondeghem LM, Yeh JZ: Evidence for two components of sodium channel block by lidocaine in isolated cardiac myocytes. Circ Res 1988; 63:869–78
75. Hondeghem LM, Katzung BG: Antiarrhythmic agents: the modulated receptor mechanism of action of sodium and calcium channel-blocking drugs. Ann Rev Pharmacol Toxicol 1984; 24:387–423
76. Hondeghem LM, Katzung BG: Time and voltage dependent interaction of antiarrhythmic drugs with cardiac sodium channels. Biochim Biophys Acta 1977; 472:373–98
77. Imaizumi Y, Gilles WR: Quinidine-induced inhibition of transient outward current in cardiac muscle. Am J Physiol 1987; 253:H704–8
78. Yang T, Roden DM: Extracellular potassium modulation of drug block of I_{Kr}. Implications for torsade de pointes and reverse use-dependence. Circulation 1996; 93:407–11
79. Grace AA, Camm AJ: Quinidine. N Engl J Med 1998; 338:35–45
80. Roden DM, Hoffman BF: Action potential prolongation and induction of abnormal automaticity by low quinidine concentrations in canine Purkinje fibers. Circ Res 1985; 56:857–67
81. Wise KR, Ye V, Campbell TJ: Action potential prolongation exhibits simple dose-dependence for sotalol, but reverse dose-dependence for quinidine and disopyramide: implications for proarrhythmia due to triggered activity. J Cardiovasc Pharmacol 1993; 21:316–22
82. Kojima M: Effects of disopyramide on transmembrane action potentials in guinea-pig papillary muscles. Eur J Pharmacol 1981; 69:11–24
83. Reiter MJ, Higgins SL, Payne AG, Mann DE: Effects of quinidine versus procainamide on the QT interval. Am J Cardiol 1986; 58:512–6
84. Campbell TJ, Wyse KR, Hemsworth PD: Effects of hyperkalemia, acidosis, and hypoxia on the depression of maximum rate of depolarization by class I antiarrhythmic drugs in guinea pig myocardium: differential actions of class Ib and Ic agents. J Cardiovasc Pharmacol 1991; 18:51–9
85. Li GR, Ferrier GR: Effects of lidocaine on reperfusion arrhythmias and electrophysiological properties in an isolated ventricular mus-

cle model of ischemia and reperfusion. J Pharmacol Exp Ther 1991; 257:997–1004

86. Ranger S, Talajic M, Lemery R, Roy D, Nattel S: Amplification of flecainide-induced ventricular slowing by exercise. A potentially significant consequence of use-dependent sodium channel blockade. Circulation 1989; 79:1000–6
87. Ranger S, Talajic M, Lemery R, Roy D, Villemaire C, Nattel S. Kinetics of use-dependent ventricular conduction slowing by antiarrhythmic drugs in humans. Circulation 1991; 83:1987-94.
88. Wang Z, Pelletier LC, Talajic M, Nattel S: Effects of flecainide and quinidine on human atrial action potentials. Role of rate-dependence and comparison with guinea pig, rabbit, and dog tissues. Circulation 1990; 82:274–83
89. The Cardiac Arrhythmia Suppression Trial (CAST) Investigators: Preliminary report of encainide and flecainide on mortality in a randomized trial of arrhythmia suppression after myocardial infarction. N Engl J Med 1989; 321:406–12
90. Levine JH, Morganroth J, Kadish AH: Mechanisms and risk factors for proarrhythmia with type Ia compared with Ic antiarrhythmic drug therapy. Circulation 1989; 80:1063–9
91. Vik-Mo H, Ohm OJ, Lund-Johansen P: Electrophysiological effects of flecainide acetate in patients with sinus nodal dysfunction. Am J Cardiol 1982; 50:1090–4
92. Boersma E, Poldermans D, Bax JJ, et al.: Predictors of cardiac events after major vascular surgery: role of clinical characteristics, dobutamine echocardiography, and beta-blocker therapy. JAMA 2001; 285:1865–73
93. Lindenauer PK, Pekow P, Wang K, Mamidi DK, Gutierrez B, Benjamin EM: Perioperative beta-blocker therapy and mortality after major noncardiac surgery. N Engl J Med 2005; 353:349–61
94. Varro A, Nanasi PP, Lathrop DA: Effects of sotalol on transmembrane ionic currents responsible for repolarization in cardiac ventricular myocytes from rabbit and guinea pig. Life Sci 1991; 49:PL7–12
95. Hohnloser SH, Woosley RL: Sotalol. N Engl J Med 1994; 331:31–8
96. Bjornstad H, Tande PM, Refsum H: Class III antiarrhythmic action of d-sotalol during hypothermia. Am Heart J 1991; 121:1429–36
97. Funck-Brentano C, Kibleur Y, Le Coz F, Poirier JM, Mallet A, Jaillon P: Rate dependence of sotalol-induced prolongation of ventricular repolarization during exercise in humans. Circulation 1991; 83:536–45
98. Pfammatter JP, Paul T, Lehmann C, Kallfelz HC: Efficacy and proarrhythmia of oral sotalol in pediatric patients. J Am Coll Cardiol 1995; 26:1002–7

99. Moray F, DiCarlo LA Jr, Krol RB, Baerman JM, Debuitler M: Acute and chronic effects of amiodarone on ventricular refractoriness, intraventricular conduction and ventricular tachycardia induction. J Am Col Cardiol 1986; 7:148–57
100. Kodama I, Kamiya K, Toyama J: Amiodarone: ionic and cellular mechanisms of action of the most promising class III agent. Am J Cardiol 1999; 84:20R–28R
101. Spinelli W, Hoffman BF: Mechanisms of termination of reentrant atrial arrhythmias by class I and class III antiarrhythmic agents. Circ Res 1989; 65:1565–79
102. Satoh H: Class III antiarrhythmic drugs (amiodarone, bretylium and sotalol) on action potentials and membrane currents in rabbit sino-atrial node preparations. Naunyn-Schmiedeberg's Arch Pharmacol 1991; 344:674–81
103. Hondeghem LM, Snyders DJ: Class III antiarrhythmic agents have a lot of potential but a long way to go. Reduced effectiveness and dangers of reverse use-dependence. Circulation 1990; 81:686–90
104. Valenzuela C, Bennett PB: Voltage- and use-dependent modulation of calcium channel current in guinea pig ventricular cells by amiodarone and des-oxo-amiodarone. J Cardiovasc Pharmacol 1991; 17:894–902
105. Mason JW, Hondeghem LM, Katzung BG: Block of inactivated sodium channels and of depolarization-induced automaticity in guinea pig papillary muscle by amiodarone. Circ Res 1984; 55:277–285
106. Honjo H, Kodama I, Kamiya K, Toyama J: Block of cardiac sodium channels by amiodarone studied by using V_{max} of action potential in single ventricular myocytes. Br J Pharmacol 1991; 102:651–6
107. Nokin P, Clinet M, Schoenfeld P: Cardiac beta adrenoceptor modulation by amiodarone. Biochem Pharmacol 1983; 32:2473–7
108. Almotrefi AA, Dzimiri N: The influence of potassium concentration on the inhibitory effect of amiodarone on guinea-pig microsomal Na^+-K^+-ATPase activity. Pharmacol Toxicol 1991; 69:140–3
109. Lalevée N, Barrère-Lemaire S, Gauthier P, Nargeot J, Richard S: Effects of amiodarone and dronedarone on voltage-dependent sodium current in human cardiomyocytes. J Cardiovasc Electrophysiol 2003; 14:885–90
110. Wegener FT, Ehrlich JR, Hohnloser SH: Dronedarone: an emerging agent with rhythm- and rate-controlling effects. J Cardiovasc Electrophysiol 2006; 17:S17–20
111. Hodeige D, Heyndrickx JP, Chatelain P, Manning A: SR 33589, a new amiodarone-like antiarrhythmic agent: anti-adrenoceptor activity in anaesthetized and conscious dogs. Eur J Pharmacol 1995; 279:25–32

112. Tákacs J, Iost N, Lengyel C, et al.: Multiple cellular electrophysiological effects of azimilide in canine cardiac preparations. Eur J Pharmacol 2003; 470:163–70
113. Foster RH, Wilde MI, Markham A: Ibutilide. A review of its pharmacological properties and clinical potential in the acute management of atrial flutter and fibrillation. Drugs 1997; 54:312–30
114. Eisenberg MJ, Brox A, Bestawros AN: Calcium channel blockers: an update. Am J Med 2004; 116:35–43
115. Karraya S, Arlock P, Katzung BG, Hondeghem LM: Diltiazem and verapamil preferentially block inactivated calcium channels. J Mol Cell Cardiol 1983; 15:145–8
116. De Paoli P, Cerbai E, Koidl B, Kirchengast M, Sartiani L, Mugelli A: Selectivity of different calcium antagonists on T- and L-type calcium currents in guinea-pig ventricular myocytes. Pharm Res 2002; 46:491–7
117. Noma A, Kotake H, Irisawa H: Slow inward current and its role mediating the chronotropic effects of epinephrine in rabbit sinoatrial nodes. Pflügers Arch 1980; 338:1–9
118. Talajic M, Papadatos D, Villemaire C, Nayebpour M, Nattel S: Antiarrhythmic actions of diltiazem during experimental atrioventricular reentrant tachycardias. Importance of use-dependent calcium channel-blocking properties. Circulation 1990; 81:334–42
119. Coetzee A, Conradie S: Calcium antagonist verapamil and reperfusion injury of the heart. J Cardiothorac Vasc Anesth 2007; 21:337–43
120. Hirota K, Ito Y, Masuda A, Momose Y: Effects of halothane on membrane ionic currents in guinea pig atrial and ventricular myocytes. Acta Anaesthesiol Scand 1989; 33:239–44
121. Bosnjak ZJ, Kampine JP: Effects of halothane, enflurane and isoflurane on the SA node. Anesthesiology 1983; 58:314–8
122. Housmans PR, Murat I: Comparative effects of halothane, enflurane, and isoflurane at equipotent anesthetic concentrations on isolated ventricular myocardium of the ferret: I. Contractility. Anesthesiology 1988; 69:451–63
123. Hanouz JL, Massetti M, Guesne G, et al.: In vitro effects of desflurane, sevoflurane, isoflurane, and halothane in isolated human right atria. Anesthesiology 2000; 92:116–24
124. Terrar DA, Victory JGG: Influence of halothane on electrical coupling in cell pairs isolated from guinea pig ventricle. Br J Pharmacol 1988; 94:509–14
125. Burt JM, Spray DC: Volatile anesthetics block intercellular communication between neonatal rat myocardial cells. Circ Res 1989; 65:829–37

126. Ozaki S, Nakaya H, Gotoh Y, Azuma M, Kemmotsu O, Kanno M: Effects of halothane and enflurane on conduction velocity and maximum rate of rise of action potential upstroke in guinea pig papillary muscles. Anesth Analg 1989; 68:219–25
127. Hüneke R, Jüngling E, Skasa M, Rossaint R, Lückhoff A: Effects of the anesthetic gases xenon, halothane, and isoflurane on calcium and potassium current in human atrial cardiomyocytes. Anesthesiology 2001; 95:999–1006
128. Hüneke R, Fabl J, Rossaint R, Lückhoff A: Effects of volatile anesthetics on cardiac ion channels. Acta Anaesthesiol Scand 2004; 48:547–61
129. Chae JE, Ahn DS, Kim MH, Lynch IIIC, Park WK: Electrophysiologic mechanism underlying action potential prolongation by sevoflurane in rat ventricular myocytes. Anesthesiology 2007; 107:67–74
130. Owczuk R, Wujtewicz MA, Sawicka W, Lasek J, Wujtewicz M: The influence of desflurane on QTc interval. Anesth Analg 2005; 101:419–22
131. Kang J, Reynolds WP, Chen XL, Ji J, Wang H, Rampe DE: Mechanisms underlying the QT interval-prolonging effects of sevoflurane and its interactions with other QT-prolonging drugs. Anesthesiology 2006; 104:1015–22
132. Whyte SD, Sanatani S, Lim J, Booker PD: A comparison of the effect on dispersion of repolarization of age-adjusted MAC values of sevoflurane in children. Anesth Analg 2007; 104:277–82
133. Aya AGM, de La Coussaye JE, Robert E, et al.: Effects of halothane and enflurane on ventricular conduction, refractoriness, and wavelength. A concentration-response study in isolated hearts. Anesthesiology 1999; 91:1873–81
134. Suzuki A, Aizawa K, Gassmayr S, Bosnjak ZJ, Kwok WM: Biphasic effect of isoflurane on the cardiac action potential. Anesthesiology 2002; 97:1209–17
135. Marijic J, Bosnjak ZJ, Stowe DF, Kampine JP: Effects and interaction of verapamil and volatile anesthetics on the isolated perfused guinea pig heart. Anesthesiology 1988; 69:914–22
136. Gallenberg LA, Stowe DF, Marijic J, Kampine JP, Bosnjak ZJ: Depression of atrial rate, atrioventricular nodal conduction, and cardiac contraction by diltiazem and volatile anesthetics in isolated hearts. Anesthesiology 1991; 74:519–30
137. Iwatsuki N, Katoh M, Ono K, Amaha K: Antiarrhythmic effect of diltiazem during halothane anesthesia in dogs and in humans. Anesth Analg 1985; 64:964–70

138. Freeman LC, Muir WW 3rd: α-adrenoceptor stimulation in the presence of halothane: effects on impulse propagation in cardiac Purkinje fibers. Anesth Analg 1991; 72:11–7
139. Weigt HU, Kwok WM, Rehmert GC, Turner LA, Bosnjak ZJ: Modulation of cardiac sodium current by α_1-stimulation and volatile anesthetics. Anesthesiology 1997; 87:1507–16
140. Weigt HU, Kwok WM, Rehmert GC, Bosnjak ZJ: Modulation of cardiac sodium current by inhalational anesthetics in the absence and presence of β-stimulation. Anesthesiology 1998; 88:114–24
141. Kroll DA, Knight PR: Antifibrillatory effects of volatile anesthetics in acute occlusion/reperfusion arrhythmias. Anesthesiology 1984; 61:657–61
142. Deutsch N, Hantler CB, Tait AR, Uprichard A, Schork MA, Knight PR: Suppression of ventricular arrhythmias by volatile anesthetics in a canine model of chronic myocardial infarction. Anesthesiology 1990; 72:1012–21
143. Coetzee A, Moolman J: Halothane and the reperfusion injury in the intact animal model. Anesth Analg 1993; 76:734–44
144. Schlack W, Preckel B, Barthel H, Obal D, Thämer V: Halothane reduces reperfusion injury after regional ischaemia in the rabbit heart in vivo. Br J Anaesth 1997; 79:88–96
145. Xiao GS, Zhou JJ, Wang GY, Cao CM, Li GR, Wong TM: In vitro electrophysiologic effects of morphine in rabbit ventricular myocytes. Anesthesiology 2005; 103:280–6
146. Blair JR, Pruett JK, Crumnine RS, Basler JS: Prolongation of QT interval in association with the administration of large doses of opiates. Anesthesiology 1987; 67:442–3
147. Blair JR, Pruett JK, Introna RPS, Adams RJ, Basler JS: Cardiac electrophysiologic effects of fentanyl and sufentanil in canine cardiac Purkinje fibers. Anesthesiology 1989; 71:565–70
148. Zaugg M, Lucchinetti E, Spahn DR, Pasch T, Garcia C, Schaub MC: Differential effects of anesthetics on mitochondrial K_{ATP} channel activity and cardiomyocyte protection. Anesthesiology 2002; 97:15–23
149. Royster RL, Keeler DK, Haisty WK, Johnston WE, Prough DS. Cardiac electrophysiologic effects of fentanyl and combination of fentanyl and neuromuscular relaxants in pentobarbital anesthetized dogs. Anesth Analg 1988; 67:15–20
150. Romero M, Laorden ML, Hernandez J, Serrano JS: Effects of morphine on isolated right atria of the rat. Gen Pharmacol 1992; 23:1135–8
151. Saini V, Carr DB, Hagestad BL, Lown B, Verrur RL: Antifibrillatory action of the narcotic agonist fentanyl. Am Heart J 1988; 115:598–605

152. Rabkin SW: Morphine and the endogenous opioid dynorphin in the brain attenuate digoxin-induced arrhythmias in guinea pigs. Pharmacol Toxicol 1992; 71:353–60
153. Pugsley MK: The diverse molecular mechanisms responsible for the actions of opioids on the cardiovascular system. Pharmacol Ther 2002; 93:51–75
154. Griffin RM, Dimich I, Jurado R, Kaplan JA: Haemodynamic effects of diltiazem during fentanyl-nitrous oxyde anaesthesia. An in vivo study in the dog. Br J Anaesth 1988; 60:655–9
155. Schmeling WT, Kampine JP, Watier DC: Negative chronotropic actions of sufentanil and vecuronium in chronically instrumented dogs pretreated with propranolol and or diltiazem. Anesth Analg 1989; 69:4–14
156. Sakai F, Hiraoka M, Amaha K: Comparative actions of propofol and thiopentone on cell membranes of isolated guinea pig ventricular myocytes. Br J Anaesth 1996; 77:508–16
157. Carnes CA, Muir WW 3rd, Van Wagoner DR: Effects of intravenous anesthetics on inward rectifier potassium current in rat and human ventricular myocytes. Anesthesiology 1997; 87:327–34
158. Martynyuk AE, Morey TE, Raatikainen JP, Seubert CN, Dennis DM: Ionic mechanisms mediating the differential effects of methohexital and thiopental on action potential duration in guinea pig and rabbit isolated ventricular myocytes. Anesthesiology 1999; 90:156–64
159. Baum VC: Distinctive effects of three intravenous anesthetics on the inward rectifier (I_{K1}) and the delayed rectifier (I_K) potassium currents in myocardium: implications for the mechanism of action. Anesth Analg 1993; 76:18–23
160. Yang CY, Wong CS, Yu CC, Luk HN, Lin CI: Propofol inhibits cardiac L-type calcium current in guinea pig ventricular myocytes. Anesthesiology 1996; 84:626–35
161. Buljubasic N, Marijic J, Berczi V, Supan DF, Kampine JP, Bosnjak ZJ: Differential effects of etomidate, propofol, and midazolam on calcium and potassium channel currents in canine myocardial cells. Anesthesiology 1996; 85:1092–9
162. Zhou W, Fontenot J, Liu S, Kennedy RH: Modulation of cardiac calcium channels by propofol. Anesthesiology 1997; 86:670–5
163. Alphin RS, Martens JR, Dennis DM: Frequency-dependent effects of propofol on atrioventricular nodal conduction in guinea pig isolated heart. Anesthesiology 1995; 83:382–94
164. Baum VC, Tecson ME: Ketamine inhibits transsarcolemmal calcium entry in guinea pig myocardium: direct evidence by single cell voltage clamp. Anesth Analg 1991; 73:804–7

165. Seagusa K, Furukawa Y, Ogiwara Y, Chiba S: Pharmacologic analysis of ketamine-induced cardiac actions in isolated, blood-perfused canine atria. J Cardiovasc Pharmacol 1986; 8:414–9
166. Hara Y, Tamagawa M, Nakaya H: The effects of ketamine on conduction velocity and maximum rate of rise of action potential upstroke in guinea pig papillary muscles: comparison with quinidine. Anesth Analg 1994; 79:687–93
167. Charbit B, Albaladejo P, Funck-Brentano C, Legrand M, Samain E, Marty J: Prolongation of QTc interval after postoperative nausea and vomiting treatment by droperidol or ondansetron. Anesthesiology 2005; 102:1094–100
168. Starr NJ, Sethna DH, Estafanou FG: Bradycardia and asystole following the rapid administration of sufentanil with vecuronium. Anesthesiology 1986; 64:521–3
169. Urquhart ML, Ramsey FM, Royster RL, Morell RS, Gerr P: Heart rate and rhythm disturbances following an edrophonium/atropine mixture for antagonism of neuromuscular blockade during fentanyl N_2O/O_2 or isoflurane N_2O/O_2 anesthesia. Anesthesiology 1987; 67:561–5
170. Bruelle P, Lefrant JY, de La Coussaye JE, et al.: Comparative electrophysiologic and hemodynamic effects of several amide local anesthetic drugs in anesthetized dogs. Anesth Analg 1996; 82:648–56
171. Aya AGM, de La Coussaye JE, Robert E, et al.: Comparison of the effects of racemic bupivacaine, levobupivacaine, and ropivacaine on ventricular conduction, refractoriness, and wavelength. An epicardial mapping study. Anesthesiology 2002; 96:641–50
172. Clarkson CW, Hondeghem ML: Mechanism for bupivacaine depression of cardiac conduction: fast block of sodium channels during the action potential with slow recovery from block during diastole. Anesthesiology 1985; 62:396–405
173. Mazoit JX, Decaux A, Bouaziz H, Edouard A: Comparative electrophysiologic effects of racemic bupivacaine, levobupivacaine, and ropivacaine in the isolate rabbit heart. Anesthesiology 2000; 93:784–92
174. Courtney KR, Kendig JJ: Bupivacaine is an effective potassium channel blocker in heart. Biochim Biophys Acta 1988; 939:163–6
175. de La Coussaye JE, Massé C, Bassoul B, Eledjam JJ, Gagnol JP, Sassine A: Bupivacaine-induced slow-inward current inhibition: a voltage clamp study in frog atrial fibres. Can J Anaesth 1990; 37:819–20
176. Sztark F, Malgat M, Dabadie P, Mazat JP: Comparison of the effects of bupivacaine and ropivacaine on heart cell mitochondrial bioenergetics. Anesthesiology 1998; 88:1340–9

177. Howie MB, Mortimer W, Candler EM, McSweeney TD, Frolicher DA: Does nifedipine enhance the cardiovascular depressive effects of bupivacaine? Reg Anesth 1989; 14:19–25
178. Timour Q, Freycz M, Couzon P, et al.: Possible role of drug interactions in bupivacaine-induced problems related to intraventricular conduction disorders. Reg Anesth 1990; 15:180–5
179. Edouard AR, Berdeaux A, Ahmad R, Samii K: Cardiovascular interactions of local anesthetics and calcium entry blockers in conscious dogs. Reg Anesth 1991; 16:95–100

James J. Lynch, MD
Gregory A. Nuttall, MD

7 Procoagulant Agents

Excessive bleeding after cardiac surgery remains a common problem, with an incidence of 11–25% in patients undergoing cardiopulmonary bypass (CPB) (1, 2). The cause of bleeding is multifactorial, and may result from inadequate surgical hemostasis, clotting factor deficiency, platelet dysfunction and deficiency, and fibrinolysis (3). Conventional treatment of postcardiac surgical coagulopathy includes the administration of allogeneic blood products including platelet concentrates, fresh frozen plasma (FFP), and cryoprecipitate. Well-known risks are associated with the use of these products, including transfusion-related lung injury, immune modulation, and disease transmission (4–6).

Both transfusion and excessive bleeding have been shown to significantly increase mortality in cardiac surgical patients (7–9). Because of the well-known risks associated with allogeneic blood product transfusion, alternative methods to treat or prevent bleeding and transfusion are highly sought after. Commonly employed techniques include modifications to the CPB circuit and technique. Examples of this include reduction of prime volume through modification of priming technique (10) and use of coated circuits (11). Autotransfusion techniques such as intraoperative cell salvage and acute normovolemic hemodilution are frequently employed as well (12, 13).

Pharmacologic agents to prevent and treat bleeding are desired by clinicians to avoid the previously mentioned risks associated with transfusion. The current pharmacologic approach to blood conservation in

Advances in Cardiovascular Pharmacology, edited by Philippe R. Housmans, MD, PhD and Gregory A. Nuttall, M.D.
Lippincott Williams & Wilkins, Baltimore © 2008.

cardiac surgery focuses predominantly on the prevention of bleeding. Adequate anticoagulation must be ensured on CPB to prevent activation of the coagulation system and thrombin production. Antifibrinolytic agents including tranexamic acid (TXA), epsilon-aminocaproic acid, and aprotinin prevent CPB-induced fibrinolysis and reduce transfusion and bleeding complications in cardiac surgery (14). These agents are discussed in Chapter 8.

A limited number of procoagulant pharmacologic agents are used to treat and prevent bleeding in patients with congenital bleeding disorders such as hemophilia A and B. With the exception of desmopressin and, more recently recombinant factor VIIa (rVIIa) (NovoSeven®, Novo Nordisk Inc.), these agents have not been extensively used or studied in cardiac surgical patients, and none of these agents have United States (US) Food and Drug Administration (FDA) approval for treating postcardiac surgical bleeding in patients without a specific coagulation disorder. This chapter will address the use of desmopressin and rVIIa in cardiac surgery, and briefly discuss other procoagulant agents currently used in the treatment of congenital bleeding disorders.

DESMOPRESSIN

Desmopressin came into clinical use in 1977 for the treatment of bleeding in patients with hemophilia A and von Willebrand disease (vWD) (15). By raising levels of factor VIII and von Willebrand factor (vWF), it has been successful in the prevention and treatment of bleeding episodes in patients with these congenital bleeding disorders. In fact, desmopressin remains the treatment of choice for patients with mild hemophilia A and type I vWD with spontaneous bleeding episodes, or who are undergoing surgical procedures (16).

Interest in desmopressin quickly expanded beyond the treatment of congenital bleeding disorders. Researchers have evaluated this drug's potential for correcting numerous acquired bleeding disorders including those resulting from renal failure, liver disease, and antiplatelet therapy. Desmopressin also has been extensively studied as an agent to reduce blood loss and transfusion in patients with previously normal coagulation undergoing surgical procedures involving large blood loss such as cardiac surgery.

Mechanism of Action and Effects of Desmopressin

Desmopressin (1-deamino-8-D-arginine vasopressin, abbreviated DDAVP) is a synthetic analogue of naturally occurring arginine vasopressin. The action of this 9-amino acid peptide replicates the action of antidiuretic hormone and leads to increased water reabsorption by the kidney. While structurally similar, desmopressin does not exhibit the vasoconstrictive effects that result from arginine vasopressin administration.

Desmopressin has been shown to increase circulating levels of factor VIII and vWF in patients with mild hemophilia, vWD, and normal coagulation (17). Factor VIII and vWF are both glycoproteins released from vascular endothelium. When activated, factor VIII promotes activation of factor X, leading to thrombin production. Von Willebrand factor promotes platelet adherence to endothelium at sites of injury, and to other platelets, through interactions with glycoprotein platelet receptors. Platelet adherence to the vessel wall is enhanced following desmopressin administration (18). Desmopressin also can shorten the bleeding time and activated partial thromboplastin time (aPTT). These tests are likely accelerated by the increased levels vWF and factor VIII (19).

Additionally, desmopressin stimulates release of tissue-type plasminogen activator into circulation. While this leads to increased plasmin generation, most of the plasmin becomes complexed with α2-antiplasmin, and does not result in significant fibrinolysis (20–22). While this effect may have little clinical significance, it has prompted several investigations to evaluate administration of desmopressin and antifibrinolytic agents in cardiac surgical patients. These will be discussed later in this chapter.

Dosing and Pharmacokinetics

Several preparations of desmopressin are available. It is most commonly administered via the intravenous and intranasal routes, however intramuscular, subcutaneous, and oral routes may be used as well. Desmopressin has very low bioavailability via oral administration; therefore an alternate route should be selected when treating acute bleeding episodes. Desmopressin is excreted by the kidneys, and about 50% is protein bound in the plasma.

The recommended intravenous dose is 0.3 mcg/kg, and should be administered slowly. Peak effect is seen in 30–60 minutes when given intravenously (23, 24). The effect on platelets in healthy volunteers lasts for about 3 hours, and can be extended with a second dose (25). In patients with hemophilia and vWD, the plasma half-life of factor VIII is 5–8 hours, and vWF is 8–10 hours (26). The dose may be repeated every 12 hours; however, tachyphylaxis may develop after several doses.

Adverse Reactions and Contraindications

Unlike arginine vasopressin, which is frequently used as a vasoconstrictor, desmopressin can be a potent vasodilator. The vasodilation is primarily a direct effect of desmopressin on vascular smooth muscle (27). Approximately one-third of patients treated with desmopressin shortly after discontinuation of CPB experience hypotension (>20% reduction of mean arterial blood pressure) that requires treatment (28, 29). Slow infusion may attenuate the vasodilation and hypotension (29).

Desmopressin leads to water reabsorption in the kidneys. Excessive water reabsorption can lead to hypervolemia, hyponatremia, and decreased plasma osmolality. Clinically significant hyponatremia (121 mEq/L) with confusion was reported after only 3 daily doses of 0.3 mcg/kg in a healthy patient (30). Sodium levels and intravascular volume status should be monitored in vulnerable patients, such as those with seizure disorders, congestive heart failure, and patients receiving multiple doses of desmopressin. Fluid restriction, diuretic therapy, and sodium supplementation may be required.

Myocardial infarction has been reported on numerous occasions in both hemophiliacs (31–33) and patients with normal coagulation (34) after receiving desmopressin. Cerebral thrombosis immediately after desmopressin administration for uremic bleeding in a patient with known atherosclerosis has been reported as well (35). While several reviews did not show a statistically significant increase in myocardial infarction (MI) with desmopressin treatment in cardiac surgical patients (36–38), one meta-analysis of desmopressin use in cardiac surgical patients reported a 2.4-fold increase in MI rate in the few trials that reported this complication (14). Desmopressin has been associated with undesired thrombotic events. While these events are infrequent, avoidance of this drug in patients with significant coronary artery disease or atherosclerosis may be prudent.

Indications and Applications

The FDA- approved uses of desmopressin are limited to congenital bleeding disorders, and use for its antidiuretic hormone effect (Table 7–1). Desmopressin has been studied and used in several acquired bleeding disorders, including bleeding associated with cardiac surgery and CPB. Treatment of acquired bleeding disorders with desmopressin is done without FDA approval. Despite routinely having normal factor VIII and vWF levels, desmopressin can successfully prevent and treat bleed-

Table 7–1. FDA Approved Indications for Desmopressin

- Mild Hemophilia A (with factor VIII levels >5%)
- Neurohypophyseal diabetes insipidus
- Primary nocturnal enuresis
- Type I von Willebrand disease

ing episodes in uremic patients undergoing surgical procedures. This may be explained by a transient normalization of bleeding time seen in 75% of these uremic patients (39). Desmopressin can also reduce bleeding time in patients with cirrhosis, and those treated with aspirin and ticlopidine (40).

The growing use of glycoprotein (GP)-IIb/IIIa inhibitors prompted investigators to examine the ability of desmopressin to reverse the platelet dysfunction induced by these agents. In one small in vitro study, desmopressin accelerated normalization of platelet function in blood samples within 1.5–2 hours, while the placebo group remained abnormal beyond 4 hours (41). Further studies are needed, including in vivo human trials, to determine if desmopressin is efficacious in restoring platelet function in patients who have received these agents.

Desmopressin in Cardiac Surgery

The first trial of desmopressin use in cardiac surgery was published in 1986. Compared with the placebo group, they reported a reduction in perioperative blood loss (~800 ml) in patients undergoing complex cardiac operations, excluding patients undergoing primary coronary artery bypass grafting (CABG) (42). It was not long before a trial showing no clear benefit of desmopressin in cardiac surgical patients appeared in the literature (43). Several negative trials followed, showing no significant reduction of total blood loss or transfusion requirement when desmopressin was given prophylactically to patients undergoing routine CABG surgery, compared with placebo (44–49). Similar negative trials were published with patients undergoing cardiac procedures not limited to CABG (50, 51).

While it can certainly be argued that desmopressin is not efficacious when administered prophylactically during routine cardiac surgery, numerous trials have reported positive findings when desmopressin is used in specific clinical situations. Results are generally positive for desmopressin in reduction of blood loss and/or transfusion in trials of cardiac surgical patients who were on aspirin therapy close to the time of surgery (52–54). Desmopressin reduced transfusion requirements in an early, but smaller trial where all patients had excessive mediastinal bleeding and an elevated bleeding time (55).

Desmopressin has also been effective in reducing blood loss in patients at risk for increased bleeding using laboratory testing after termination of CPB. Despotis et al. randomized patients with abnormal hemoSTATUS (Medtronic Blood Management) clot-ratios to receive desmopressin or placebo (56). Similarly, Mongan and Hosking randomized patients with a reduced mean amplitude on thromboelastogram (TEG) (Hellige Thromboelastograph, Haemoscope Corporation) after

CPB (57). The test results selected in both groups identify patients with platelet dysfunction. In both trials, the desmopressin-treated group had significantly less blood loss and transfusion requirements.

Some authors suggest that the lack of efficacy shown in many desmopressin trials results from the release of tissue plasminogen activator, which may contribute to fibrinolysis and bleeding in the post-CPB period. One trial has shown that tranexamic acid administration with desmopressin reduces fibrinolysis, bleeding, and transfusion requirements, compared to desmopressin alone (58). However, without placebo group in this trial, it is not know if there was any fibrinolysis associated with desmopressin therapy itself. In another trial, aprotinin significantly reduced blood loss, transfusion, and fibrinolysis compared to desmopressin and placebo groups (59). Although desmopressin was no more efficacious than placebo in reducing blood loss and transfusion, mean D-dimer levels in the desmopressin group were lower than the placebo group throughout the perioperative period. Although not analyzed statistically, this suggests there was no increased fibrinolysis that resulted from desmopressin administration (59). An earlier trial of 163 patients undergoing a variety of cardiac surgical procedures showed no significant benefit of desmopressin when administered with TXA (60). It is likely that desmopressin does not cause clinically significant fibrinolysis, but also that desmopressin offers little or no benefit if the patient is already receiving an antifibrinolytic agent.

Two meta-analyses examine the effect of desmopressin on blood loss or transfusion in cardiac surgical patients. Cattaneo et al. analyzed results from 17 randomized trials, including 1171 patients. They found a 9% reduction of postoperative blood loss with desmopressin, but no significant difference in transfusion compared to the placebo group. When limiting their analysis to trials with higher blood loss in the placebo group (>1109 ml/24 hr), reduction of blood loss with desmopressin increased to 34%. They conclude that desmopressin only reduces blood loss in cardiac operations that induce excessive blood loss (61).

The other meta-analysis, by Carless et al., included 18 trials with 1295 patients and looked at transfusion outcome with desmopressin. They found reductions in the desmopressin-treated patients, using weighted mean difference, of 114 ml for total blood loss, and 0.34 units for allogeneic red blood cell (RBC) transfusions. Neither of these findings was statistically significant, and the authors conclude there is no convincing evidence that desmopressin reduces perioperative allogeneic RBC transfusion (36).

Other meta-analyses have shown that aprotinin and lysine analogues are superior in reducing perioperative RBC transfusions (37) and blood loss (14) when compared to desmopressin in cardiac surgical patients, and that little benefit was seen in patients treated with desmopressin. However, one did show a significant blood loss reduction when desmopressin was given if all patients in the trial were taking aspirin (37).

Desmopressin in Pediatric and Congenital Cardiac Surgery

Three separate randomized double-blind trials using desmopressin after CPB in pediatric and congenital cardiac surgical patients showed no reduction in postoperative blood loss or transfusion in patients treated with desmopressin (62–64). This lack of effect may partly be explained by a reduced ability of infants and children to release factor VIII and vWF from storage sites (62, 63). The routine use of desmopressin is not advised in this patient population.

Summary

After 30 years, DDAVP remains the treatment of choice for bleeding disorders resulting from mild hemophilia A and type I vWD. Current evidence does not support the routine use of desmopressin in cardiac surgical patients. The recent Society of Thoracic Surgeons (STS) and Society of Cardiovascular Anesthesiologists (SCA) Clinical Practice Guidelines concluded that routine use of desmopressin as prophylaxis is not recommended, but its use is reasonable in patients with demonstrated platelet dysfunction that may be responsive to the drug (65). Desmopressin is probably best used selectively in cardiac surgical patients, as an adjunct to blood component therapy in patients with active bleeding or who are at high risk for bleeding from platelet dysfunction resulting from CPB, uremia, and aspirin therapy. There may be a slight risk of MI associated with desmopressin use; therefore, it should be used with caution in patients with coronary artery disease.

RECOMBINANT ACTIVATED FACTOR VII

Recombinant factor VIIa is a procoagulant agent that gained FDA approval in 1999 for treatment of bleeding episodes in hemophilia A and B patients with inhibitors to factors VIII or IX. In 2005 the indications were expanded to include prevention of bleeding episodes from invasive procedures in hemophilia patients with inhibitors. Additionally, it gained approval for treatment and prevention of bleeding episodes for patients with congenital factor VII deficiency. Recent years have seen an abundance of literature describing off-label use of rVIIa in various acquired bleeding disorders, with many of these listed in Table 7–2. Not surprisingly, there has been great interest in rVIIa as a non-transfusion treatment for bleeding associated with cardiac surgery.

Table 7–2. Common Non-FDA Approved Applications of Recombinant Factor VIIa

- Acute intracerebral hemorrhage (66)
- Critical bleeding in trauma patients (67)
- Bleeding from quantitative and qualitative platelet disorders (68)
- Coagulopathy from advanced liver disease (69)
- Bleeding during liver transplantation (70)
- Reversal of warfarin anticoagulation (71, 72)
- Obstetrical hemorrhage (73)

Mechanism of rVIIa

Tissue factor (TF) is expressed on vessel wall cell membranes in response to vascular injury. Normally activated factor VII binds to the exposed TF, resulting in activation of factor X and a small amount of thrombin production. This thrombin then promotes activation of factors V and VIII and platelets. The TF-VIIa complex also activates factor IX, which binds to activated platelets forming a tenase complex (74). This factor IXa, along with factor VIIIa, activate factor X on the surface of the activated platelet. Factor Xa complexes with factor Va, leading to a burst thrombin production. This mechanism is illustrated in Figure 7–1. Factor VIIa also has effects independent of TF as shown in Figure 7–2. It directly activates factors IX and X on the surface of activated platelets, leading to a thrombin burst mentioned above.

Although the exact mechanism of rVIIa is not completely understood, it is known that rVIIa works similarly to natural factor VIIa, only requiring higher concentrations than normally seen in blood (75). Supraphysiologic factor VII levels (1000 times normal) result from pharmacologic doses of rVIIa (76). While debate continues as to whether the TF-dependent or TF-independent mechanism is most important to the effect of rVIIa, there seems to be a shift of emphasis in the literature toward the TF-independent effects on activated platelets (74, 77). The hemostatic effect in hemophiliac patients with inhibitors requires activation of coagulation by bypassing either factor VIII or IX. Recombinant factor VIIa accomplishes this by enhancing thrombin production by activating factor X in TF pathways shown in Figure 7–1, and directly on activated platelets shown in Figure 7–2 (78). Neither pathway requires involvement factors VIII or IX.

Dosing and Pharmacokinetics

The recommended dose of rVIIa for hemophiliac patients with inhibitors is 90 mcg/kg. A lower dose of 15–40 mcg/kg may be sufficient for treat-

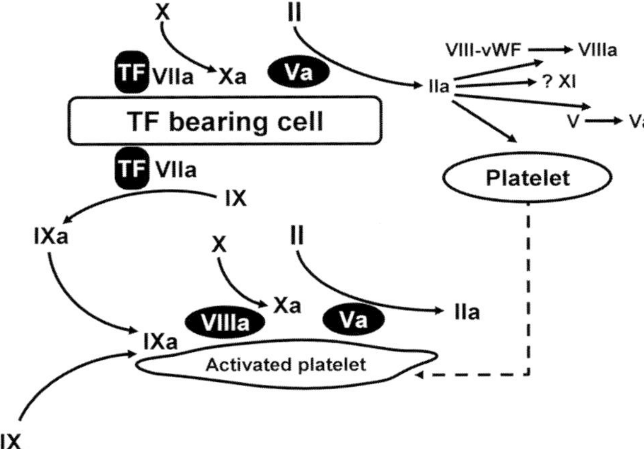

FIGURE 7–1. Cell-based model of hemostasis demonstrating actions of tissue factor-bound VIIa. (TF = tissue factor, vWF = von Willebrand factor). Reproduced with permission from Hoffman, M, Monroe DM 3rd, Roberts, HR: Activated factor VII activates factors IX and X on the surface of activated platelets: thoughts on the mechanism of action of high-dose activated factor VII. Blood Coagul Fibrinolysis 1998: 9 Suppl 1:S61–5

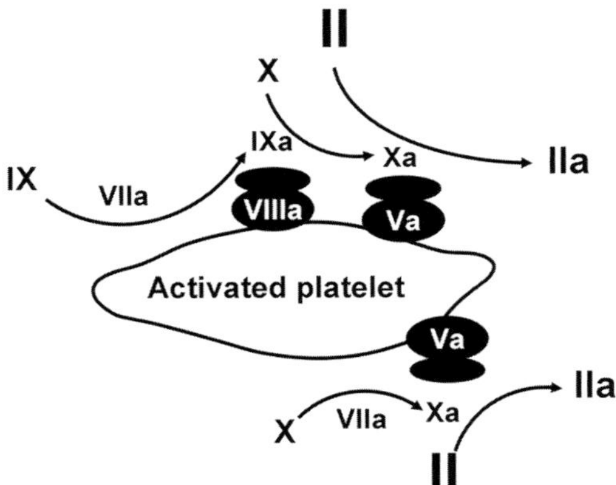

FIGURE 7–2. Actions of VIIa on surface of activated platelet, independent of tissue factor. Reproduced with permission from Roberts HR, Monroe, DM 3rd, Hoffman, M: Safety profile of recombinant factor VIIa. Semin Hematol 2004; 41:101–8

ing factor VII deficiency. The drug is given as an intravenous bolus, although a continuous infusion may be considered for patients who will require numerous scheduled doses. The mean half-life of rVIIa in hemophiliac patients is 2.9 hours in non-bleeding episodes, and 2.3 hours in patients with active bleeding (79). Because of the short half-life of the drug, repeated doses are given every 2 hours with active bleeding or to prevent surgical bleeding in hemophilia patients (80).

Cost of rVIIa Treatment

Currently rVIIa is a very expensive drug, and costs between $1.00 and $1.50 per microgram in the US. A typical dose of 70 mcg/kg, for a 70-kg adult, would cost $5000–$6000. This can result in a significant financial burden to hospitals, especially when multiple doses are given. In addition to safety concerns with off-label indications, cost remains one of the main reasons that rVIIa use is often scrutinized.

Safety and Efficacy of rVIIa in Adult Cardiac Surgical Patients

The earliest publications in the cardiac surgical literature are case reports and small case series describing successful off-label use of rVIIa as rescue therapy, when there was excessive bleeding after CPB that was refractory to standard treatment (81–83). Since then, there have been well over 20 publications describing rVIIa use in cardiac surgical patients, with the majority of these retrospective in nature. A recent review of the Australian Haemostasis Registry reported an efficacy of 84% in stopping or decreasing bleeding in 266 cardiac surgical patients with critical bleeding (84). Like this review, most retrospective case series report that rVIIa was effective in reducing bleeding or preventing surgical reexploration in 80–100% of patients when used as rescue therapy (85–89). While this is encouraging, retrospective reports are subject to significant reporting bias, therefore true efficacy can not be defined from these publications.

The use of rVIIa is considered safe in hemophiliacs, with a very low incidence of thrombotic complications (90). As with any procoagulant agent, there may be potential for creating excessive thrombosis, and the risk of rVIIa in patients without a preexisting coagulation disorder is not known. The majority of thromboembolic complications from rVIIa reported to the FDA have resulted from off-label use, and occurred in patients with active bleeding. Reported events included stroke, myocardial infarction, arterial and venous thrombosis, pulmonary embolism, and device occlusion (91). A large randomized trial of rVIIa for acute intracerebral hemorrhage in non-hemophiliac patients showed a 7% incidence of serious thromboembolic events in the rVIIa group compared with 2% in the placebo group. While this was not statistically significant, further analysis limited to only arterial thromboembolic events showed a significantly higher rate in the rVIIa patients (5%) with no arterial events in the placebo group ($P = 0.01$) (66).

Cardiac surgical patients may have increased thrombotic risk from rVIIa therapy. These patients often have significant coronary artery disease, as well as aortic and peripheral atherosclerotic disease. Disruption of a vulnerable or unstable atherosclerotic plaque can lead to exposure of TF to the circulation (92). With cardiac surgery and CPB there is upregulation of TF at surgical sites, and on monocytes in the systemic circulation. The increased TF expression leads to activation of the extrinsic coagulation cascade, and may induce a hypercoagulable state (93, 94). Exposed TF provides a location for rVIIa to bind and promote thrombus formation. While the TF exposed at surgical sites contributes to surgical hemostasis, expression in other locations, such as disrupted atherosclerotic plaques, may increase the potential for thrombosis in those locations. It is postulated that rVIIa administration in the presence of widespread TF expression after CPB may increase the risk of undesired thrombotic complications (95). Antifibrinolytic therapy is commonly employed to reduce bleeding associated with cardiac surgery. It is not known if concomitant administration of antifibrinolytics, or other agents that augment the coagulation system, raises the thrombotic potential of rVIIa.

Thromboembolic complications have been reported in many series of cardiac surgical patients and have been as high as 25%, (89) while no thromboembolic events were seen in others (86–88, 96, 97). Many of the reported thromboembolic events can be attributed to high-risk surgical procedures, (89, 98) need for ventricular assist device support (99) and concomitant administration with other procoagulant agents other than traditional blood component transfusions (89, 100). It is likely that certain cardiac surgical patients may have increased thrombotic risk from the drug, but randomized trials will be needed to help identify those at risk.

Reported mortality rates with rescue therapy also vary significantly. While many case reports and smaller series reported no mortality, several of the larger series had rates between 19% and 38% (87–89, 97, 98). Study design, however, prohibits making any association between rVIIa administration and actual risk of mortality or other complications from these publications.

Understanding that limited conclusions about efficacy and safety can be made from retrospective case series, several authors have attempted to provide more useful evidence in a growing number of retrospective studies with matched control patients looking at rVIIa as rescue therapy for excessive bleeding, (96, 97, 101–103) as well as 2 small randomized trials where rVIIa was given prophylactically (104, 105). Most trials with a matched control group show a significant reduction of bleeding and/or transfusion immediately after rVIIa administration compared with control patients (96, 97, 101, 103). Similarly, rVIIa-treated patients often had less blood loss and transfusions in the 24-hour period after rVIIa was given (96, 102). One study that showed immediate improvement after rVIIa administration found no difference in 24-hour blood loss or transfusion requirements in the treatment group (97).

Differing results were also seen in the two small randomized trials of prophylactic rVIIa. Diprose et al. showed a significant reduction in transfusion requirement and percentage of patients transfused in a small trial of repeat non-coronary surgery in adults (104). A larger trial of infants receiving rVIIa after protamine administration found no reduction of blood loss, transfusions, or time to chest closure in the treatment group (105). While it can be postulated that the difference in efficacy between the two randomized trials was dose-related (90 mcg/kg vs. 40 mcg/kg), this conclusion cannot be made because of the very different study groups.

Most of these publications showed no differences in thrombotic complications compared with the control group (103, 104), or had no thrombotic events in the treatment group (96, 97, 105). In the largest series with matched controls, Karkouti et al. reported a significant increase in acute renal dysfunction, but no difference in acute renal failure. While 4 strokes were seen in the rVIIa-treated patients and only 1 in control patients, this finding did not achieve statistical significance (101).

There was no evidence of increased mortality with rVIIa administration, with rates being no different from the control group (96, 97, 101, 103), or no mortality in the treatment group (104, 105). Karkouti and colleagues subsequently published a much larger experience of their rVIIa usage in refractory blood loss in 115 cardiac surgical patients, comparing complications of rVIIa-treated patients with a large control group defined as having excessive bleeding after cardiac surgery. After risk-adjustment for predictors for adverse events, there was no increase in adverse event rates in the patients treated with rVIIa. The authors do suggest that early treatment with rVIIa may lead to better outcomes, compared to late treatment (106).

Despite the numerous publications on this topic, many questions regarding rVIIa use in adult cardiac surgical patients remain unanswered. There is no consensus on the optimal dose or timing of rVIIa treatment. While most publications suggest that rVIIa was efficacious in reducing bleeding, at least in the short-term, the true risk of thrombotic and other adverse events from rVIIa therapy is unknown. Larger randomized prospective trials are needed to determine the optimal usage and safety profile of rVIIa.

Use of rVIIa in Pediatric Cardiac Surgical Patients

Compared with the adult literature, significantly less rVIIa use in pediatric cardiac surgical patients has been reported. Most of the publications, including case reports/series (107–110) and 1 unmatched case-control study (111), show decreased blood loss or resolution of bleeding after rVIIa administration, with no thrombotic events noted. Another series showed that rVIIa prevented surgical reexploration in 7 of 8 bleeding pediatric patients who met criteria for re-exploration (112). The only prospective randomized trial, including 76 pediatric cardiac surgical patients, showed no benefit of rVIIa (40 mcg/kg) when administered prophylactically to patients (n = 40) after protamine administration. While there was a significant reduction of prothrombin time (PT) in the rVIIa-treated patients, there was no improvement of blood loss, time to chest closure, or transfusion requirements compared with the control group. No thrombotic events were noted in either group (105).

Several publications have described rVIIa usage in 20 pediatric patients on extracorporeal membrane oxygenation (ECMO) support. While the drug reduced or stopped bleeding after a single dose on many occasions (111, 113, 114), most patients received multiple doses for persistent or recurrent bleeding (111, 114–116). Very high cumulative doses were reported in 2 patients, with a 3-year-old receiving 700 mcg/kg from 2 doses (115) and a 13-year-old receiving 10 doses of 90 mcg/kg, totaling 900 mcg/kg in less than 24 hours (116), both without any circuit thrombosis.

Based on the current literature about use of rVIIa in pediatric cardiac surgical patients, the only thrombotic events reported have occurred in patients on ECMO, and included 2 patients on ECMO during the early postoperative period after modified Norwood stage 1 repair (111). One received 50 mcg/kg 4 hours postoperatively and required an emergent circuit change due to clots in the circuit 8 hours later. The other received 2 doses, each 40 mcg/kg. The latter patient developed a femoral arterial thrombosis at the site of attempted arterial line insertion, along with an atrial thrombus. This patient was weaned from ECMO, and required a left atrial thrombectomy and, ultimately, a below-the-knee amputation. It is unclear if either of these patients was receiving any anticoagulation at the time of rVIIa administration.

While the low rate of undesirable thrombosis in pediatric cardiac surgical patients is encouraging, there is not enough evidence to know if rVIIa is truly safe in these patients. The thrombotic events reported resulted in significant morbidity, and could potentially have been fatal for these neonates. The management of neonates and pediatric patients with excessive bleeding can be very difficult. While rVIIa can be an appealing treatment option for these patients, it must be used with caution until its safety profile is known. Perhaps it should be avoided in the early postoperative period in neonates requiring ECMO.

Use of rVIIa to Control Bleeding Resulting from Direct Thrombin Inhibitors

Recombinant factor VIIa also has been used to treat bleeding in patients receiving a direct thrombin inhibitor (DTI). Patients with heparin-induced thrombocytopenia type II (HIT) presenting for cardiac surgery are at high risk for thrombosis if they are exposed to heparin when they have circulating antibodies to heparin-platelet factor 4 complexes (117). In antibody-positive patients, a DTI is used for anticoagulation for CPB. Unlike heparin, the DTIs have no reversal agent, and excessive bleeding is common after termination of CPB (118). Bleeding after CPB is typically treated with blood component transfusion. Dialysis or ultrafiltration techniques may also be attempted to accelerate drug removal.

While rVIIa has been shown to improve bleeding time in animals treated with DTI, the effect was less pronounced than that seen with activated prothrombin complex concentrate (APCC) administration (119). Young and colleagues recently reported improvement of TEG parameters when rVIIa was added to blood from humans receiving DTI therapy (120). Their findings suggest the effect may be dose-related, with less improvement seen with their higher bivalirudin concentration, which is still much lower than that required for CPB anticoagulation.

The case reports describing rVIIa administration after CPB with excessive bleeding resulting from DTI therapy report variable efficacy. Bleeding quickly improved in 2 patients who had already received significant blood component transfusion prior to rVIIa administration (121, 122), with one of the patients requiring an additional dose of rVIIa despite undergoing 90 minutes of modified ultrafiltration after the first dose (122). An infant receiving 2 doses of 90 mcg/kg showed no apparent benefit from the drug (123). Another patient receiving rVIIa 20 hours postoperatively had resolution of bleeding over a few hours (124). These reports suggest that rVIIa may help correct bleeding when used in combination with blood component therapy, but is not always effective. Further evaluation of dialysis techniques to remove the DTI from circulation, and other pharmacologic agents such as APCC to reverse the DTI effects, may offer more insight to help clinicians treat this difficult problem.

Summary

Based on the current literature, both the STS and SCA Clinical Practice Guidelines on blood conservation and the Proceedings of the Canadian Consensus Conference on the role of rVIIa in on-pump cardiac surgery conclude that although there is no strong evidence supporting its use, rVIIa is reasonable to consider when bleeding remains unresponsive to routine hemostatic therapy (65, 125).

Recombinant factor VIIa is an expensive procoagulant drug approved for use in hemophiliac patients with inhibitors, and patients with factor VII deficiency. The efficacy and safety profiles of its off-label use in cardiac surgical patients remain unclear. Prospective, randomized studies will be needed to help define when rVIIa use is likely to be efficacious, and which patients are at increased risk for undesirable thrombosis. Until these studies are completed, it is reasonable to consider rVIIa for when bleeding is excessive, and resistant to traditional blood component therapy. It should be avoided if DIC, advanced atherosclerosis, or sepsis are present. Extreme caution should be used if considering rVIIa in the presence of other procoagulant agents.

OTHER PROCOAGULANT AGENTS: PROTHROMBIN COMPLEX CONCENTRATE AND ACTIVATED PROTHROMBIN COMPLEX CONCENTRATE

Several procoagulant agents are used for the treatment of patients with hemophilia A and hemophilia B, with deficiencies of factor VIII and IX, respectively. Coagulation factor concentrates and recombinant preparations of factor VIII and IX are available to treat documented deficiencies of these factors in patients without inhibitors. Chronic exposure to these coagulation factor concentrates can lead to development of inhibitors, or antibodies to the deficient coagulation factor (126). The presence of significant levels of inhibitors requires alternate therapies that bypass the inhibitor in the coagulation process.

There are 3 agents for patients with hemophilia with inhibitors. Recombinant factor VIIa was discussed earlier in this chapter. A second agent is prothrombin complex concentrate (PCC) (Beriplex® P/N, CSL Behring, and Octaplex®, Octapharma) which is a partially purified factor IX concentrate obtained from plasma obtained from human donors. PCC also contains variable amounts of factors II, VII, and X (127). The third agent is activated prothrombin complex concentrate (APCC), also known as anti-inhibitor coagulant complex, and factor VIII inhibitor bypassing fraction (FEIBA®) (FEIBA® VH and Autoplex® T, Baxter AG). Similar to PCC, APCC contains concentrates of factors II, VII, IX, and X from human plasma. During the preparation process these factors are activated; therefore, APCC contains both active and precursor forms of the vitamin K-dependent clotting factors. The preparations are either heat-treated (Autoplex® T) or vapor-heated (FEIBA® VH) for viral inactivation, (128) although there is still a small risk of viral transmission.

Prothrombin complex concentrate is indicated for prevention or treatment of bleeding episodes in patients with factor IX deficiency and patients with inhibitors to factor VIII. APCC is indicated in hemophiliac patients with inhibitors to factor VIII or IX, and in patients with acquired inhibitors to factor VIII, XI, and XII. APCC should not be used in patients with coagulation factor deficiencies without inhibitors (128). These agents normalize hemostasis by either replacing deficient coagulation factors or bypassing the need factors for VIII and IX in thrombin production and clot formation (129). Therapy with APCC in hemophiliacs is considered safe, with a recent review of >4500 infusions showing a <0.04% rate of adverse events and no thrombotic complications (130). It is also suggested that the thrombotic risk of APCC (FEIBA) is less than that of rVIIa (131).

The majority of literature describing use of these agents in nonhemophiliacs comes from outside the United States. As with rVIIa, there is increasing interest in use of PCC in patients requiring rapid reversal of vitamin K-antagonist anticoagulation. Reports describe rapid normalization of the International Normalized Ratio (INR) within 3–10 minutes, even in over-anticoagulated patients (132, 133). A few thrombotic events have been reported with this application (134). Additionally, no randomized trials have been published comparing PCC and rVIIa for rapid reversal of oral anticoagulant reversal in humans, and the optimal agent for this use remains undecided (135).

Two animal studies have described the use of APCC to antagonize anticoagulation resulting from direct thrombin inhibitors (DTI). Both report a reduction in bleeding time with APCC administration (119, 136). In the most recent study, authors showed that APCC was superior to rVIIa in reducing the bleeding time associated with high-dose DTI treatment (119). The effect on bleeding time by APCC in these studies is encouraging; however, studies in humans will be required to determine if APCC therapy is safe and efficacious therapy for patients experiencing hemorrhage after CPB related these anticoagulants.

These agents should be used with caution, and should not be used in patients with increased thrombotic risk, including those with disseminated intravascular coagulation, liver disease, and sepsis (137). Further study of PCC and APCC in patients without hemophilia is necessary to help define efficacy and safety of these agents and determine if there is a role for there use in cardiac surgical patients.

CONCLUSIONS

Effective and safe procoagulant agents are highly sought after for treatment of congenital and acquired bleeding disorders. An ideal agent would be inexpensive, efficacious without causing undesired thrombosis, carry no infectious risk, and treat a wide variety of bleeding disorders. Unfortunately such an agent does not exist. Desmopressin therapy is hindered by limited efficacy. Recombinant factor VIIa is very expensive, without large prospective randomized trials to determine efficacy and safety of off-label usage in cardiac surgical patients. While the future may provide additional treatment options, clinicians should focus their efforts on blood conservation and the prevention of bleeding at this time.

References

1. Nuttall GA., et al.: Determination of normal versus abnormal activated partial thromboplastin time and prothrombin time after cardiopulmonary bypass. J Cardiothorac Vasc Anesth 1995: 9: 355–61
2. Despotis GJ, Grishaber JE, Goodnough LT: The effect of an intraoperative treatment algorithm on physicians' transfusion practice in cardiac surgery. Transfusion 1994; 34:290–6
3. Hartmann M. et al.: Effects of cardiac surgery on hemostasis. Transfus Med Rev 2006; 20: 230–41
4. American Society of Anesthesiologists Task Force on Blood Component Therapy: Practice guidelines for blood component therapy: a report by the American Society of Anesthesiologists Task Force on Blood Component Therapy. Anesthesiology 1996; 84: 732–47
5. Schreiber GB, et al.: The risk of transfusion-transmitted viral infections. The Retrovirus Epidemiology Donor Study. N Engl J Med 1996; 334:1685–90
6. Shander A: Emerging risks and outcomes of blood transfusion in surgery. Semin Hematol 2004; 41(1 Suppl 1): 117–24
7. Engoren MC, et al.: Effect of blood transfusion on long-term survival after cardiac operation. Ann Thorac Surg 2002; 74: 1180–6
8. Karkouti K, et al.: The independent association of massive blood loss with mortality in cardiac surgery. Transfusion 2004; 44:1453–62
9. Spiess BD, et al.: Platelet transfusions during coronary artery bypass graft surgery are associated with serious adverse outcomes. Transfusion 2004; 44:1143–8
10. Shapira OM, et al.: Reduction of allogeneic blood transfusions after open heart operations by lowering cardiopulmonary bypass prime volume. Ann Thorac Surg 1998; 65:724–30
11. Kreisler KR, et al.: Heparin-bonded cardiopulmonary bypass circuits reduce the rate of red blood cell transfusion during elective coronary artery bypass surgery. J Cardiothorac Vasc Anesth 2005; 19:608–11.
12. Cross MH: Autotransfusion in cardiac surgery. Perfusion 2001; 16:391–400
13. McGill N, et al.: Mechanical methods of reducing blood transfusion in cardiac surgery: randomised controlled trial. BMJ 2002; 324:1299

14. Levi M, et al.: Pharmacological strategies to decrease excessive blood loss in cardiac surgery: a meta-analysis of clinically relevant endpoints. Lancet 1999; 354:1940–7
15. Mannucci PM, et al.: 1-Deamino-8-d-arginine vasopressin: a new pharmacological approach to the management of haemophilia and von Willebrands' diseases. Lancet 1977; 1:869–72
16. Mannucci PM: Hemostatic drugs. N Engl J Med 1998; 339:245–53
17. Mannucci PM: Nontransfusional hemostatic agents. In: Lascalzo J, Schafer AI, eds: Thrombosis and Hemorrhage.Lippincott Williams & Wilkins: Philadelphia. 2002;915–928
18. Sakariassen KS, et al.: DDAVP enhances platelet adherence and platelet aggregate growth on human artery subendothelium. Blood 1984; 64:229–36
19. Mannucci PM, et al.: Studies on the prolonged bleeding time in von Willebrand's disease. J Lab Clin Med 1976; 88:662–71
20. Cash JD, Gader, AM, da Costa J: Proceedings: The release of plasminogen activator and factor VIII to lysine vasopressin, arginine vasopressin, I-desamino-8-d-arginine vasopressin, angiotensin and oxytocin in man. Br J Haematol 1974; 27:363–4
21. Levi M, et al.: Plasminogen activation in vivo upon intravenous infusion of DDAVP. Quantitative assessment of plasmin-alpha 2-antiplasmin complex with a novel monoclonal antibody based radioimmunoassay. Thromb Haemost 1992: 67:111–6
22. Mannucci PM, et al.: Mechanism of plasminogen activator and factor VIII increase after vasoactive drugs. Br J Haematol 1975; 30:81–93
23. Kohler M, et al.: Comparative study of intranasal, subcutaneous and intravenous administration of desamino-D-arginine vasopressin (DDAVP). Thromb Haemost 1986; 55: 108–11
24. Lethagen S, et al.: Intranasal and intravenous administration of desmopressin: effect on FVIII/vWF, pharmacokinetics and reproducibility. Thromb Haemost 1987; 58:1033–6
25. Lethagen S, et al.: Effect kinetics of desmopressin-induced platelet retention in healthy volunteers treated with aspirin or placebo. Haemophilia 2000; 6:15–20
26. Mannucci PM: Desmopressin (DDAVP) in the treatment of bleeding disorders: the first 20 years. Blood 1997; 90:2515–21
27. Johns RA: Desmopressin is a potent vasorelaxant of aorta and pulmonary artery isolated from rabbit and rat. Anesthesiology 1990; 72:858–64
28. Frankville DD, et al.: Hemodynamic consequences of desmopressin administration after cardiopulmonary bypass. Anesthesiology 1991; 74:988–96

29. Reich DL, et al.: Desmopressin acetate is a mild vasodilator that does not reduce blood loss in uncomplicated cardiac surgical procedures. J Cardiothorac Vasc Anesth 1991; 5:142–5
30. Humphries JE. Siragy H: Significant hyponatremia following DDAVP administration in a healthy adult. Am J Hematol 1993; 44:12–5
31. Bond L, Bevan D: Myocardial infarction in a patient with hemophilia treated with DDAVP. N Engl J Med 1988; 318:121
32. Hartmann S. Reinhart W: Fatal complication of desmopressin. Lancet 1995; 345:1302–3
33. Virtanen R, Kauppila M, Itala M: Percutaneous coronary intervention with stenting in a patient with haemophilia A and an acute myocardial infarction following a single dose of desmopressin. Thromb Haemost 2004; 92:1154–6
34. McLeod BC: Myocardial infarction in a blood donor after administration of desmopressin. Lancet 1990; 336:1137–8
35. Byrnes JJ, Larcada A, Moake JL: Thrombosis following desmopressin for uremic bleeding. Am J Hematol 1988; 28:63–5
36. Carless PA, et al.: Desmopressin for minimising perioperative allogeneic blood transfusion. Cochrane Database Syst Rev 2004:CD001884
37. Laupacis A, Fergusson, D: Drugs to minimize perioperative blood loss in cardiac surgery: meta-analyses using perioperative blood transfusion as the outcome. The International Study of Peri-operative Transfusion (ISPOT) Investigators. Anesth Analg 1997: 85:1258–67
38. Mannucci PM, Carlsson S, Harris, AS: Desmopressin, surgery and thrombosis. Thromb Haemost 1994; 71:154–5
39. Mannucci PM, et al.: Deamino-8-D-arginine vasopressin shortens the bleeding time in uremia. N Engl J Med 1983; 308:8–12
40. Mannucci PM, et al.: Controlled trial of desmopressin in liver cirrhosis and other conditions associated with a prolonged bleeding time. Blood 1986; 67:1148–53
41. Reiter RA, et al.: Desmopressin antagonizes the in vitro platelet dysfunction induced by GPIIb/IIIa inhibitors and aspirin. Blood 2003; 102:4594–9
42. Salzman EW, et al.: Treatment with desmopressin acetate to reduce blood loss after cardiac surgery. A double-blind randomized trial. N Engl J Med 1986; 314:1402–6
43. Rocha E, et al.: Does desmopressin acetate reduce blood loss after surgery in patients on cardiopulmonary bypass? Circulation 1988; 77:1319–23
44. Andersson TL, et al.: Effects of desmopressin acetate on platelet aggregation, von Willebrand factor, and blood loss after cardiac surgery with extracorporeal circulation. Circulation 1990; 81:872–8

45. Hackmann T, et al.: A trial of desmopressin (1-desamino-8-D-arginine vasopressin) to reduce blood loss in uncomplicated cardiac surgery. N Engl J Med 1989; 321:1437–43
46. Hedderich GS, et al.: Desmopressin acetate in uncomplicated coronary artery bypass surgery: a prospective randomized clinical trial. Can J Surg 1990; 33:33–6
47. Lazenby WD, et al.: Treatment with desmopressin acetate in routine coronary artery bypass surgery to improve postoperative hemostasis. Circulation 1990; 82: IV413–9
48. Marquez J, et al.: Repeated dose administration of desmopressin acetate in uncomplicated cardiac surgery: a prospective, blinded, randomized study. J Cardiothorac Vasc Anesth 1992; 6:674–6
49. Ozkisacik E, et al.: Desmopressin usage in elective cardiac surgery. J Cardiovasc Surg (Torino) 2001; 42:741–7
50. Ansell J, et al.: Does desmopressin acetate prophylaxis reduce blood loss after valvular heart operations? A randomized, double-blind study. J Thorac Cardiovasc Surg 1992; 104:117–23
51. Temeck BK, et al.: Desmopressin acetate in cardiac surgery: a double-blind, randomized study. South Med J 1994; 87:611–5
52. Dilthey G, et al.: Influence of desmopressin acetate on homologous blood requirements in cardiac surgical patients pretreated with aspirin. J Cardiothorac Vasc Anesth 1993; 7:425–30
53. Gratz I, et al.: The effect of desmopressin acetate on postoperative hemorrhage in patients receiving aspirin therapy before coronary artery bypass operations. J Thorac Cardiovasc Surg 1992; 104:1417–22
54. Sheridan DP, et al.: Use of desmopressin acetate to reduce blood transfusion requirements during cardiac surgery in patients with acetylsalicylic-acid-induced platelet dysfunction. Can J Surg 1994; 37:33–6
55. Czer LS, et al.: Treatment of severe platelet dysfunction and hemorrhage after cardiopulmonary bypass: reduction in blood product usage with desmopressin. J Am Coll Cardiol 1987; 9:1139–47
56. Despotis GJ, et al.: Use of point-of-care test in identification of patients who can benefit from desmopressin during cardiac surgery: a randomised controlled trial. Lancet 1999; 354:106–10
57. Mongan PD, Hosking MP: The role of desmopressin acetate in patients undergoing coronary artery bypass surgery. A controlled clinical trial with thromboelastographic risk stratification. Anesthesiology 1992; 77:38–46
58. Ozal E, et al.: Does tranexamic acid reduce desmopressin-induced hyperfibrinolysis? J Thorac Cardiovasc Surg 2002; 123:539–43
59. Casas JI, et al.: Aprotinin versus desmopressin for patients undergoing operations with cardiopulmonary bypass. A double-blind

placebo-controlled study. J Thorac Cardiovasc Surg 1995; 110:1107–17

60. Horrow JC, et al.: Hemostatic effects of tranexamic acid and desmopressin during cardiac surgery. Circulation 1991; 84:2063–70
61. Cattaneo M, et al.: The effect of desmopressin on reducing blood loss in cardiac surgery-a meta-analysis of double-blind, placebo-controlled trials. Thromb Haemost 1995; 74:1064–70
62. Oliver WC, Jr., et al.: Desmopressin does not reduce bleeding and transfusion requirements in congenital heart operations. Ann Thorac Surg 2000; 70:1923–30
63. Reynolds LM, et al.: Desmopressin does not decrease bleeding after cardiac operation in young children. J Thorac Cardiovasc Surg 1993; 106:954–8
64. Seear MD, et al.: The effect of desmopressin acetate (DDAVP) on postoperative blood loss after cardiac operations in children. J Thorac Cardiovasc Surg 1989; 98:217–9
65. Ferraris VA, et al.: Perioperative blood transfusion and blood conservation in cardiac surgery: the Society of Thoracic Surgeons and The Society of Cardiovascular Anesthesiologists clinical practice guideline. Ann Thorac Surg 2007; 83: S27–86
66. Mayer SA, et al.: Recombinant activated factor VII for acute intracerebral hemorrhage. N Engl J Med 2005; 352:777–85
67. Cameron P, et al.: The use of recombinant activated factor VII in trauma patients: Experience from the Australian and New Zealand haemostasis registry. Injury 2007; 38:1030–8
68. Poon, MC: The evidence for the use of recombinant human activated factor VII in the treatment of bleeding patients with quantitative and qualitative platelet disorders. Transfus Med Rev 2007; 21:223–36
69. Ramsey G: Treating coagulopathy in liver disease with plasma transfusions or recombinant factor VIIa: an evidence-based review. Best Pract Res Clin Haematol 2006; 19:113–26
70. Lodge JP, et al.: Efficacy and safety of repeated perioperative doses of recombinant factor VIIa in liver transplantation. Liver Transpl 2005; 11:973–9
71. Levi M, Bijsterveld NR, Keller TT: Recombinant factor VIIa as an antidote for anticoagulant treatment. Semin Hematol 2004; 41:65–9
72. Sorensen B, et al.: Reversal of the International Normalized Ratio with recombinant activated factor VII in central nervous system bleeding during warfarin thromboprophylaxis: clinical and biochemical aspects. Blood Coagul Fibrinolysis 2003; 14:469–77

73. Franchini M, Lippi G, Franchi M: The use of recombinant activated factor VII in obstetric and gynaecological haemorrhage. BJOG 2007; 114:8–15
74. Hedner U: Mechanism of action of recombinant activated factor VII: an update. Semin Hematol 2006; 43:S105–7
75. Monroe DM, et al.: Platelet activity of high-dose factor VIIa is independent of tissue factor. Br J Haematol 1997; 99:542–7
76. Roberts HR, Monroe DM 3rd, Hoffman M: Safety profile of recombinant factor VIIa. Semin Hematol 2004; 41:101–8
77. Hoffman M, Monroe DM, 3rd, Roberts HR: Activated factor VII activates factors IX and X on the surface of activated platelets: thoughts on the mechanism of action of high-dose activated factor VII. Blood Coagul Fibrinolysis 1998; 9 Suppl 1: S61–5
78. Roberts HR, et al.: Newer concepts of blood coagulation. Haemophilia 1998; 4:331–4
79. Lindley CM, et al.: Pharmacokinetics and pharmacodynamics of recombinant factor VIIa. Clin Pharmacol Ther 1994; 55:638–48
80. Shapiro AD, et al.: Prospective, randomised trial of two doses of rFVIIa (NovoSeven) in haemophilia patients with inhibitors undergoing surgery. Thromb Haemost 1998; 80:773–8
81. Al Douri M, et al.: Effect of the administration of recombinant activated factor VII (rFVIIa; NovoSeven) in the management of severe uncontrolled bleeding in patients undergoing heart valve replacement surgery. Blood Coagul Fibrinolysis 2000; 11 Suppl 1: S121–7
82. Hendriks HG, et al.: An effective treatment of severe intractable bleeding after valve repair by one single dose of activated recombinant factor VII Anesth Analg 2001; 93:287–9, 2nd contents page
83. Stratmann G, Russell IA, Merrick SH: Use of recombinant factor VIIa as a rescue treatment for intractable bleeding following repeat aortic arch repair. Ann Thorac Surg 2003; 76:2094–7
84. Isbister J, et al.: Recombinant activated factor VII in critical bleeding: experience from the Australian and New Zealand Haemostasis Register. Intern Med J. 2008; 38:156–65
85. Aggarwal A, et al.: Recombinant activated factor VII (rFVIIa) as salvage treatment for intractable hemorrhage. Thromb J 2004; 2:9
86. Bishop CV, et al.: Recombinant activated factor VII: treating postoperative hemorrhage in cardiac surgery. Ann Thorac Surg 2006; 81:875–9
87. Filsoufi F, et al.: Effective management of refractory postcardiotomy bleeding with the use of recombinant activated factor VII Ann Thorac Surg 2006; 82:1779–83
88. Halkos ME, et al.: Early experience with activated recombinant factor VII for intractable hemorrhage after cardiovascular surgery. Ann

Thorac Surg 2005; 79:1303–6
89. Raivio P, Suojaranta-Ylinen R, Kuitunen AH: Recombinant factor VIIa in the treatment of postoperative hemorrhage after cardiac surgery. Ann Thorac Surg 2005; 80:66–71
90. Lloyd Jones M, et al.: Control of bleeding in patients with haemophilia A with inhibitors: a systematic review. Haemophilia, 2003; 9:464–520
91. O'Connell KA, et al.: Thromboembolic adverse events after use of recombinant human coagulation factor VIIa. JAMA 2006; 295:293–8
92. Corti R, et al.: Evolving concepts in the triad of atherosclerosis, inflammation and thrombosis. J Thromb Thrombolysis 2004; 17:35–44
93. Chung JH, et al.: Pericardial blood activates the extrinsic coagulation pathway during clinical cardiopulmonary bypass. Circulation 1996; 93:2014–8
94. Ernofsson M, Thelin S, Siegbahn A: Monocyte tissue factor expression, cell activation, and thrombin formation during cardiopulmonary bypass: a clinical study. J Thorac Cardiovasc Surg 1997; 113:576–84
95. Dietrich W, Spannagl M: Caveat against the use of activated recombinant factor VII for intractable bleeding in cardiac surgery. Anesth Analg 2002; 94:1369–70; author reply 1370–1
96. Gelsomino S, et al.: Treatment of refractory bleeding after cardiac operations with low-dose recombinant activated factor VII (NovoSeven®): a propensity score analysis. Eur J Cardiothorac Surg. 2008; 33:64–71
97. von Heymann C, et al.: Recombinant activated factor VII for refractory bleeding after cardiac surgery—a retrospective analysis of safety and efficacy. Crit Care Med 2005; 33:2241–6
98. McCall P, Story DA, Karapillai D: Audit of factor VIIa for bleeding resistant to conventional therapy following complex cardiac surgery. Can J Anaesth 2006; 53:926–33
99. Gandhi MJ, et al.: Use of activated recombinant factor VII for severe coagulopathy post ventricular assist device or orthotopic heart transplant. J Cardiothorac Surg 2007; 2: 32
100. Bui JD, et al.: Fatal thrombosis after administration of activated prothrombin complex concentrates in a patient supported by extracorporeal membrane oxygenation who had received activated recombinant factor VII J Thorac Cardiovasc Surg 2002; 124:852–4
101. Karkouti K, et al.: Recombinant factor VIIa for intractable blood loss after cardiac surgery: a propensity score-matched case-control analysis. Transfusion 2005; 45:26–34

102. Romagnoli S, et al.: Small-dose recombinant activated factor VII (NovoSeven) in cardiac surgery. Anesth Analg 2006; 102:1320–6
103. Tritapepe L, et al.: Recombinant activated factor VII for refractory bleeding after acute aortic dissection surgery: a propensity score analysis. Crit Care Med 2007; 35:1685–90
104. Diprose P, et al.: Activated recombinant factor VII after cardiopulmonary bypass reduces allogeneic transfusion in complex non-coronary cardiac surgery: randomized double-blind placebo-controlled pilot study. Br J Anaesth 2005; 95:596–602
105. Ekert H, et al.: Elective administration in infants of low-dose recombinant activated factor VII (rFVIIa) in cardiopulmonary bypass surgery for congenital heart disease does not shorten time to chest closure or reduce blood loss and need for transfusions: a randomized, double-blind, parallel group, placebo-controlled study of rFVIIa and standard haemostatic replacement therapy versus standard haemostatic replacement therapy. Blood Coagul Fibrinolysis 2006; 17:389–95
106. Karkouti K, et al.: Determinants of complications with recombinant factor VIIa for refractory blood loss in cardiac surgery. Can J Anaesth 2006; 53:802–9
107. Brady KM, Easley RB, Tobias JD: Recombinant activated factor VII (rFVIIa) treatment in infants with hemorrhage. Paediatr Anaesth 2006; 16:1042–6
108. Leibovitch L, et al.: Recombinant activated factor VII for life-threatening pulmonary hemorrhage after pediatric cardiac surgery. Pediatr Crit Care Med 2003; 4:444–6
109. Razon Y, et al.: Recombinant factor VIIa (NovoSeven) as a hemostatic agent after surgery for congenital heart disease. Paediatr Anaesth 2005; 15:235–40
110. Tobias JD, et al.: Recombinant factor VIIa to control excessive bleeding following surgery for congenital heart disease in pediatric patients. J Intensive Care Med 2004; 19:270–3
111. Agarwal HS, et al.: Recombinant factor seven therapy for postoperative bleeding in neonatal and pediatric cardiac surgery. Ann Thorac Surg 2007; 84:161–8
112. Pychynska-Pokorska M, et al.: The use of recombinant coagulation factor VIIa in uncontrolled postoperative bleeding in children undergoing cardiac surgery with cardiopulmonary bypass. Pediatr Crit Care Med 2004; 5:246–50
113. Verrijckt A, et al.: Activated recombinant factor VII for refractory bleeding during extracorporeal membrane oxygenation. J Thorac Cardiovasc Surg 2004; 127:1812–3

114. Wittenstein B, et al.: Recombinant factor VII for severe bleeding during extracorporeal membrane oxygenation following open heart surgery. Pediatr Crit Care Med 2005; 6:473–6
115. Davis MC, et al.: Use of thromboelastograph and factor VII for the treatment of postoperative bleeding in a pediatric patient on ECMO after cardiac surgery. J Extra Corpor Technol 2006; 38:165–7
116. Dominguez TE, et al.: Use of recombinant factor VIIa for refractory hemorrhage during extracorporeal membrane oxygenation. Pediatr Crit Care Med 2005; 6:348–51
117. Arepally G, Cines DB: Pathogenesis of heparin-induced thrombocytopenia and thrombosis. Autoimmun Rev 2002; 1:125–32
118. Nuttall GA, et al.: Patients with a history of type II heparin-induced thrombocytopenia with thrombosis requiring cardiac surgery with cardiopulmonary bypass: a prospective observational case series. Anesth Analg 2003; 96:344–50, table of contents
119. Elg M, Carlsson S, Gustafsson D: Effect of activated prothrombin complex concentrate or recombinant factor VIIa on the bleeding time and thrombus formation during anticoagulation with a direct thrombin inhibitor. Thromb Res 2001; 101:145–57
120. Young G, et al.: Recombinant activated factor VII effectively reverses the anticoagulant effects of heparin, enoxaparin, fondaparinux, argatroban, and bivalirudin ex vivo as measured using thromboelastography. Blood Coagul Fibrinolysis 2007; 18:547–53
121. Oh JJ, et al.: Recombinant factor VIIa for refractory bleeding after cardiac surgery secondary to anticoagulation with the direct thrombin inhibitor lepirudin. Pharmacotherapy 2006; 26:569–77
122. Stratmann G, et al.: Reversal of direct thrombin inhibition after cardiopulmonary bypass in a patient with heparin-induced thrombocytopenia. Anesth Analg 2004; 98:1635–9, table of contents
123. Malherbe S, et al.: Argatroban as anticoagulant in cardiopulmonary bypass in an infant and attempted reversal with recombinant activated factor VII Anesthesiology 2004; 100:443–5
124. Hein OV, et al.: Protracted bleeding after hirudin anticoagulation for cardiac surgery in a patient with HITII and chronic renal failure. Artif Organs 2005; 29:507–10
125. Karkouti K, et al.: The role of recombinant factor VIIa in on-pump cardiac surgery: proceedings of the Canadian Consensus Conference. Can J Anaesth 2007; 54:573–82
126. Key NS: Inhibitors in congenital coagulation disorders. Br J Haematol 2004; 127:379–91
127. Romisch J, Bonik K, Miller HG: Comparative in vitro investigation of prothrombin complex concentrates. Semin Thromb Hemost 1998; 24:175–81

128. FEIBA VH Anti-Inhibitor Coagulant Complex Vapor Heated [package insert]. Deerfield, IL: Baxter; 2005.
129. Turecek PL, et al.: FEIBA: mode of action. Haemophilia 2004; 10 Suppl 2: 3–9
130. Dimichele D, Negrier C: A retrospective postlicensure survey of FEIBA efficacy and safety. Haemophilia 2006; 12:352–62
131. Aledort LM: Comparative thrombotic event incidence after infusion of recombinant factor VIIa versus factor VIII inhibitor bypass activity. J Thromb Haemost 2004; 2:1700–8
132. Riess HB, et al.: Prothrombin complex concentrate (Octaplex®) in patients requiring immediate reversal of oral anticoagulation. Thromb Res 2007; 121:9–16
133. Vigue B, et al.: Ultra-rapid management of oral anticoagulant therapy-related surgical intracranial hemorrhage. Intensive Care Med 2007; 33:721–5
134. Bertram M, et al.: Managing the therapeutic dilemma: patients with spontaneous intracerebral hemorrhage and urgent need for anticoagulation. J Neurol 2000; 247:209–14
135. Aguilar MI, et al.: Treatment of warfarin-associated intracerebral hemorrhage: literature review and expert opinion. Mayo Clin Proc 2007; 82:82–92
136. Diehl KH, et al.: Investigation of activated prothrombin complex concentrate as potential hirudin antidote in animal models. Haemostasis 1995; 25:182–92
137. Preston FE, et al.: Rapid reversal of oral anticoagulation with warfarin by a prothrombin complex concentrate (Beriplex): efficacy and safety in 42 patients. Br J Haematol 2002; 116:619–24

Paul E. Stensrud, MD
Gregory A. Nuttall, MD

8 Pharmacology of Antifibrinolytic Agents

INTRODUCTION

Significant hemorrhage may result from trauma (surgical or otherwise) and/or disorders of blood coagulation. Significant hemorrhage results in patient morbidity and increased cost of care, both in terms of cost of treatment of morbidity as well as in cost of transfusion therapy (1, 2). Additionally, transfusion therapy may itself result in complications (i.e., infection, allergic reaction, lung injury), further increasing morbidity and cost. Hemorrhage is recognized as a significant risk associated with certain surgical procedures, including major orthopedic procedures, major hepatic procedures (including orthotopic liver transplantation), major vascular procedures, and, notably, cardiac surgical procedures requiring cardiopulmonary bypass. Excessive perioperative hemorrhage results in poor patient outcomes and greatly increases economic cost of care.

Adequate perioperative hemostasis depends on a complex relationship between many factors. Inadequate surgical hemostasis may be present. Nonsurgical treatment of hemorrhage will be ineffective in the absence of adequate surgical hemostasis. Defects in coagulation may result in bleeding despite otherwise adequate surgical hemostasis. Coagulopathies may be due to preexisting patient conditions, medications, anesthetic variables, hemodilution, patient temperature, interaction with devices supporting circulation such as the cardiopulmonary bypass machine, as well as other factors. Defining the cause of ongoing hemorrhage is crucial to instituting proper therapy.

Advances in Cardiovascular Pharmacology, edited by Philippe R. Housmans, MD, PhD and Gregory A. Nuttall, M.D.
Lippincott Williams & Wilkins, Baltimore © 2008.

Fibrinolysis is an important mechanism in modulation of coagulation. Pharmacologic therapy inhibiting fibrinolysis may effectively increase coagulation and hemostasis by reducing the breakdown of thrombus and clearing pro-thrombotic substances from the body. Antifibrinolytic compounds may be administered in response to documented excessive fibrinolytic activity suspected of contributing to hemorrhage, or they may be administered prophylactically to high-risk patients who are considered likely to benefit from antifibrinolytic therapy. Agents used in the United States for this purpose include ε-aminocaproic acid, tranexamic acid, and aprotinin.

HEMOSTATIC MECHANISMS

Initial hemostasis is achieved by platelet aggregation in the area of vascular injury. At the injury site, von Willebrand Factor (vWF) interaction with exposed endothelial substrate reveals platelet binding sites for the GPIb platelet receptors (Figure 8–1). Platelets then adhere to the injured area, and complex feedback mechanisms encourage further platelet adhesion and spread, forming a weak platelet plug that results in initial hemostasis.

Strengthening of the initial platelet plug is accomplished by the coagulation cascade, which produces thrombin. The thrombin produced converts fibrinogen to fibrin, which cross-links the loosely adhered platelets in the initial plug, strengthening the platelet plug and improv-

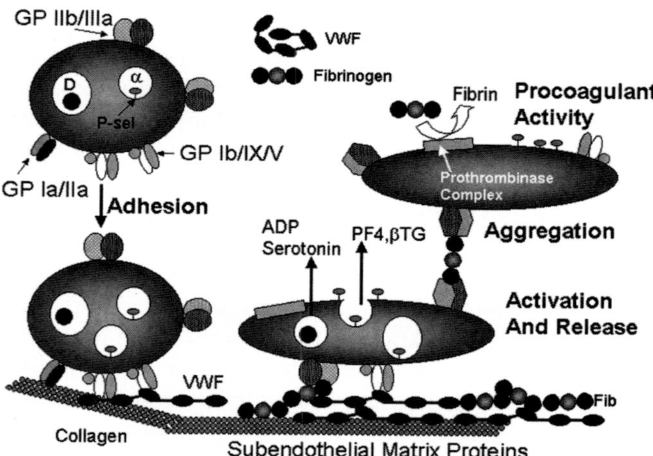

FIGURE 8–1. Platelet adhesion and aggregation. GP = glycoprotein, VWF = von Willebrand Factor, D = platelet dense granule, α = platelet α granule, P-sel = P selectin, ADP = adenosine diphosphate, PF4 = platelet factor 4, β TG = β thromboglobulin, fib = fibrin. From http://referencelab.clevelandclinic.org/images/PlateletAdhesionActivitationAggregation.jpg. Accessed 6 December 2007.

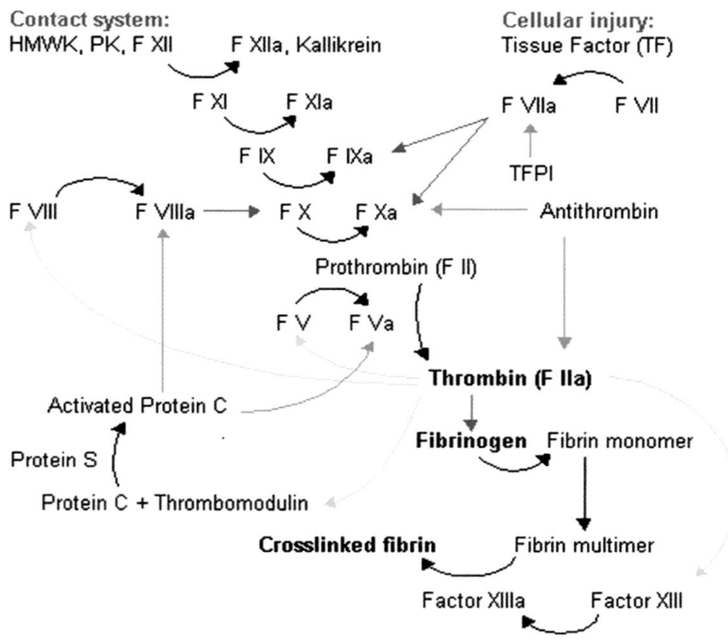

FIGURE 8–2. **The enzymatic coagulation cascade. HWMK = High molecular weight kininogen, PK = Prekallikrein, TFPI = Tissue factor pathway inhibitor.**
Black arrow = the conversion/activation of coagulation factor.
Red arrows = the action of inhibitors of coagulation factors.
Blue arrows = the reactions catalyzed by the activated factor.
Grey arrow = the various functions of thrombin, activated factor II.
 From http://www.biocrawler.com/encyclopedia/Coagulation. Accessed 6 December, 2007.

ing hemostasis. The coagulation cascade is made up of serine proteases, which interact in a complex fashion.

The extrinsic pathway of coagulation begins with the interaction of exposed tissue factor (TF) with factors VII and VIIa (Figure 8–2). The TF-VIIa complex, in the presence of calcium, activates factor X, generating factor Xa. The intrinsic pathway begins with the activation of factor XII to factor XIIa by kallikrein on damaged endothelium or foreign surfaces. Factor XIIa in turn converts factor XI to factor XIa. In the presence of calcium, factor XIa converts factor IX to factor IXa. Factor IXa forms a complex with tissue-bound factor VIIIa. The resulting enzymatic complex then acts to convert factor X to factor Xa, and the common coagulation pathway begins with this merging of extrinsic and intrinsic pathways.

Patients with defects in components of the intrinsic pathway of coagulation demonstrate no clinical bleeding disorders. However, this portion of the coagulation cascade may play a role in wound healing and modulation of hemostatic mechanisms.

In the common pathway of coagulation, factor Xa combines with factor Va, phospholipid, and calcium to form the prothrombinase complex. This complex then converts prothrombin to thrombin. Thrombin converts fibrinogen to fibrin, activates factor XIII which cross-links fibrin, and activates factors V and VIII, which are cofactors for earlier portions of the pathway. Thrombin also causes platelet aggregation.

REGULATING HEMOSTASIS

Activity within the coagulation cascade activates negative feedback mechanisms, which serve to limit coagulation and prevent excessive coagulation that might result in deleterious intravascular thrombosis (Figure 8–2). Thrombin is inhibited by binding to endothelial thrombomodulin. The reaction converts thrombin to an activator of Protein C. Activated Protein C then inactivates factors Va and VIIIa, preventing thrombin formation. Antithrombin inhibits thrombin and factor Xa, among others. This inhibition is slow in the absence of heparin, which greatly accelerates these reactions. Further negative feedback is provided by endothelial-bound tissue factor pathway inhibitor, which inactivates factor Xa, and the resulting enzymatic complex inactivates factor VIIa within the TF-VIIa complex.

The fibrinolytic system is an important modulator of hemostasis (Figure 8–3). Fibrinolysis begins with the conversion of plasminogen to plasmin by plasminogen activators. Plasmin breaks down fibrin and inactivates factors Va and VIIIa and inhibits platelet function. Additionally, plasmin facilitates the formation of more plasmin. Complex interactions regulate fibrinolysis, including feedback relationships between various components of fibrinolysis as well as controlled synthesis of plasminogen activators and plasminogen activator inhibitors.

Fibrinolysis is blocked by plasminogen activator inhibitors, which include tissue plasminogen activator (t-PA) and other plasminogen activators. In the body, t-PA mainly is responsible for clearing fibrin from the circulation. Tissue-bound α_2-antiplasmin inhibits plasmin directly, but does not effectively inhibit fibrin-bound plasmin, which can still demonstrate significant fibrinolytic activity.

PERIOPERATIVE USE OF ANTIFIBRINOLYTIC AGENTS

There are two classes of United States Food and Drug Administration (FDA)-approved antifibrinolytics: lysine analogues and aprotinin. They

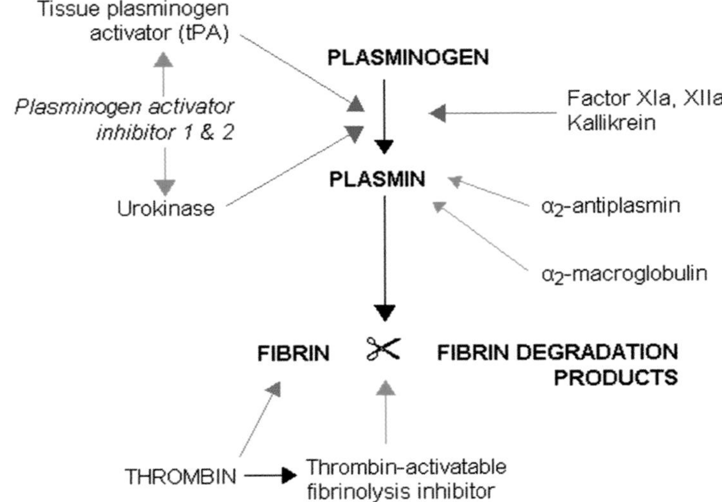

FIGURE 8–3. The fibrinolytic pathway. Scissors = plasmin breaking down fibrin to fibrin degradation products.
Black arrow = the conversion/activation of the factor.
Red arrows = the action of inhibitors of the factors.
Blue arrows = the reactions catalyzed by the activated factor.
Grey arrow = the various functions of thrombin, activated factor II.
Permission granted from: Wikipedia. This article is licensed under the GNU Free Documentation License. It uses material from the Wikipedia article "Fibrinolysis." From http://content.answers.com/main/content/wp/en/0/0e/Fibrinolysis.png. Accessed 6 December, 2007.

are both helpful in controlling bleeding from the action of plasmin. These agents are useful in a variety of conditions or procedures that are associated with excess fibrinolysis such as cardiac surgery with cardiopulmonary bypass (CPB) or liver transplantation, or surgery on tissues in the body that contain high concentrations of t-PA.

The lysine analogues and aprotinin have been used in cardiac surgery for a number of years and have been shown to decrease blood loss and transfusion requirements associated with CPB (1, 3–7). The use of the antifibrinolytic started with proteinase inhibitor, aprotinin, during cardiac operations requiring CPB. The beneficial effects of prophylactic aprotinin on blood loss and transfusion requirements in cardiac surgery were first reported in 1987 by Royston et al. (8). Since this publication, a multitude of studies and several meta-analyses have confirmed the benefits of prophylactic aprotinin in reducing blood loss and transfusion in cardiac surgery with CPB. Aprotinin also had the distinct advantage of statistically reducing reexploration for bleeding and at least some of studies demonstrated superiority with respect to a reduction in either blood loss or transfusion (7, 9). A recent meta-analysis study has even demonstrated aprotinin to be superior over lysine analogue antifibrinolytic drugs in reducing blood loss and transfusion (10). Similar benefits of prophylactic aprotinin use have been reported in orthopedic and liver surgeries (11). Given the high cost of aprotinin and the presumed mechanism of action of aprotinin as an antifibrinolytic, cheaper lysine analogue antifibrinolytics started to be used for the same purpose.

Antifibrinolytic drugs also have been used to decrease bleeding during surgical procedures that involve tissues of the body that contain high concentrations of t-PA. The release of t-PA increases local fibrinolysis due to increased plasmin activity, which can result in excessive bleeding. The organs of the human body that contain high concentrations of t-PA are: the saliva of the mouth, the brain, the gastric mucosa, and the prostate gland. The clinical situations where antifibrinolytic drugs have been used to prevent bleeding are: as a mouth wash in hemophilia patients undergoing dental surgery, in patients with a subarachnoid hemorrhage, in those patients with gastritis or peptic ulcer disease, and in those undergoing surgery on the prostate gland (12).

Of the antifibrinolytic agents, aprotinin is the only FDA-approved agent for preventing bleeding associated with coronary bypass graft surgery. As a result of the publications of Mangano et al. and Karkouti et al. that demonstrated increased complications with the use of aprotinin (13, 14), the FDA in 2006 revised the labeling of aprotinin to strengthen its safety warning and limit its approved usage to patients at an increased risk for blood loss and blood transfusion during coronary bypass graft surgery. On November 5, 2007, the FDA requested that the manufacturer of aprotinin suspend shipments of aprotinin due to excessive mortality being reported by the data safety monitoring board for the trial of antifibrinolytic therapy entitled Blood Conservation using Antifibrinolytics: A Randomized Trial in High-Risk Cardiac Surgery Patients (BART) in the patient group receiving aprotinin (15). The manufacturer of aprotinin has suspended marketing and distribution of aprotinin.

The two synthetic antifibrinolytic lysine analogues are ε-aminocaproic acid and tranexamic acid. Both agents have chemical structure that is similar to the amino acid lysine, thus the name lysine analog. Both agents bind reversibly to both plasminogen and to plasmin, which results in a conformational change in both molecules (Figure 8–4). The binding of the lysine analogue drugs to plasmin prevents plasmin from binding to the lysine moiety of fibrinogen or fibrin, thus preventing the proteolytic digestion of fibrinogen or fibrin to fibrin degradation products. Many recent studies have demonstrated that prophylactic administration of tranexamic acid and ε-aminocaproic acid can reduce blood

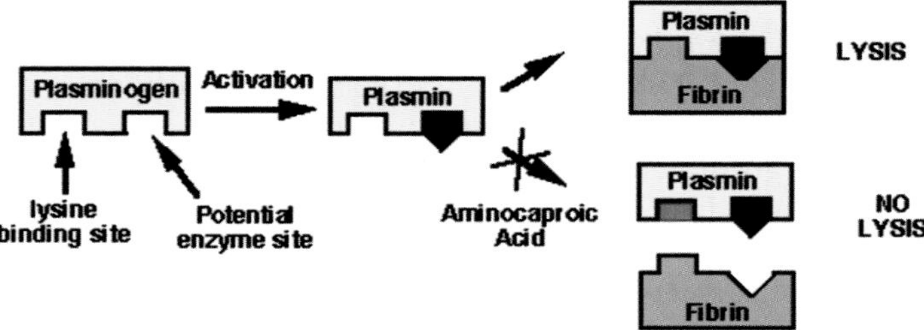

FIGURE 8–4. The mechanism of lysine analog antifibrinolytics. Red rectangle = lysin analog antifibrinolytic, Lysis = fibrinolysis.

loss and/or transfusion requirement in cardiac (11, 16, 17), liver (18), and orthopedic (19) surgeries. Their low cost and rare risks of complications and side effects make lysine analogues (particularly tranexamic acid) attractive prophylactic regents to promote hemostasis in surgeries.

PHARMACOLOGY OF ANTIFIBRINOLYTIC AGENTS

ε-Aminocaproic Acid

The lysine analogue ε-aminocaproic acid (EACA) is a potent inhibitor of plasminogen and plasmin. Inhibition is by means of a competitive blockade of the ability of the fibrinolytic enzymes to bind the lysine sites of fibrinogen (20). The reported dosing schedules of EACA for prophylaxis of cardiac surgical patients vary widely. Ray and O'Brien compared single-dose EACA (20 g) to single-dose aprotinin in patients undergoing CPB (21). In the report of Eaton and Deeb, the dose of EACA varied from a total 5–40 g prebypass as a bolus followed by infusion or multiple boluses (22). A current multicenter randomized trial uses a 10 g loading dose of EACA, followed by 2 g/h infusion during cardiopulmonary bypass (23). Butterworth et al. have calculated that published dosing schemes for EACA in cardiac surgical patients would theoretically result in sustained plasma concentrations of EACA of 250–790 mcg/ml during CPB (24).

The molecular weight of EACA is 131.17 and its pH is approximately 6.8 (25, 26). It is not protein-bound (27). Volume of distribution after intravenous dosing is approximately 30 L, although this measurement was determined in healthy volunteers (26). EACA undergoes hepatic metabolism, with 14–35% of the dose being so metabolized (28). Excretion is 85% renal, with 65% of the drug recovered unchanged (28). Butterworth et al. noted significantly prolonged EACA kinetics in patients with renal failure (24). The elimination half-life of EACA is variable, ranging from 1 to 5 hours (29, 30). EACA may be cleared by both peritoneal and hemodialysis, and dosing may need to be adjusted to account for this (27, 29). CPB is thought to alter the volume of distribution of EACA, but dosing protocols obviously have not been standardized (24). This group felt that a 2-compartment pharmacokinetic model best fit the data on EACA, although earlier investigators felt that EACA pharmacokinetics were best explained by a 3-compartment model (29).

Adverse effects associated with EACA have been reported mainly in patients receiving long-term therapy. Morbilliform rash has been reported in association with EACA therapy (31, 32). Hyperkalemia has occurred, which is suspected to be due to extracellular potassium shift, and plasma potassium levels should be monitored (33). Diarrhea and abdominal pain are common (26). Prolonged high-dose therapy has been reported to be associated with a drug-induced myopathy as well as muscular necrosis (34–38). Myoglobinuria is common (39). Dizziness, confusion, headache, and seizures have been reported (26, 40, 41). Renal failure associated with EACA is possibly due to drug interference with urokinase, causing thrombus retention within the kidney (42–44). However, a study of a series of more than 1500 patients undergoing coronary artery bypass grafting who received EACA perioperatively failed to demonstrate postoperative reduction in creatine clearance (45). Bradycardia has been reported with rapid intravenous administration of EACA (26). Modest hypotension is also reported with intravenous administration (46).

As might be expected, thromboembolic complications are reported in association with EACA therapy. Fibrinolytic activity does not return to normal for 3–4 days after EACA administration (47). Cerebral sinus thrombosis has occurred in patients receiving prolonged EACA (48, 49). Renal artery thrombosis has been reported in patients receiving EACA (50). Interestingly, very high doses of EACA may prolong bleeding time and increase bleeding in patients with subarachnoid hemorrhage (51). Fatal pulmonary microthrombus formation has been reported in patients undergoing cardiac surgery for end-stage heart failure who received antifibrinolytic therapy perioperatively. One of these patients received EACA (52).

Tranexamic Acid

Tranexamic acid (trans-4-aminomethylcyclohexane-1-carboxylic acid), a synthetic lysine analogue, is a competitive inhibitor of plasmin and plasminogen (53). Effects of tranexamic acid (TXA) is more potent and long-lasting than EACA in vitro and it is generally used more widely (11). The dose of tranexamic acid administered prophylactically to prevent excessive bleeding associated with cardiac surgery and CPB varies greatly between institutions. Published dosing schedules for tranexamic acid range between 150 mg/kg loading dose (54) to 10 mg/kg loading dose followed by a 1 mg/kg/hr infusion (55). There is a very large multicenter prospective randomized trial, Blood Conservation using Antifibrinolytics: A Randomized Trial in High-Risk Cardiac Surgery Patients (BART), comparing tranexamic acid therapy, ε-aminocaproic acid therapy, and aprotinin therapy ongoing in Canada (23). The dose of TXA in this study is 30 mg/kg load, 2 mg/kg pump prime, and 16 mg/kg/hr infusion. The concentration of TXA that is needed to reduce t-PA activity by 80% in vitro is 10 μg/ml (56). Tranexamic acid may also abolish plasmin-induced platelet activation in vitro at 16 μg/ml (57). Most studies of TXA pharmacokinetics have been performed in normal volunteers, patients with chronic renal failure, or noncardiac surgical patients (58–61). At therapeutic concentrations, TXA is only minimally bound to plasma proteins (approximately 3%), primarily plasminogen. The initial volume of distribution for TXA is about 9–12 L (Prod Info Cyclokapron®, 2000). The apparent volume of distribution for TXA at steady-state is 0.39 L/kg. The volume of distribution of the central compartment is 0.18 L/kg (62). The renal clearance of TXA is 110–116 ml/m with the percent renal excretion being 39–95% (58). The elimination characteristics of TXA are dependent on whether it is given intravenously or by mouth. Following intravenous administration, about 95% of a dose of TXA is excreted unchanged in the urine (58). Another study found that 45% of a 10-mg/kg intravenous dose is excreted in the urine during the first 3 hours, with 90% being excreted over 24 hours (63). The elimination half-life of TXA is 2 hours (58, 62).

Cardiac surgery with CPB is thought to alter TXA pharmacokinetics. Dowd et al. (64) examined the effects of CPB on TA plasma concentrations and elimination kinetics in 30 adult patients undergoing elective coronary artery bypass grafting, valve surgery, or repair of atrial septal defect received after induction of anesthesia. Three intravenous doses of TXA were used: TXA 50 mg/kg, TXA 100 mg/kg, or TXA 10 mg/kg over 15 minutes, with 1 mg $\cdot$ kg$^{-1}\cdot$ hr^{-1} maintenance infusion for 10 hours. They performed pharmacokinetic modeling using a mixed effects technique. Models of increasing complexity were compared using Schwarz-Bayesian Criterion (SBC). They found that TXA concentrations rapidly fell in all three groups. The data that were generated fit well to a 2-compartment model, and adjustments for CPB were supported by SBC. Their model estimated a central compartment's volume of distribution for TXA of 10.3 l before CPB for a patient with 80 kg body weight and 11.9 l during and after CPB; remaining compartment volumes of distribution of 8.5 l before CPB and 9.8 l during and after CPB. Their model estimated clearance of TXA of 0.15 l/s before CPB, 0.11 l/s during CPB, and 0.17

l/s after CPB; and clearance of TXA from remaining compartment volumes of distribution of 0.18 l/s before CPB and 0.21 l/s during and after CPB. Based on simulation of previous studies of TXA efficacy, Dowd et al. estimated possibly improved dosing regimens for TXA.

Adverse effects have been reported in association with TA therapy. Hypotension is sometimes noted with rapid intravenous administration of TA (65). Diarrhea and nausea associated with TA therapy are more common with oral versus intravenous dosing (66–68). Cerebral ischemia and infarction have been noted in patients receiving TA for subarachnoid hemorrhage (66, 67, 69). Central venous stasis retinopathy has been reported in two patients who received TA (70). Thrombocytopenia in patients receiving TA is rare, as are prolonged bleeding times and coagulation defects (71).

TA therapy has been associated with thromboembolic disorders. These include massive pulmonary thromboembolism (72) and arterial thrombosis (66, 73). Glomerular thrombosis resulting in acute renal cortical necrosis has been (74, 75). Hepatic venous occlusion has been reported in patients receiving TA who underwent stem cell transplantation (76).

Nafamostat

Nafamostat (6-amidino-2-naphthyl para-guanidinobenzoate) is a synthetic serine protease inhibitor. It has been noted to have a wide range of effects, including anticoagulant, antifibrinolytic, and antiplatelet effects (77, 78). It is not yet FDA-approved for use in the United States. Nafamostat inhibits thrombin, factors Xa and XIIa, kallikrein, plasmin, and complement (20). Nafamostat has been reported to reduce blood loss in cardiac surgery (79–81). Antifibrinolytic activity of nafamostat is by way of inhibiting plasmin activity (81). Fifty percent inhibition of thrombin activity is achieved at in vitro concentrations of 0.01 micromol/L (82). Nafamostat prolongs activated partial thromboplastin time, thrombin time, and prothrombin time (77).

Murase et al. report the dose of nafamostat in patients undergoing cardiopulmonary bypass is 40 mg/h infusion via central venous line, beginning with heparin administration and continuing throughout bypass (81). This group suggests that plasma levels of 1–10 nmol/L are sufficient to inhibit platelet aggregation, fibrinolysis, and coagulation. Blood concentrations achieved with the 40 mg/h infusion of nafamostat in this study were 51 ng/ml at initiation of CPB, 2050 ng/ml during hypothermia, and 166 ng/ml following rewarming after CPB.

Nafamostat undergoes rapid esterase hydrolysis in the blood, followed by glucuronidation of metabolites by the liver (77, 83). Metabolites are mainly excreted in the urine, with a small amount excreted in bile (84). The elimination half-life of nafamostat is approximately 8 minutes (84, 85).

Nafamostat metabolites are reported to inhibit renal cortical collecting tubule sodium conductance, resulting in decrease in potassium excretion with subsequent hyperkalemia (85, 86). Nausea and vomiting are rare (87). Bleeding complications with nafamostat were lower than those observed with heparin or low-molecular-weight heparin in dialysis patients (88). A single case of anaphylactoid reaction to nafamostat is reported (87).

Aprotinin

Aprotinin is a naturally occurring inhibitor of serine protease enzymes that is derived from bovine lung tissue. Mechanism of action of aprotinin is complicated and still incompletely understood, though it inhibits several important serine proteases, including kallikrein, plasmin, thrombin, elastase, trypsin, and chymotrypsin (89). Aprotinin does bind to plasmin and thus prevents the degradation of fibrin and fibrinogen. Aprotinin also may help to preserve platelet function by preventing plasmin-induced degradation of the platelet glycoprotein 1b receptor. The glycoprotein 1b receptor mediates platelet adhesion to vWF. At higher doses, aprotinin also inhibits both tissue and plasma kallikrein. Kallikrein is able to activate and attract neutrophils and cleaves high-molecular weight kininogen to bradykinin and activated high-molecular weight kininogen. Both bradykinin and activated high-molecular weight kininogen stimulate inflammation in leukocytes. Since kallikrein participates in contact activation of Factor XII, inhibition of kallikrein by aprotinin decreases the amount of thrombin generated. A side effect of this action is that aprotinin falsely prolongs both the activated partial thromboplastin time and the activated clotting time, especially in the presence of heparin. As a result of the above drug actions, aprotinin possesses antifibrinolytic, anti-inflammatory, and platelet-sparing effects.

Aprotinin-plasmin binding is approximately 30 times stronger than kallikrein (90, 91), so a higher blood level is necessary to inhibit the activity of kallikrein. Aprotinin concentration is measured in kallikrein inhibitory units (KIU). One KIU is defined as that amount of aprotinin that decreases the activity of two biological kallikrein units by 50% (90). Plasmin is inhibited (ED_{50}) in vitro at a plasma aprotinin concentration of 125 KIU/ml, while in vitro kallikrein inhibition (ED_{50}) occurs at 200–250 KIU/ml. The quoted target concentration of aprotinin is 200 KIU/ml (92–94). Aprotinin is a costly agent administered to adults by a fixed dosage regardless of the patient's weight, gender, and the presence of renal impairment or other disease states. A full dose is a loading dose of 2×10^6 KIU (280 mg) followed by a maintenance infusion of 500 000

KIU/hr (70 mg/hr), with a bypass prime of 2x10^6 KIU (280 mg) (95). The half-dose regimen uses half of each of these doses.

Following intravenous administration of aprotinin, aprotinin plasma levels decline rapidly due to distribution into extracellular fluid with 80–90% of a dose being temporarily stored in proximal renal tubular epithelium prior to elimination (96). Plasma aprotinin concentrations decrease in biphasic manner, with distribution half-life of 0.32–0.5 hours and elimination half-life of 5.35–8.28 hours (97). About 80–85% of aprotinin is metabolized by the kidney with 25–40% of aprotinin being removed by way of glomerular filtration. The elimination half-life of aprotinin is 13.3–14.9 hours in patients with chronic renal insufficiency (98). The pharmacokinetics of aprotinin were determined preoperatively when doses of 500,000 and 1,000,000 KIU were administered as an infusion over 30 minutes to 28 patients. Plasma aprotinin concentrations were measured for 48 hours using a sandwich-enzyme-linked immunosorbent assay. A 3-compartment model was fit to the measured aprotinin concentrations using extended nonlinear least-squares regression (99). They found that plasma aprotinin concentrations at the end of the 30-minute infusion were 147 ± 61 KIU/ml for the 1,000,000-KIU dose, and 60 ± 19 KIU/ml for the 500,000-KIU dose. Elimination clearance of aprotinin was 35.5 ml/min, and volume of distribution at steady state was 26.5 l.

The pharmacokinetics of aprotinin has been well determined before CPB (99) and the elimination clearance has been determined during and after CPB (100). CPB influences the achievement of steady state pharmacokinetics in terms of aprotinin elimination. A study of 14 patients who received full-dose aprotinin during cardiac surgery with CPB found plasma aprotinin concentrations of 234 ± 30 KIU/mL at pre-CPB; 229 ± 35 KIU/mL at CPB + 30; 184 ± 27 KIU/mL at CPB + 90; and 179 ± 22 KIU/mL at end CPB (92). In a study of 30 adult cardiac surgical patients receiving either full- or half-dose aprotinin, the mean plasma aprotinin concentration peaked 5 minutes following initiation of CPB (full 401 ± 92 KIU/ml, half 226 ± 56 KIU/ml) (101). After 60 minutes of CPB, the mean plasma aprotinin concentration was less (full 236 ± 81 KIU/ml, half 160 ± 63 KIU/ml). There was large variation in the aprotinin concentration between patients for both full- and half-dose regimens. There was a statistically significant correlation between aprotinin concentration and patient weight ($r^2 = 0.67$, $p < 0.05$).

A single dose of aprotinin has been reported to reduce the levels of serum cholinesterase by 25% (102), although this result has been questioned (103). Others have reported that aprotinin inhibits the action of serum cholinesterase by 5–16% (104). This effect is probably not significant unless the patient has underlying defects in plasma cholinesterase levels or activity.

Adverse effects associated with aprotinin include the thromboembolic disorders discussed earlier, which have resulted in the current suspension of aprotinin shipment. Other adverse effects have been reported. Skin rash and urticaria have been noted (96, 105). Disseminated intravascular coagulation has been reported in association with aprotinin therapy (106). There is a risk of anaphylaxis due to aprotinin due to its polypeptide structure (96, 107). The risk is highest with re-exposure to the drug; the risk is less than 1% with initial exposure and increases to as much as 10% in cases of repeat administration (105, 108, 109). The risk of anaphylaxis with re-exposure to aprotinin is highest within 6 months of initial administration, with the incidence decreasing thereafter (110). The risk of development of IgG antibodies to aprotinin is highest when patients are exposed to both intravenous aprotinin and aprotinin in topical fibrin glue preparations (111). Additionally, significant antibody response may be elicited by topical fibrin glue preparations containing aprotinin, even when the patient receives no intravenous aprotinin (112). Rapid intravenous administration of aprotinin may release histamine (109). Bronchospasm is rarely noted with aprotinin (113). A single case of acute respiratory distress syndrome associated with aprotinin therapy has been reported (114). The authors suggested that the pulmonary reaction may have been due to an anaphylactoid reaction or to microthrombosis within pulmonary arterioles. There is a concern that aprotinin therapy may lead to a subclinical hypercoagulable state resulting in an increased incidence of postoperative graft thrombosis and other thromboembolic phenomena (115, 116). Aprotinin use with hypothermic circulatory arrest has been associated with diffuse venous thromboembolism in a cardiac surgical patient with factor V Leiden (117).

Aprotinin has been noted to have adverse effects on renal function. Karkouti et al. demonstrated increased incidence of renal dysfunction in patients receiving aprotinin relative to that in patients receiving TA for cardiac surgery (14). Mangano et al. demonstrated increased risk of renal dysfunction following CABG in patients receiving aprotinin (13). However, other studies designed specifically to study renal function have shown no relationship between aprotinin and postoperative renal dysfunction in cardiac surgical patients (109, 118).

CONCLUSION

Antifibrinolytic agents have been increasingly used to reduce perioperative transfusion requirements in various types of major surgery, including cardiac surgery. EACA, TA, and aprotinin have been extensively studied and found effective in reducing transfusion requirements related to these surgeries. However, this effect is not without risk, as demonstrated by the more recent reports related to aprotinin and outcome, which have resulted in the current withdrawal of aprotinin from the market. The risks and benefits of using antifibrinolytic agents in any given situation must be weighed carefully.

References

1. Munoz JJ, Birkmeyer NJ, Birkmeyer JD, O'Connor GT, Dacey LJ: Is epsilon-aminocaproic acid as effective as aprotinin in reducing bleeding with cardiac surgery?: a meta-analysis. Circulation 1999; 99:81–9
2. Goodnough LT, Soegiarso RW, Birkmeyer JD, Welch HG: Economic impact of inappropriate blood transfusion in coronary artery bypass graft surgery. Am. J. Med 1993; 94:509–14
3. Laupacis A, Fergusson D: Drugs to minimize perioperative blood loss in cardiac surgery: meta-analyses using perioperative blood transfusion as the outcome. The International Study of Perioperative Transfusion (ISPOT) Investigators. Anesth Analg 1997; 85:1258–67
4. Levi M, Cromheecke M, de Jonge E, Prins M, de Mol B, Briet E, Buller H: Pharmacological strategies to decrease excessive blood loss in cardiac surgery: a meta-analysis of clinically relevant endpoints. Lancet 1999; 354:1940–7
5. Sedrakyan A, Treasure T, Elefteriades J: Effect of aprotinin on clinical outcomes in coronary artery bypass graft surgery: a systematic review and meta-analysis of randomized clinical trials. J Thorac Cardiovasc Surg 2004; 128:442–8
6. Carless P, Moxey A, Stokes B, Henry D: Are antifibrinolytic drugs equivalent in reducing blood loss and transfusion in cardiac surgery? A meta-analysis of randomized head-to-head trials. BMC Cardiovasc Disord 2005; 5:19
7. Brown JR, Birkmeyer NJ, O'Connor GT: Meta-analysis comparing the effectiveness and adverse outcomes of antifibrinolytic agents in cardiac surgery. Circulation 2007; 115:2801–13
8. Royston D, Bidstrup BP, Taylor KM, Sapsford RN: Effect of aprotinin on need for blood transfusion after repeat open-heart surgery. Lancet 1987; 2:1289–91
9. Henry D, Moxey A, Carless P, O'Connell D, McClelland B, Henderson K, Sly K, Laupacis A, Fergusson D: Anti-fibrinolytic use for minimising perioperative allogeneic blood transfusion. Cochrane Database Syst Rev 2001; 4:CD001886
10. Carless P, Moxey A, Stokes B, Henry D: Are antifibrinolytic drugs equivalent in reducing blood loss and transfusion in cardiac surgery? A meta-analysis of randomized head-to-head trials. BMC Cardiovasc Disord 2005; 5:1–12

11. Ozier Y, Schlumberger S: Pharmacological approaches to reducing blood loss and transfusions in the surgical patient. Can J Anaesth 2006; 53(6 Suppl): S21–9
12. Sindet-Pedersen S, Ramstrom G, Bernvil S, Blomback M: Hemostatic effect of tranexamic acid mouthwash in anticoagulant-treated patients undergoing oral surgery. New Engl J Med 1989; 320:840–843
13. Mangano DT, Tudor IC, Dietzel C; Multicenter Study of Perioperative Ischemia Research Group; Ischemia Research and Education Foundation.: The risk associated with aprotinin in cardiac surgery. N Engl J Med 2006; 354:353–65
14. Karkouti K, Beattie W, Dattilo K, et al.: A propensity score case-control comparison of aprotinin and tranexamic acid in high-transfusion-risk cardiac surgery. Transfusion 2006; 46:327–38
15. FDA: FDA requests marketing suspension of Trasylol. FDA News, November 5, 2007
16. Casati V, Guzzon D, Oppizzi M, et al.: Hemostatic effects of aprotinin, tranexamic acid and epsilon-aminocaproic acid in primary cardiac surgery. Ann Thorac Surg 1999; 68:2252–6; discussion 2256–7
17. Kristeller JL, Stahl RF, Roslund BP, Roke-Thomas M: Aprotinin use in cardiac surgery patients at low risk for requiring blood transfusion. Pharmacotherapy 2007; 27:988–94
18. Dalmau A, Sabate A, Acosta F, et al.: Tranexamic acid reduces red cell transfusion better than epsilon-aminocaproic acid or placebo in liver transplantation. Anesth Analg 2000; 91:29–34
19. Camarasa M, Olle G, Serra-Prat M, et al.: Efficacy of aminocaproic, tranexamic acids in the control of bleeding during total knee replacement: a randomized clinical trial. Br J Anaesth 2006; 96:576–82
20. Mahdy AM, Webster NR: Perioperative systemic haemostatic agents. Br J Anaesth 2004; 93:842–58
21. Ray MJ, O'Brien MF: Comparison of epsilon-aminocaproic acid and low-dose aprotinin in cardiopulmonary bypass: efficiency, safety and cost. Ann Thorac Surg 2001; 71:838–43
22. Eaton MP, Deeb GM: Aprotinin versus epsilon-aminocaproic acid for aortic surgery using deep hypothermic circulatory arrest. J Cardiothorac Vasc Anesth 1998; 12:548–52
23. Mazer D, Fergusson D, Hebert P, et al.: Incidence of massive bleeding in a blinded randomized controlled trial of antifibrinolytic drugs in high risk cardiac surgery [abstract]. Anesth Analg 2006; 102:SCA95

24. Butterworth J, James RL, Lin Y, Prielipp RC, Hudspeth AS: Pharmacokinetics of epsilon-aminocaproic acid in patients undergoing aortocoronary bypass surgery. Anesthesiology 1999; 90:1624–35
25. Fleeger C: USAN and the USP dictionary of drug names. Rockville, MD: U. S. Pharmacopeial Convention, Inc., 1994
26. Product Information: Amicar®, aminocaproic acid. Florence, KY: Xanodyne Pharmacal, Inc.; 2001
27. Fish SS, Pancorbo S, Berkseth R: Pharmacokinetics of epsilon-aminocaproic acid during peritoneal dialysis. J Neurosurg 1981; 54:736–9
28. Pagliaro LA, Benet LZ: Critical compilation of terminal half-lives, percent excreted unchanged, and changes of half-life in renal and hepatic dysfunction for studies in humans with references. J Pharmacokinet Biopharm 1975; 3:333–83
29. Frederiksen MC, Bowsher DJ, Ruo TI, et al.: Kinetics of epsilon-aminocaproic acid distribution, elimination, and antifibrinolytic effects in normal subjects. Clin Pharmacol Ther 1984; 35:387–93
30. Porte RJ, Leebeek FW: Pharmacological strategies to decrease transfusion requirements in patients undergoing surgery. Drugs 2002; 62:2193–211
31. Villarreal O: Systemic dermatitis with eosinophilia due to epsilon-aminocaproic acid. Contact Dermatitis 1999; 40:114
32. Chakrabarti A, Collett KA: Purpuric rash due to epsilon-aminocaproic acid. Br Med J 1980; 281:197–8
33. Perazella MA, Biswas P: Acute hyperkalemia associated with intravenous epsilon-aminocaproic acid therapy. Am J Kidney Dis 1999; 33:782–5
34. Frank MM, Sergent JS, Kane MA, Alling DW: Epsilon aminocaproic acid therapy of hereditary angioneurotic edema. A double-blind study. N Engl J Med 1972; 286:808–12
35. Shaw MD, Miller JD: Letter: Epsilon-aminocaproic acid and subarachnoid haemorrhage. Lancet 1974; 2:847–8
36. Lane RJ, McLelland NJ, Martin AM, Mastaglia FL: Epsilon aminocaproic acid (EACA) myopathy. Postgrad Med J 1979; 55:282–5
37. Morris CD, Jacobs P, Berman PA, Rutherfoord GS: Epsilon-aminocaproic acid-induced myopathy. A case report. S Afr Med J 1983; 64:363–6
38. Biswas CK, Milligan DA, Agte SD, Kenward DH, Tilley PJ: Acute renal failure and myopathy after treatment with aminocaproic acid. Br Med J 1980; 281:115–6
39. Rizza RA, Sclonick S, Conley CL: Myoglobinuria following aminocaproic acid administration. JAMA 1976; 236:1845–6

40. Rabinovici R, Heyman A, Kluger Y, Shinar E: Convulsions induced by aminocaproic acid infusion. DICP 1989; 23:780–1
41. Feffer SE, Parray HR, Westring DW: Seizure after infusion of aminocaproic acid. JAMA 1978; 240:2468
42. Pitts TO, Spero JA, Bontempo FA, Greenberg A: Acute renal failure due to high-grade obstruction following therapy with epsilon-aminocaproic acid. Am J Kidney Dis 1986; 8:441–4
43. Lindgardh G, Andersson L: Clot retention in the kidneys as a probable cause of anuria during treatment of haematuria with epsilon-aminocaproic acid. Acta Med Scand 1966; 180:469–73
44. Charytan C, Purtilo D: Glomerular capillary thrombosis and acute renal failure after epsilon-amino caproic acid therapy. N Engl J Med 1969; 280:1102–4
45. Stafford-Smith M, Phillips-Bute B, Reddan DN, Black J, Newman MF: The association of epsilon-aminocaproic acid with postoperative decrease in creatinine clearance in 1502 coronary bypass patients. Anesth Analg 2000; 91:1085–90
46. Swartz C, Onesti G, Ramirez O, Shah N, Brest AN: Cardiac and renal hemodynamic effects of the antifibrinolytic agent, epsilon aminocaproic acid. Curr Ther Res Clin Exp 1966; 8:336–42
47. Burchiel KJ, Schmer G: A method for monitoring antifibrinolytic therapy in patients with ruptured intracranial aneurysms. J Neurosurg 1981; 54:12–5
48. Hoffman EP, Koo AH: Cerebral thrombosis associated with Amicar therapy. Radiology 1979; 131:687–9
49. Achiron A, Gornish M, Melamed E: Cerebral sinus thrombosis as a potential hazard of antifibrinolytic treatment in menorrhagia. Stroke 1990; 21:817–9
50. Tubbs RR, Benjamin SP, Dohn DE: Recurrent subarachnoid hemorrhage associated with aminocaproic acid therapy and acute renal artery thrombosis. Case report. J Neurosurg 1979; 51:94–7
51. Glick R, Green D, Ts'ao C, Witt WA, Yu AT, Raimondi AJ: High dose epsilon-aminocaproic acid prolongs the bleeding time and increases rebleeding and intraoperative hemorrhage in patients with subarachnoid hemorrhage. Neurosurgery 1981; 9:398–401
52. Cooper JR, Jr., Abrams J, Frazier OH, et al.: Fatal pulmonary microthrombi during surgical therapy for end-stage heart failure: possible association with antifibrinolytic therapy. J Thorac Cardiovasc Surg 2006; 131:963–8
53. Royston D: Blood-sparing drugs: aprotinin, tranexamic acid, and epsilon-aminocaproic acid. Int Anesthesiol Clin 1995; 33:155–179
54. Karski J, Dowd N, Joiner R, et al.: The effect of three different doses of tranexamic acid on blood loss after cardiac surgery with mild

systemic hypothermia (32 degrees C). J Cardiothorac Vasc Anesth 1998; 12:642–6

55. Horrow J, Van Riper D, Strong M, Grunewald K, Parmet J: The dose-response relationship of tranexamic acid. Anesthesiology 1995; 82:383–392
56. Andersson L, Nilsoon I, Colleen S, et al.: Role of urokinase and tissue activator in sustaining bleeding and the management thereof with EACA and AMCA. Ann N YAcad Sci 1968; 146:642–658
57. Soslau G, Horrow J, Brodsky I: Effect of tranexamic acid on platelet ADP during extracorporeal circulation. Am J Hematol 1991; 38:113–9
58. Pilbrant A, Schannong M, Vessman J: Pharmacokinetics and bioavailability of tranexamic acid. Eur J Clin Pharmacol 1981; 20:65–72
59. Nilsson I: Clinical pharmacology of aminocaproic and tranexamic acids. J Clin Pathol 1980; 33 (suppl 14):41–7
60. Andersson L, Eriksson O, Hedlund P, Kjellman H, Lindqvist B: Special considerations with regard to the dosage of tranexamic acid in patients with chronic renal diseases. Urol Res 1978; 6:83–8
61. Benoni G, Bjorkman S, Fredin H: Application of pharmacokinetic data from healthy volunteers for the predication of plasma concentrations of tranexamic acid in surgical patients. Clin Drug Invest 1995; 10:280–7
62. Puigdellivol E, Carral ME, Moreno J, Pla-Delfina JM, Jane F: Pharmacokinetics and absolute bioavailability of intramuscular tranexamic acid in man. Int J Clin Pharmacol Ther Toxicol 1985; 23:298–301
63. Verstraete M: Clinical application of inhibitors of fibrinolysis. Drugs 1985; 29:236–61
64. Dowd NP, Karski JM, Cheng DC, et al.: Pharmacokinetics of tranexamic acid during cardiopulmonary bypass. Anesthesiology 2002; 97:390–9
65. Product Information: Cyklokapron®, trenexamic acid. Kalamazoo, MI: Pharmacia and Upjohn Company; 2001
66. Fodstad H, Forssell A, Liliequist B, Schannong M: Antifibrinolysis with tranexamic acid in aneurysmal subarachnoid hemorrhage: a consecutive controlled clinical trial. Neurosurgery 1981; 8:158–65
67. Vermeulen M, Lindsay KW, Murray GD, et al.: Antifibrinolytic treatment in subarachnoid hemorrhage. N Engl J Med 1984; 311:432–7
68. Munch EP, Weeke B: Non-hereditary angioedema treated with tranexamic acid. A 6-month placebo controlled trial with follow-up 4 years later. Allergy 1985; 40:92–7

69. Agnelli G, Gresele P, De Cunto M, Gallai V, Nenci GG: Tranexamic acid, intrauterine contraceptive devices and fatal cerebral arterial thrombosis. Case report. Br J Obstet Gynaecol 1982; 89:681–2
70. Snir M, Axer-Siegel R, Buckman G, Yassur Y: Central venous stasis retinopathy following the use of tranexamic acid. Retina 1990; 10:181–4
71. Adams HP, Jr.: Current status of antifibrinolytic therapy for treatment of patients with aneurysmal subarachnoid hemorrhage. Stroke 1982; 13:256–9
72. Woo KS, Tse LK, Woo JL, Vallance-Owen J: Massive pulmonary thromboembolism after tranexamic acid antifibrinolytic therapy. Br J Clin Pract 1989; 43:465–6
73. Davies D, Howell DA: Tranexamic acid and arterial thrombosis. Lancet 1977; 1:49
74. Koo JR, Lee YK, Kim YS, Cho WY, Kim HK, Won NH: Acute renal cortical necrosis caused by an antifibrinolytic drug (tranexamic acid). Nephrol Dial Transplant 1999; 14:750–2
75. Levin MD, Betjes MG, TH VdK, Wenberg BL, Leebeek FW: Acute renal cortex necrosis caused by arterial thrombosis during treatment for acute promyelocytic leukemia. Haematologica 2003; 88:ECR21
76. Mori T, Aisa Y, Shimizu T, et al.: Hepatic veno-occlusive disease after tranexamic acid administration in patients undergoing allogeneic hematopoietic stem cell transplantation. Am J Hematol 2007; 82:838–9
77. Matsuo T, Kario K, Nakao K, Yamada T, Matsuo M: Anticoagulation with nafamostat mesilate, a synthetic protease inhibitor, in hemodialysis patients with a bleeding risk. Haemostasis 1993; 23:135–41
78. Shimada M, Matsumata T, Shirabe K, Kamakura T, Taketomi A, Sugimachi K: Effect of nafamostat mesilate on coagulation and fibrinolysis in hepatic resection. J Am Coll Surg 1994; 178:498–502
79. Sato T, Tanaka K, Kondo C, et al.: Nafamostat mesilate administration during cardiopulmonary bypass decreases postoperative bleeding after cardiac surgery. ASAIO Trans 1991; 37:M194–5
80. Tanaka K, Kondo C, Takagi K, et al.: Effects of nafamostat mesilate on platelets and coagulofibrinolysis during cardiopulmonary bypass surgery. ASAIO J 1993; 39:M545–9
81. Murase M, Usui A, Tomita Y, Maeda M, Koyama T, Abe T: Nafamostat mesilate reduces blood loss during open heart surgery. Circulation 1993; 88:II432–6
82. Hu ZJ, Iwama H, Suzuki R, Kobayashi S, Akutsu I: Time course of activated coagulation time at various sites during continuous

haemodiafiltration using nafamostat mesilate. Intensive Care Med 1999; 25:524–7
83. Usui A, Hiroura M, Kawamura M, et al.: Nafamostat mesilate reduces blood-foreign surface reactions similar to biocompatible materials. Ann Thorac Surg 1996; 62:1404–11
84. Nagaya M, Futamura M, Kato J, Niimi N, Fukuta S: Application of a new anticoagulant (Nafamostat Mesilate) to control hemorrhagic complications during extracorporeal membrane oxygenation—a preliminary report. J Pediatr Surg 1997; 32:531–5
85. Iwama H, Nakane M, Ohmori S, et al.: Nafamostat mesilate, a kallikrein inhibitor, prevents pain on injection with propofol. Br J Anaesth 1998; 81:963–4
86. Kitagawa H, Chang H, Fujita T: Hyperkalemia due to nafamostat mesylate. N Engl J Med 1995; 332:687
87. Maruyama H, Miyakawa Y, Gejyo F, Arakawa M: Anaphylactoid reaction induced by nafamostat mesilate in a hemodialysis patient. Nephron 1996; 74:468–9
88. Kubota T, Miyata A, Maeda A, Hirota K, Koizumi S, Ohba H: Continuous haemodiafiltration during and after cardiopulmonary bypass in renal failure patients. Can J Anaesth 1997; 44:1182–6
89. Hess PJ, Jr.: Systemic inflammatory response to coronary artery bypass graft surgery. Am J Health Syst Pharm 2005; 62:S6–9
90. Wiman B: On the reaction of plasmin or plasmin-streptokinase complex with aprotinin or alpha 2-antiplasmin. Thromb Res 1980; 17:143–152
91. Nakahara M: Inhibitory effect of aprotinin and gabexate mesilate on human plasma kallikrein. Arzneimittel-Forschung 1983; 33:969–971
92. Bennett-Guerrero E, Sorohan JG, Howell ST, et al.: Maintenance of therapeutic plasma aprotinin levels during prolonged cardiopulmonary bypass using a large-dose regimen. Anesth Analg 1996; 83:1189–92
93. Dietrich W, Spannagl M, Jochum M, et al.: Influence of high-dose aprotinin treatment on blood loss and coagulation patterns in patients undergoing myocardial revascularization. Anesthesiology 1990; 73:1119–26
94. Royston D: High-dose aprotinin therapy: a review of the first five years' experience. J. Cardiothorac Vasc Anesth 1992; 6:76–100
95. Royston D, von Kier S: Reduced haemostatic factor transfusion using heparinase-modified thrombelastography during cardiopulmonary bypass. Br J Anaesth 2001; 86:575–8
96. Hardy JF, Desroches J: Natural and synthetic antifibrinolytics in cardiac surgery. Can J Anaesth 1992; 39:353–65

97. Peters DC, Noble S: Aprotinin: an update of its pharmacology and therapeutic use in open heart surgery and coronary artery bypass surgery. Drugs 1999; 57:233–60
98. Muller FO, Schall R, Hundt HK, et al.: Pharmacokinetics of aprotinin in two patients with chronic renal impairment. Br J Clin Pharmacol 1996; 41:619–20
99. Levy JH, Bailey JM, Salmenpera M: Pharmacokinetics of aprotinin in preoperative cardiac surgical patients. Anesthesiology 1994; 80:1013–8
100. O'Connor CJ, Brown DV, Avramov M, Barnes S, O'Connor HN, Tuman KJ: The impact of renal dysfunction on aprotinin pharmacokinetics during cardiopulmonary bypass. Anesth Analg 1999; 89:1101–7
101. Beath SM, Nuttall GA, Fass DN, Oliver WC, Jr., Ereth MH, Oyen LJ: Plasma aprotinin concentrations during cardiac surgery: full-versus half-dose regimens. Anesth Analg 2000; 91:257–64
102. Chasapakis G, Augustaki O, Kekis N, et al.: The influence of the kallikrein-trypsin inactivator Trasylol on the serum cholinesterase. Br J Anaesth 1968; 40:456–8
103. Ambrus JL, Wilkens H, Ambrus CM, Back N: Effect of the protease inhibitor Trasylol on cholinesterase levels and on susceptibility to succinylcholine. Res Commun Chem Pathol Pharmacol 1970; 1:141–8
104. Doenicke A, Gesing H, Krumey I, Schmidinger S: Influence of aprotinin (Trasylol) on the action of suxamethonium. Br J Anaesth 1970; 42:948–60
105. Freeman JG, Turner GA, Venables CW, Latner AL: Serial use of aprotinin and incidence of allergic reactions. Curr Med Res Opin 1983; 8:559–61
106. Milne AA, Drummond GB, Paterson DA, Murphy WG, Ruckley CV: Disseminated intravascular coagulation after aortic aneurysm repair, intraoperative salvage autotransfusion, and aprotinin. Lancet 1994; 344:470–1
107. Dietrich W, Ebell A, Busley R, Boulesteix AL: Aprotinin and anaphylaxis: analysis of 12,403 exposures to aprotinin in cardiac surgery. Ann Thorac Surg 2007; 84:1144–50
108. Ong BC, Tan SS, Tan YS: Anaphylactic reaction to aprotinin. Anaesth Intensive Care 1999; 27:538
109. Blauhut B, Gross C, Necek S, Doran JE, Spath P, Lundsgaard-Hansen P: Effects of high-dose aprotinin on blood loss, platelet function, fibrinolysis, complement, and renal function after cardiopulmonary bypass. J Thorac Cardiovasc Surg 1991; 101:958–67

110. Dietrich W: Incidence of hypersensitivity reactions. Ann Thorac Surg 1998; 65:S60–4; discussion S74–6
111. Scheule AM, Beierlein W, Wendel HP, Jurmann MJ, Eckstein FS, Ziemer G: Aprotinin in fibrin tissue adhesives induces specific antibody response and increases antibody response of high-dose intravenous application. J Thorac Cardiovasc Surg 1999; 118:348–53
112. Scheule AM, Beierlein W, Wendel HP, Eckstein FS, Heinemann MK, Ziemer G: Fibrin sealant, aprotinin, and immune response in children undergoing operations for congenital heart disease. J Thorac Cardiovasc Surg 1998; 115:883–9
113. Ceriana P, Maurelli M, Locatelli A, Bianchi T, Maccario R, De Amici M: Anaphylactic reaction to aprotinin. J Cardiothorac Vasc Anesth 1995; 9:477–8
114. Vucicevic Z, Suskovic T: Acute respiratory distress syndrome after aprotinin infusion. Ann Pharmacother 1997; 31:429–32
115. Cosgrove Dr, Heric B, Lytle B, et al.: Aprotinin therapy for reoperative myocardial revascularization: a placebo-controlled study. Ann Thorac Surg 1992; 54:1031–6
116. Okita Y, Takamoto S, Ando M, Morota T, Yamaki F, Kawashima Y: Is use of aprotinin safe with deep hypothermic circulatory arrest in aortic surgery? Investigations on blood coagulation. Circulation 1996; 94:II177–81
117. Shore-Lesserson L, Reich DL: A case of severe diffuse venous thromboembolism associated with aprotinin and hypothermic circulatory arrest in a cardiac surgical patient with factor V Leiden. Anesthesiology 2006; 105:219–21
118. Schweizer A, Hohn L, Morel DR, Kalangos A, Licker M: Aprotinin does not impair renal haemodynamics and function after cardiac surgery. Br J Anaesth 2000; 84:16–22

William J. Mauermann, MD
Roxann D. Barnes, MD

9 Diuretics and Cardiovascular Anesthesia

INTRODUCTION

Diuretics continue to be one of the pharmacologic pillars by which patients with cardiovascular disease are managed. They are often a standard part of the medical regimen for patients with hypertension (1) and are used to control volume status in patients with congestive heart failure secondary to valvular or ventricular dysfunction (2).

Diuretics are also extensively used in the perioperative period, especially in patients undergoing cardiac and major vascular surgery. It is well known that cardiac surgery with extracorporeal circulation induces a systemic inflammatory response (3, 4). As part of this response, a capillary leak syndrome commonly results with third spacing of fluid into both the peripheral tissues and the pulmonary bed (5). Diuresis may be needed to decrease lung water such that patients will tolerate tracheal extubation. Diuretics are also commonly used with the goal of either protecting the kidneys from perioperative insults or managing volume and electrolyte status when significant renal injury has occurred.

Many patients presenting for cardiac surgery will already be using diuretics and nearly all patients undergoing cardiac surgery will encounter these drugs at some point during the perioperative period. Thus, it is important that cardiac anesthesiologists have an understanding of these commonly used medications. This chapter will provide a brief review of renal function and the principles of diuretics. We will discuss pertinent aspects of the pharmacokinetics and pharmacodynamics

Advances in Cardiovascular Pharmacology, edited by Philippe R. Housmans, MD, PhD and Gregory A. Nuttall, M.D.

of the various classes of diuretics, classifying these medications by their mechanism of action. We will also discuss the clinical relevance and use of each of the diuretics classes. Lastly, we will review the literature surrounding diuretic use in the perioperative period with particular attention to the potential benefits and risks to postoperative renal function.

RENAL FUNCTION AND PRINCIPLES OF DIURETIC USE

The kidneys, or more accurately, the nephrons, are essential for maintaining homeostatic volume states as well as regulating acid-base and electrolyte balance. Large amounts of plasma are filtered into the renal tubule. Modification of the urine content then occurs by reabsorbing substances that need to be conserved and allowing waste products to be excreted. Certain substances may be actively reabsorbed or excreted according the current needs of the organism. When it comes to reabsorbing salt and water, the kidney is extremely effective. Healthy humans filter approximately 180 liters of plasma and 25,000 mEq of sodium chloride (NaCl) a day with 99% of this filtered load being reabsorbed (6, 7). This efficient reclamation of filtered salt and water comes at an enormous energy expense. While the kidneys make up 0.5% of the body's weight, they are responsible for 7% of total-body oxygen consumption.

Diuretics are intuitively thought of as agents that increase the volume and rate of urine excretion. In reality they must also increase the amount of sodium (Na^+) that is excreted in order to be useful. Sodium is the major determinant of serum osmolality and thus, intravascular fluid volume. In the kidney, solutes may pass from the renal tubule into the tubular cells or interstitial space by active or passive mechanisms. However, the movement of water out the renal tubule is always passive and in relation to the osmotic gradient created by the reabsorption of solutes, with NaCl being the most important. To decrease extracellular water, urinary excretion of water must be increased and this must occur with a concomitant increase in NaCl excretion. Thus, the goal of diuretic therapy is really natriuresis (increase in Na^+ excretion) with water passively following.

The nephron is the basic urine-forming unit of the kidney. At the proximal aspect of the nephron is the glomerulus with its filtering mechanism. Attached to the glomerulus is the renal tubule which is responsible for modification of the urine contents. Physiologists have now divided the nephron into 14 segments based on function and cellular morphology (8), but for simplicity, the tubule elements can still be thought of as 4 segments: the proximal tubule, the Loop of Henle, the distal tubule, and the collecting ducts. Salt, and thus water, move out of the renal tubule and into the tubule cells across the tubule cell's apical membrane (membrane between the cell and renal tubule). The exact mechanisms of transport vary between the segments but are always dependent on an electrochemical gradient that favors Na^+ movement. This gradient is created by the Na^+, K^+-ATPase found exclusively in the basolateral membrane (cell membrane opposite to the apical membrane). The Na^+, K^+-ATPase pump serves to move Na^+ out of the cell and into the blood and moves K^+ into the cell. As the Na^+ concentration in the cell is now low, the chemical gradient favors the flux of Na^+ from the renal tubule into the tubule cell. The differing mechanisms of Na^+ transport in the nephron segments provide specific targets for the actions of diuretics and account for their relatively isolated sites of action (Figure 9-1).

The proximal tubule reabsorbs approximately 65% of the filtered salt and water load. Na^+ is transported with bicarbonate ($HCO3^-$) in the early portion and primarily with chloride ions (Cl^-) in the latter portions. The Loop of Henle is responsible for about 25% of salt and 15% of water reabsorption. Here, 1 Na^+ is transported into the cell with 1 potassium (K^+) and two Cl^- via a symporter. A Na^+-H^+ (hydrogen ion) antiporter in the apical membrane is also present in both of these segments. These two segments are relatively "load dependent" in that they reclaim Na^+ in relative proportion to the amount delivered (6). The dis-

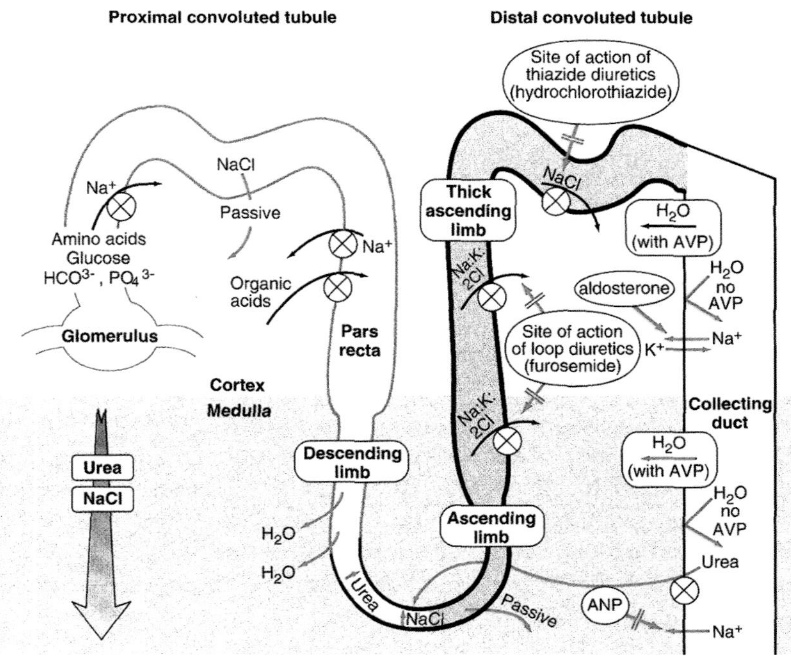

FIGURE 9-1. From Harrison's Principles of Internal Medicine, 16th Edition, © 2005.

tal tubule (via a Na^+-Cl^- symporter) and the collecting ducts (Na^+ absorption, K^+ excretion) combine to reclaim ~7% of the filtered Na^+ load. The distal tubule is impermeable to water. In the collecting ducts 8–17% of the filtered water is passively reabsorbed depending on the plasma concentration of antidiuretic hormone.

CLASSES OF DIURETICS

Inhibitors of Carbonic Anhydrase

First discovered in the 1950's, acetazolamide is the prototypical agent in this class (6). In the proximal tubule, a Na^+-H^+ exchanger transports H^+ into the tubular lumen in exchange for Na^+. The H^+ combines with the filtered HCO_3^- to form H_2CO_3 which dissociates to CO_2 and H_20 (9). The decomposition of H_2CO_3 to CO_2 and water is usually slow; however, carbonic anhydrase (CA) found in the luminal and basolateral membranes of the proximal renal tubules (7) accelerates this reaction significantly. CO_2 then diffuses into the epithelial cells where it combines with H_20 to form H_2CO_3—a reaction induced by cytoplasmic CA. As the proton concentration in the epithelial cell is low, H_2CO_3 dissociates quickly into H^+ and HCO_3^-. A Na^+-HCO_3^- symporter then transports $NaHCO_3$ into the interstitial space (9). The net effect is the transfer of $NaHCO_3$ from the tubule lumen to the interstitial space, with water passively following. Thus, CA is critically important in the reabsorption of $NaHCO_3$ and in acid secretion. Inhibition of CA prevents reabsorption of HCO_3^- in the proximal tubule and leads to increased $NaHCO_3$, chloride, and phosphorus excretion (7). These effects of carbonic anhydrase inhibitors on the excretion of HCO_3^- are self limited as the resulting metabolic acidosis decreases the amount of filtered HCO_3^- delivered to the tubules.

While carbonic anhydrase inhibitors enjoyed early enthusiasm as diuretics after their initial discovery, their clinical usefulness is limited. The inhibition of sodium ion reabsorption is limited to the proximal tubule and is overcome by sodium reabsorption in the more distal tubule segments as these segments see an increased solute delivery (7). In addition, by increasing the delivery of solutes to the macula densa, tubuloglomerular feedback leads to increased afferent arteriolar resistance, thus reducing glomerular filtration rate (GFR) and renal blood flow (RBF). Nonetheless, at least one study has shown acetazolamide to be an effective diuretic when given in combination with diuretics that block Na^+ resorption in the distal tubules (10).

Acetazolamide may be helpful in preventing and/or treating high altitude mountain sickness (11) and in the treatment of patients with familial periodic paralysis (12). It also may be useful for treating metabolic alkalosis caused by diuretic induced H^+ excretion. Orally administered azetazolamide (200–375 mg/day) has a half-life of 6–9 hours and is primarily renally excreted.

Osmotic Diuretics

Of the four agents in this class (mannitol, glycerin, isosorbide, and urea), mannitol is the most commonly utilized in clinical practice. Oral absorption is poor, and thus it must be given intravenously (13). It is available in concentrations of 5–25% and the dose ranges from 0.5–3 gms/kg/24-hour period (14).

Mannitol has multiple actions and effects, most of which are mediated by its ability to increase the osmolality of plasma and renal tubular fluid. Mannitol is frequently used to decrease intracranial pressure (15) and intraocular pressure (16). An osmotic increase in extracellular fluid volume decreases blood viscosity and has important rheologic effects. Mannitol also has significant effects on renal function and perfusion, and its extensive use in cardiac and vascular surgery makes it important to the anesthesiologist.

The site of action of the osmotic diuretics in the kidney has been controversial. Early evidence pointed to the proximal tubule as the primary site of action. Osmotic diuretics are nonresorbable solutes and it was suspected that they limited the osmotic movement of water into the interstitial space from the renal tubule. By confining free water to the tubular lumen, Na^+ concentration was reduced and Na^+ reabsorption was blunted or ceased (9). More recent evidence suggests the Loop of Henle to be the primary site of action. Oncotic mediated increases in extracellular fluid volume and decreased blood viscosity lead to inhibition of renin release. Subsequently, RBF increases and washes NaCl and urea from the renal medulla, thus decreasing the oncotic gradient that favors free water movement from the tubule to the interstitial space (9). Increased prostaglandin production, with its resultant vasodilation of the renal vasculature, also may contribute to an increase in RBF (17).

Mannitol has been proposed to have renal protective effects. Given in adequate doses, it reliably increases urine output in patients with adequate renal function and renal perfusion. Hematuria often occurs during cardiac surgery secondary to anticoagulation, and myoglobinuria occurs secondary to hemolysis caused by extracorporeal circulation. Hemoglobin and especially myoglobin are known to be nephrotoxic (14, 18). It has been proposed that by increasing renal tubular flow rates, these nephrotoxins may be diluted and/or more efficiently removed. Augmented RBF by dilation of the afferent arteriole may be protective. By increasing oncotic pressure, mannitol potentially reduces swelling of renal elements due to the inflammatory reaction caused by cardiopulmonary bypass

(19). Mannitol is a free radical scavenger with antioxidant properties (20) that have been proposed to confer end organ protection.

Loop Diuretics

Furosemide, ethacrynic acid, bumetanide, and torsemide are the loop diuretics in common clinical use. These agents are the most consistently efficacious diuretics due to their site of action in the thick ascending limb of the Loop of Henle. The thick ascending limb absorbs approximately 25% of the filtered Na^+ load, and renal tubule cells distal to this point lack the capacity to reabsorb a significantly increased Na^+ load (9). This strategic site of action makes the loop diuretics very effective.

Loop diuretics are highly protein-bound and reach the Loop of Henle by active secretion from the blood into the proximal renal tubule (21). They exert their effects by blocking the Na-K-2Cl transporter (22, 23). The loop diuretics are anions with a high affinity for the Na-K-2Cl transporter and are capable of nearly complete blockade of this transporter. The net effect on urine excretion is a substantial increase in Na^+ and Cl^- excretion (up to 25% of the filtered load (6)), and an increase in K^+, H^+, Ca^{2+} and Mg^{2+} excretion (Table 9–1). In healthy adults, an intravenous dose of 40 mg of furosemide or 1 mg of bumetanide causes a maximal response that results in the excretion of 200–250 mEq of sodium in 3–4 liters of urine over 3–4 hours (24). The sodium content of the resulting urine approximates that of 0.5% normal saline (25).

If intravascular volume is adequate, the loop diuretics generally increase renal blood flow. This effect may be partially mediated by prostaglandins and is attenuated by nonsteroidal anti-inflammatory drugs (7, 9). Loop diuretics, especially furosemide, also increase venous compliance and decrease systemic vascular resistance acutely (26). The vascular effects are likely prostaglandin mediated. These effects are important in patients with decompensated heart failure, as a decrease in afterload may benefit the failing left ventricle and the increase in venous capacitance often confers at least partial relief to patients suffering from pulmonary edema even before diuresis has occurred. While these agents appear to have relaxing properties on the vascular system, they also are strong stimulators of renin and aldosterone production (27). This effect occurs independently of, but may be augmented by, intravascular hypovolemia and resultant baroreceptor activity (6). As a result of the relatively short half-life of the loop diuretics (approximately 1 hour for bumetanide, 1.5–2 hours for furosemide (25)) a rebound in salt and water conservation may occur after plasma levels of the diuretic have fallen to ineffective levels but while renin and aldosterone levels remain high (28). While this is of little consequence in the operating room where patients' fluid intake can be carefully controlled, it may be clinically very

TABLE 9–1.

	Cations					Anions			Uric Acid		Renal Hemodynamics			
	Na^+	K^+	H^+†	Ca^{2+}	Mg^{2+}	Cl^-	HCO_3^-	$H_2PO_4^-$	Acute	Chronic	RBF	GFR	FF	TGF
Inhibitors of carbonic anhydrase (primary site of action is proximal tubule)	+	++	–	NC	V	(+)	++	++	I	–	–	–	NC	+
Osmotic diruetics (primary site of action loop of Henle)	++	+	I	+	++	+	+	+	+	I	+	NC	–	I
Inhibitors of Na^+–K^+–$2Cl^-$ symport (primary site of action is thick, descending limb)	++	++	+	++	++	++	+‡	+‡	+	–	V (+)	NC	V(–)	–
Inhibitors of Na^+–$2Cl^-$ symport (primary site of action is distal convoluted tubule)	+	++	+	V(–)	V(+)	+	+‡	+‡	+	–	NC	V(–)	V(–)	NC
Inhibitors of renal epithelial sodium channels (primary site of action is late distal tubule and collecting duct)	+	–	–	–	–	+	(+)	NC	I	–	NC	NC	NC	NC
Antagonists of mineralocorticoid receptors (primary site of action is late distal tubule and collecting duct)	+	–	–	I	–	+	(+)	I	I	–	NC	NC	NC	NC

Except for uric acid, changes are for acute effects of diruretics in the absence of significant volume depletion, which would trigger complex physiological adjustments; ++, +, (+), –, NC, V, V(+), V(–), and I indicate marked increase, mild to moderate increase, slight increase, decrease, no change, variable effect, variable increase, variable decrease, and insufficient data, respectively. For cations and anions, the indicated effects refer to absolute changes in fractional excretion. RBF, renal blood flow; GFR, glomerular filtration rate; FF, filtration fraction; TGF, tubuloglomerular feedback.

†H^+, titratable acid and NH_4^+.

‡In general, these effects are restricted to those individual agents that inhibit carbonic anhydrase. However, there are notable exceptions in which symport inhibitors: increase bicarbonate and phosphate (e.g., metolazone, bumetanide) (see Puschett and Winaver, 1992).

important in the awake patient recovering on the hospital ward who is given free access to salt-containing foods and free water.

A logical approach to combating the problem of peaks and troughs in plasma levels of loop diuretics and the resultant rebound in salt and water retention secondary to elevated renin and aldosterone levels would be a continuous infusion of loop diuretics. Copeland and colleagues studied the effects of dosing 0.3 mg/kg of furosemide twice on postoperative day one (total daily dose of 0.6 mg/kg) or delivering an infusion of 0.05 mg/kg/hr of furosemide for 12 hours (total dose 0.6 mg/kg) (29). The authors found no differences between the groups in the total amounts of urine, sodium, or potassium excreted during the 12-hour study period. In 1994, Martin and Danziger reviewed the available literature on the continuous infusion of loop diuretics in critically ill patients (30). These authors concluded that while there is a relative paucity of literature on this subject, the continuous infusion of loop diuretics may confer some advantages over bolus administration in terms of total drug required and diuretic response. Importantly, the incidence of adverse effects with this approach appears to be minimal.

Aside from the acute rebound in sodium and water reabsorption that occurs after a single dose of loop diuretics, long-term tolerance is also known to occur. In the acute setting, renal tubule segments distal to the Loop of Henle are unable to significantly reclaim the increased sodium load that is delivered after the administration of loop diuretics. However, with time, the distal collecting duct cells hypertrophy and their ability to reabsorb sodium is greatly increased (31–33). This finding is consistent with the common clinical scenario whereby patients on chronic therapy with loop diuretics require higher doses to induce diuresis than do patients without prior exposure. The increased sodium absorption in the collecting ducts can be overcome by concomitantly administering a thiazide diuretic (see next section) which often results in a synergistic response in diuresis (34, 35).

Renal function also appears to play a role in individual responses to loop diuretics. In healthy patients without prior exposure, 40 mg of intravenous furosemide appears to exert a maximal effect with little additional diuretic efficacy above this dose. However, the loop diuretics rely on active secretion into the renal tubule to exert their effects. Patients with renal insufficiency and a reduced number of normally functioning nephrons likely secrete less drug into the tubules. Brater and colleagues have shown that patients with chronic renal failure secrete only about 10% of furosemide into the urine versus approximately 70% in healthy patients (36). These investigators found that in patients with severe renal disease, a dose of 160 mg of furosemide is needed to reach maximal efficacy (36).

While all of the diuretics have significant effects on electrolyte balance (Table 9–1), the high efficacy of the loop diuretics has the potential to cause severe metabolic derangement. Their use, particularly in high doses, in the perioperative period mandates careful monitoring. Calcium, magnesium, sodium, and potassium levels in particular must be monitored to avoid adverse cardiovascular effects, especially with regard to cardiac arrhythmias. In addition, it should be noted that the loop diuretics can cause ototoxicity. This is most common with furosemide and usually seen after high doses administered intravenously, but has occurred with doses as low as 40 mg.

Thiazide Diuretics (Inhibitors of Sodium-Chloride Symport)

The thiazide diuretics (metolazone and hydrochlorothiazide being most common) exert their effects in the distal tubule where they inhibit the Na^+-Cl^- symporter that is normally responsible for reclaiming 3–6% of the filtered Na^+ load (6, 37, 38). As 90% of filtered sodium is reabsorbed before reaching the distal tubule, the thiazides are relatively weak diuretics. The exception is when they are used with chronic administration of loop diuretics. The net effect of acute thiazide administration is a small increase in sodium and chloride excretion with an increase in potassium and hydrogen ion excretion. The effects on renal blood flow are minimal.

While the thiazides are relatively weak diuretics, they often are a part of the medical regimen of many patients presenting for cardiac surgery, as they are commonly used to treat hypertension. Indeed, they have been the most studied antihypertensive during the past 4 decades and were involved in the first trials showing that controlling hypertension decreased morbidity and mortality (39). Despite the thiazides' long history of use in the management of hypertension, they are constantly being reevaluated against the newer agents, including angiotensin-converting enzyme (ACE) inhibitors, angiotensin receptor blockers, and calcium channel blockers. Recently, two large trials have shown that a thiazide-based antihypertensive regimen is at least as good, if not superior with regard to specific situations, in preventing adverse outcomes from hypertensive disease (40, 41).

As with all diuretics, the thiazides have the potential to produce adverse effects on electrolyte balance. Indeed, this has been a criticism of their use as antihypertensives (42). Hypokalemia is known to occur with chronic use and if not treated with adequate potassium supplementation, may attenuate the antihypertensive and cardioprotective effects (43, 44). Hyperglycemia can also be seen with thiazide use. The mechanism behind this hyperglycemia is unknown but may be mediated in part by hypokalemia, as it improves if potassium stores are replaced (44).

These potential side effects should be noted by the anesthesiologist and their magnitude should be identified by preoperative blood analysis.

Antagonists of Mineralocorticoid Receptors (Potassium Sparing Agents)

Spironolactone is the most commonly utilized agent in this class. It acts in the distal tubule which accounts for 90% of the renally excreted potassium (7). Normally, aldosterone binds to receptors in the epithelial cells of the distal tubule. This results in the synthesis of proteins that increase the conductance of Na^+ across the tubule lumen into the epithelial cells and accelerates the function of the Na^+ pump in the basolateral membrane. The net effect is to remove Na^+ from the tubule lumen in exchange for K^+ and H^+ ions. Spironolactone binds to the aldosterone receptor and inhibits production of the required proteins. Of note, because spironolactone's site of action is the epithelial cells, it is the only diuretic that does not require entrance in the tubule lumen to be effective (9).

The effects of spironolactone are directly proportional to the amount of aldosterone present in a given individual (i.e., the effects are most potent in patients with high endogenous levels of aldosterone). This may be due to a primary hyperaldosterone condition (adrenal adenomas, adrenal hyperplasia) or a secondary cause of increased aldosterone levels (hepatic cirrhosis, heart failure, nephritic syndrome). Used alone in patients with heart failure, it is a relatively weak diuretic. Thus, it is most often used as adjunctive therapy with a loop or thiazide diuretic where it helps prevent hypokalemia. When added to medical regimens for heart failure, spironolactone decreases ventricular arrhythmias and morbidity and mortality (45, 46).

DIURETICS IN CARDIAC AND VASCULAR SURGERY

Diuretics are a ubiquitous part of the practice of cardiovascular anesthesiology and surgery. Many patients will present to the operating room with a history of diuretic use as a part of their medical regimen, either for the treatment of hypertension or for the control of volume status. These medications have important effects on electrolyte balance, and preoperative laboratory work should be noted when available. When interviewing these patients it is important to note when the last dose of diuretic was taken, as the use of these agents in the face of nil per os orders may leave the patient significantly volume-depleted. Diuretics are undoubtedly useful for managing volume status in surgical patients. However, despite evidence of efficacy, they also continue to be used with the goal of preventing perioperative renal dysfunction.

Despite many advances in the care of the cardiac and vascular surgery patient, postoperative renal injury continues to be a common and dreaded complication. When it occurs, renal failure increases morbidity, mortality, length of hospital and ICU stay, and cost of care. Estimates of acute renal failure (ARF) after cardiac surgery are complicated by the varying definitions used by different investigator groups. However, an incidence of up to 30% is not uncommon in many series (47). At least one analysis has shown ARF to be the most potent predictor of outcome after cardiac surgery with an adjusted odds ratio for death of 7.8 in patients who develop ARF postoperatively (48). The incidence of ARF after aortic surgery is no less alarming, with an occurrence of approximately 15–25% after thoracoabdominal aortic aneurysm repairs (49). Godet et al. showed a 20–25% incidence of ARF after aortic surgery in 475 patients over a 12- year period (50). In this study, the incidence of ARF remained stable over the study period despite advances in patient management and surgical technique.

While numerous investigators have focused their efforts on reducing the occurrence of renal injury during cardiac and vascular surgery, there have been few significant improvements. As the body of literature on this subject continues to evolve, it is becoming ever clearer that the etiology of renal function is multifactorial. Preexisting renal impairment, periods of reduced renal perfusion or ischemia, perioperative exposure to nephrotoxic agents, atherosclerotic disease, inflammatory processes, and genetic predisposition are likely all responsible for the occurrence of postoperative renal dysfunction. As such, it is logical that there is no one "magic bullet" that will significantly reduce the incidence of this complication. However, osmotic and loop diuretics have been a focus of study for their potential renal protective properties.

The effects of osmotic and loop diuretics on the kidneys make them attractive as renal protective agents. The osmotic actions of mannitol decrease cellular edema in other tissue beds and it is logical to believe that it would do the same in the renal tubules after an insult. In addition, it is a free radical scavenger that may be protective in the presence of tissue injury. Furosemide increases renal blood flow increasing production of prostaglandins (47) and has been reported to reduce tubular oxygen consumption and improve renal tolerance to hypoxia by inhibiting Na^+ reabsorption (51, 52). Both agents dilute the urine and increase urine output, which potentially expedites the removal of hemoglobin and myoglobin (both of which are nephrotoxic (14, 18)) and other debris if present.

Literature touting the benefits of diuretics in cardiac and major vascular surgery dates to the 1960's (53). While successes have been reported in animal models and uncontrolled human case series, the number of well done, randomized trials is few. Lasnigg and colleagues randomized

126 patients with normal preoperative renal function undergoing cardiac surgery to receive either "renal-dose" dopamine (2 mcg/kg/min), furosemide (0.5 mcg/kg/min), or placebo infusions for 48 hours beginning with the commencement of surgery (47). They showed no difference in renal outcome parameters between the dopamine and placebo groups. More importantly, they showed statistically significant worse outcomes in the patients receiving furosemide. Patients in the furosemide group were more likely to have a significant increase in serum creatinine (>0.5 mg/dl), a higher maximum increase in creatinine, and lower creatinine clearance during the study period. Also important to note, the only two patients requiring renal replacement therapy were both in the furosemide group. One hypothesis these authors proposed for the negative effects of furosemide on renal function is that while this agent may produce prostaglandin mediated increases in renal blood flow, there also may be maldistribution of flow away from the vulnerable renal medulla.

This is not the only study reporting the negative effects of furosemide on renal function. Lombardi et al. reported a case series of 50 patients with serum creatinine levels less than 1.5 mg/dL undergoing cardiac surgery (54). All patients received 1 mg/kg of furosemide and 3 ml/kg of 20% mannitol at the beginning of cardiopulmonary bypass. Additional doses of furosemide were administered as needed to control volume status and hemodilution. All patients showed a decline in renal function after operation and 11.5% developed a creatinine level >2 mg/dl. Using multivariate analysis, the predictors of developing a postoperative creatinine level >2mg/dl were a slightly higher baseline creatinine (1.01 mg/dL versus 1.26 mg/dL) and higher total doses of intraoperative furosemide (96.5 + 20 mg versus 140 + 49 mg; p=0.001).

Carcoana and colleagues published a trial in 2003 evaluating the effects of mannitol and dopamine on renal function in cardiac surgery (55). One hundred patients were randomized to one of four groups: placebo, mannitol 1g/kg added to CPB prime, dopamine 2 mcg/kg/min from induction of anesthesia to 1 hour post-CPB, or mannitol plus dopamine. The primary outcome in this study was the urinary excretion of β_2-microblobulin (β_2M), a reportedly sensitive marker of proximal renal tubular function. This group found that dopamine infusions increased the excretion of β_2-M postoperatively and that there was no difference in excretion between the placebo and mannitol groups. Furthermore, mannitol conferred no advantage in terms of creatinine clearance or highest serum creatinine versus placebo.

In a small study, Nicholson et al. randomized 28 patients undergoing aortic aneurysm repair to receive either 0.3 g/kg of mannitol or saline before aortic cross-clamping (56). They found no differences in postoperative blood urea levels, serum creatinine concentrations, or creatinine clearance between the groups. As these authors note, these markers are relatively insensitive measures of renal injury. Thus, they also studied urinary concentrations of albumin and N-acetyl glucosaminidase, which have been reported to be sensitive markers of renal injury. These investigators did show decreased urinary levels of these markers in the patients receiving mannitol and used these findings to support the claim that mannitol reduces subclinical renal injury after infrarenal aortic aneurysm repair.

The above studies suggest that diuretics have little to offer in the way of renal protection and may, in fact, be harmful. Diuretics are given for multiple reasons in the operating room and ICU. One common reason for administering diuretics in the operating room is the presence of what is felt to be inadequate urine output. While urine output in the operating room may be a marker of adequate end organ perfusion, and thus a marker of adequate hemodynamic status, it does not correlate with renal outcome (47, 54, 57). Simply giving diuretics to observe increased urine output confers no benefit to patients in terms of renal outcome, and may be harmful. The potential negative effects of furosemide have been discussed. Mannitol, while not conclusively shown to be renal protective, is thought of as a benign medication that may be helpful. But even mannitol has the potential to do damage if the diuresis induced is not adequately replaced with intravascular fluids and leaves the kidney in a prerenal, intravascularly depleted state. Certainly there always will be a role for diuretics in cardiovascular anesthesia, but, as with any medication, the reasons for administering them should be evidence-based and not a reflexive action to decreased urine output.

VASOACTIVE AGENTS FOR DIURESIS

While not classified as diuretics, some vasoactive medications are used with the goal of increasing Na^+ and water excretion. Any vasoactive agent may have important effects on renal function and urine output depending on how it affects renal blood flow. An agent that increases perfusion to the kidneys, either by an increase in cardiac output or vasodilation, is likely to exert some diuretic effect, although the effect will be attenuated by autoregulation of the renal vasculature and other inhibitory mechanisms. Medications that cause vasoconstriction of the renal vasculature will decrease renal perfusion and may decrease urine output. Three agents that are often discussed in terms of their effects on renal blood flow and urine output will be reviewed here: dopamine, fenoldopam, and nesiritide.

Dopamine

Despite a recent preponderance of evidence indicating that dopamine lacks renal protective qualities, "renal dose dopamine" continues to be used with the goal of preventing postoperative renal failure. While dopamine likely does not prevent renal failure, it does have effects on renal blood flow and salt and water excretion.

By binding to dopaminergic-1 receptors in the renal vasculature, dopamine increases renal blood flow (58). At the proximal tubule, Loop of Henle, and collecting ducts, dopamine inhibits sodium and water reabsorption (47). These effects have been hypothesized to reduce renal oxygen consumption (47). Dopamine also increases the formation of prostaglandins which dilate medullary blood vessels and have been proposed to further decrease renal oxygen consumption.

Studies in cardiac surgical patients (47, 59) as well as a meta-analysis involving over 900 patients (60) have confirmed what has long been contended by many authors: that renal dose dopamine does not protect the kidneys from injury. Even renal doses (2–3 mcg/kg/min) may increase myocardial oxygen consumption which is clearly detrimental to patients recovering from cardiac surgery. Thus, dopamine should not be used with the intention of "protecting the kidneys." Despite its lack of renal protective qualities, dopamine is occasionally helpful for diuresis.

Fenoldopam

Fenoldopam is the first selective dopamine-1 receptor agonist and has been approved by the Food and Drug Administration for treatment of hypertensive emergencies. Studies indicate that fenoldopam improves renal function when renal blood flow is reduced due to severe hypertension (61, 62). The effects appear to be due to increased blood flow to both the renal cortex and medulla (63). These findings have sparked an interest in the use of fenoldopam for renal protection in cardiac and major vascular surgery.

The first randomized study of fenoldopam in cardiac surgery was performed by Caimmi and colleagues (64). In this study, 160 patients were randomized to receive either fenoldopam infusions (0.1–0.3 mcg/kg/min) during CPB and in the early postoperative period or during conventional management. Enrolled patients had a baseline serum creatinine of >1.5 mg/dl and underwent uncomplicated operations. Patients receiving dopamine, dobutamine, or epinephrine were excluded from the study group. Furosemide and dopamine were used to treat urine outputs of <0.5 ml/kg/hr. Patients receiving fenoldopam infusions showed a reduction in serum creatinine levels from preoperative measurements versus the control patients who had an elevation in their postoperative creatinine levels. Creatinine clearance was also improved in the study patients versus controls. The authors concluded that administration of fenoldopam is appropriate in patients with impaired renal function during cardiac surgery.

Unfortunately, these results could not be replicated in a more rigorously controlled trial by Bove et al. (63). These investigators enrolled patients at high risk for renal failure (as determined by the Continuous Improvement in Cardiac Surgery Program scores) undergoing cardiac surgery. Patients were randomized to receive either 0.05 mcg/kg/min of fenoldopam or 2.5 mcg/kg/min of dopamine commencing after the induction of anesthesia and continuing for 24 hours. In this study the incidence of acute renal failure (increase in serum creatinine levels of ≥25% above baseline) was similar in both groups (42.5% in the fenoldopam group versus 40% in the dopamine group, $p=0.9$). Peak postoperative serum creatinine levels also were similar between groups.

The results by Bove et al. in cardiac surgery were echoed by a similar study in patients undergoing major vascular surgery. Oliver and colleagues compared the use of fenoldopam with sodium nitroprusside and dopamine in patients undergoing abdominal aortic surgery utilizing an aortic cross clamp (65). In this study there was no difference in indices of renal function including increases in serum creatinine of ≥0.5 mg/dl, urine output, creatinine clearance, or ARF between the two groups.

While there was early enthusiasm for the potential benefits of fenoldopam on renal function in cardiac and major vascular surgery based on small case series and animal data, carefully conducted studies in cardiac and vascular surgery now indicate that there likely is no renal protection conferred by fenoldopam.

Nesiritide

Nesiritide is a recombinant form of human B-type natriuretic peptide (BNP). Endogenous BNP is released from the ventricular walls in response to ventricular dysfunction and wall stress and is a marker of acute heart failure (66). BNP binds to receptors in the vasculature, including the kidney, where it has natriuretic and diuretic properties (67, 68). In health, nesiritide increases glomerular filtration rate (GFR) and induces natriuresis and diuresis (69–71). In heart failure patients, it at least maintains renal blood flow and/or GFR (72) and maintains or increases renal Na^+ and water excretion (71, 73, 74).

The NAPA trial recently evaluated the effects of nesiritide infusions on renal function in patients with left ventricular (LV) dysfunction undergoing coronary artery bypass grafting (CABG) surgery with cardiopulmonary bypass (72). In this prospective, double- blind trial, patients with an LV ejection fraction ≤40% were randomized to receive an infusion of nesiritide (0.01 mcg/kg/min without bolus) or placebo. The infusion was started before incision and continued for at least 24 hours, and up to 96 hours at the discretion of the attending physician. In this study serum creatinine increased in both the study and control groups postoperatively. However, this increase was attenuated in the patients receiving nesiritide and these patients recovered to a baseline creatinine level much sooner. The decrease in GFR at the time of hospital discharge (or by day 14, whichever came sooner) was also less in the nesiritide group. These effects were particularly pronounced in patients with preexisting renal dysfunction defined as a preoperative creatinine level >1.2 mg/dl. Perhaps most importantly, survival at 180 days was significantly higher in the nesiritide group (6.6% mortality in nesiritide group versus 14.7% mortality in the control group, P=0.046).

As the authors note, this study has limitations (72). Other aspects of patient care were not controlled for and the 180-day mortality end point was added late. This was an exploratory study but its positive results will undoubtedly spark further research in the use of nesiritide for renal protection in the perioperative period. In the interim it may be a useful agent for both its diuretic properties and in optimizing the volume status of patients with heart failure before elective cardiac surgery or transplantation.

CONCLUSIONS

Diuretics have a long history of use and continue to be a ubiquitous part of the practice of cardiac surgery and anesthesia. In particular, the loop and osmotic diuretics are useful in the acute setting for controlling patients' volume status. There is little evidence to support the concept that they protect the kidneys from injury in the perioperative period, despite continued use with this intention. The intravenous agents dopamine, fenoldopam, and nesiritide also have important diuretic and naturetic properties. Emerging evidence suggests that nesiritide may be a useful agent for attenuating renal insult during cardiac surgery.

References

1. Rosendorff C, Black HR, Cannon CP, et al.: Treatment of hypertension in the prevention and management of ischemic heart disease: a scientific statement from the American Heart Association Council for High Blood Pressure Research and the Councils on Clinical Cardiology and Epidemiology and Prevention. Circulation 2007; 115:2761–88
2. Hunt SA, Abraham WT, Chin MH, et al.: ACC/AHA 2005 guideline update for the diagnosis and management of chronic heart failure

in the adult: a report of the American College of Cardiology/American Heart Association Task Force on Practice Guidelines (Writing Committee to Update the 2001 Guidelines for the Evaluation and Management of Heart Failure): developed in collaboration with the American College of Chest Physicians and the International Society for Heart and Lung Transplantation: endorsed by the Heart Rhythm Society. Circulation 2005; 112:e154–235
3. Hall RI, Smith MS, Rocker G: The systemic inflammatory response to cardiopulmonary bypass: pathophysiological, therapeutic, and pharmacological considerations. Anesth Analg 1997; 85:766–82
4. Wan S, LeClerc JL, Vincent JL: Inflammatory response to cardiopulmonary bypass: mechanisms involved and possible therapeutic strategies. Chest 1997; 112:676–92
5. Boldt J, Kling D, Scheld HH, Hempelmann G: Lung management during cardiopulmonary bypass: influence on extravascular lung water. J Cardiothorac Anesth 1990; 4:73–9
6. Antes LM, Fernandez PC: Principles of diuretic therapy. Dis Mon 1998; 44:254–68
7. Morrison RT: Edema and principles of diuretic use. Med Clin North Am 1997; 81:689–704
8. Kriz W, Bankir L: A standard nomenclature for structure of the kidney. The Renal Commission of the International Union of Physiological Sciences (IUPS). Anat Embryol (Berl) 1988; 178:N1–8
9. Jackson EK: Diuretics. 11th ed. New York: McGraw-Hill.
10. Knauf H, Mutschler E: Sequential nephron blockade breaks resistance to diuretics in edematous states. J Cardiovasc Pharmacol 1997; 29:367–72
11. Hackett PH, Roach RC: High-altitude illness. N Engl J Med 2001; 345:107–14
12. Links TP, Zwarts MJ, Oosterhuis HJ: Improvement of muscle strength in familial hypokalaemic periodic paralysis with acetazolamide. J Neurol Neurosurg Psychiatry 1988; 51:1142–5
13. Laker MF, Bull HJ, Menzies IS: Evaluation of mannitol for use as a probe marker of gastrointestinal permeability in man. Eur J Clin Invest 1982; 12:485–91
14. Poullis M: Mannitol and cardiac surgery. Thorac Cardiovasc Surg 1999; 47:58–62
15. Warren SE, Blantz RC: Mannitol. Arch Intern Med 1981; 141:493–7
16. van Hengel P, Nikken JJ, de Jong GM, et al.: Mannitol-induced acute renal failure. Neth J Med 1997; 50:21–4
17. Johnston PA, Bernard DB, Perrin NS, Levinsky NG: Prostaglandins mediate the vasodilatory effect of mannitol in the hypoperfused rat kidney. J Clin Invest 1981; 68:127–33

18. Heyman SN, Greenbaum R, Shina A, et al.: Myoglobinuric acute renal failure in the rat: a role for acidosis? Exp Nephrol 1997; 5:210–6
19. Utley JR, Stephens DB, Wachtel C, et al.: Effect of albumin and mannitol on organ blood flow, oxygen delivery, water content, and renal function during hypothermic hemodilution cardiopulmonary bypass. Ann Thorac Surg 1982; 33:250–7
20. Cox DL, Riley B, Chang P, et al.: Effects of molecular oxygen, oxidation-reduction potential, and antioxidants upon in vitro replication of Treponema pallidum subsp. pallidum. Appl Environ Microbiol 1990; 56:3063–72
21. Odlind B, Beermann B: Renal tubular secretion and effects of furosemide. Clin Pharmacol Ther 1980; 27:784–90
22. Burg MB: Tubular chloride transport and the mode of action of some diuretics. Kidney Int 1976; 9:189–97
23. Forbush B, 3rd, Palfrey HC: [3H]bumetanide binding to membranes isolated from dog kidney outer medulla. Relationship to the Na, K, Cl co-transport system. J Biol Chem 1983; 258:11787–92
24. Brater DC: Diuretic therapy. N Engl J Med 1998; 339:387–95
25. Shankar SS, Brater DC: Loop diuretics: from the Na-K-2Cl transporter to clinical use. Am J Physiol-Renal Physiol 2003; 284:F11–21
26. Dormans TP, van Meyel JJ, Gerlag PG, et al.: Diuretic efficacy of high dose furosemide in severe heart failure: bolus injection versus continuous infusion. J Am Coll Cardiol 1996; 28:376–82
27. Imbs JL, Schmidt M, Giesen-Crouse E: Pharmacology of loop diuretics: state of the art. Adv Nephrol Necker Hosp 1987; 16:137–58
28. Wilcox CS, Mitch WE, Kelly RA, et al.: Response of the kidney to furosemide. I. Effects of salt intake and renal compensation. J Lab Clin Med 1983; 102:450–8
29. Copeland JG, Campbell DW, Plachetka JR, et al.: Diuresis with continuous infusion of furosemide after cardiac surgery. Am J Surg 1983; 146:796–9
30. Martin SJ, Danziger LH: Continuous infusion of loop diuretics in the critically ill: a review of the literature. Crit Care Med 1994; 22:1323–9
31. Ellison DH, Velazquez H, Wright FS: Adaptation of the distal convoluted tubule of the rat. Structural and functional effects of dietary salt intake and chronic diuretic infusion. J Clin Invest 1989; 83:113–26
32. Kaissling B, Stanton BA: Adaptation of distal tubule and collecting duct to increased sodium delivery. I. Ultrastructure. Am J Physiol 1988; 255:F1256–68
33. Stanton BA, Kaissling B. Adaptation of distal tubule and collecting duct to increased Na delivery. II. Na+ and K+ transport. Am J Physiol 1988; 255:F1269–75

34. Ellison DH: The physiologic basis of diuretic synergism: its role in treating diuretic resistance. Ann Intern Med 1991; 114:886–94
35. Sica DA, Gehr TW: Diuretic combinations in refractory oedema states: pharmacokinetic-pharmacodynamic relationships. Clin Pharmacokinet 1996; 30:229–49
36. Brater DC, Anderson SA, Brown-Cartwright D: Response to furosemide in chronic renal insufficiency: rationale for limited doses. Clin Pharmacol Ther 1986; 40:134–9
37. Beaumont K, Vaughn DA, Fanestil DD: Thiazide diuretic drug receptors in rat kidney: identification with [3H]metolazone. Proc Natl Acad Sci USA 1988; 85:2311–4
38. Ellison DH, Velazquez H, Wright FS: Thiazide-sensitive sodium chloride cotransport in early distal tubule. Am J Physiol 1987; 253:F546–54
39. Sawicki PT, McGauran N: Have ALLHAT, ANBP2, ASCOT-BPLA, and so forth improved our knowledge about better hypertension care? Hypertension 2006; 48:1–7
40. Major cardiovascular events in hypertensive patients randomized to doxazosin vs chlorthalidone: the antihypertensive and lipid-lowering treatment to prevent heart attack trial (ALLHAT). ALLHAT Collaborative Research Group. JAMA 2000; 283:1967–75
41. Wing LM, Reid CM, Ryan P, et al.: A comparison of outcomes with angiotensin-converting-enzyme inhibitors and diuretics for hypertension in the elderly. N Engl J Med 2003; 348:583–92
42. McInnes GT, Yeo WW, Ramsay LE, Moser M: Cardiotoxicity and diuretics: much speculation-little substance. J Hypertens 1992; 10:317–35
43. Franse LV, Pahor M, Di Bari M, et al.: Hypokalemia associated with diuretic use and cardiovascular events in the Systolic Hypertension in the Elderly Program. Hypertension 2000; 35:1025–30
44. Wilcox CS, Welch WJ, Schreiner GF, Belardinelli L: Natriuretic and diuretic actions of a highly selective adenosine A1 receptor antagonist. J Am Soc Nephrol 1999; 10:714–20
45. Pitt B, Zannad F, Remme WJ, et al.: The effect of spironolactone on morbidity and mortality in patients with severe heart failure. Randomized Aldactone Evaluation Study Investigators. N Engl J Med 1999; 341:709–17
46. Ramires FJ, Mansur A, Coelho O, et al.: Effect of spironolactone on ventricular arrhythmias in congestive heart failure secondary to idiopathic dilated or to ischemic cardiomyopathy. Am J Cardiol 2000; 85:1207–11

47. Lassnigg A, Donner E, Grubhofer G, et al.: Lack of renoprotective effects of dopamine and furosemide during cardiac surgery. J Am Soc Nephrol 2000; 11:97–104
48. Chertow GM, Levy EM, Hammermeister KE, et al.: Independent association between acute renal failure and mortality following cardiac surgery. Am J Med 1998; 104:343–8
49. Swaminathan M, Stafford-Smith M: Renal dysfunction after vascular surgery. Curr Opin Anaesthesiol 2003; 16:45–51
50. Godet G, Fleron MH, Vicaut E, et al.: Risk factors for acute postoperative renal failure in thoracic or thoracoabdominal aortic surgery: a prospective study. Anesth Analg 1997; 85:1227–32
51. Brezis M, Rosen S, Silva P, Epstein FH: Transport activity modifies thick ascending limb damage in the isolated perfused kidney. Kidney Int 1984; 25:65–72
52. Schoenwald PK: Intraoperative management of renal function in the surgical patient at risk. Focus on aortic surgery. Anesthesiol Clin North America 2000; 18:719–37
53. Etheredge EE, Levitin H, Nakamura K, Glenn WW: Effect of mannitol on renal function during open-heart surgery. Ann Surg 1965; 161:53–62
54. Lombardi R, Ferreiro A, Servetto C: Renal function after cardiac surgery: adverse effect of furosemide. Ren Fail 2003; 25:775–86
55. Carcoana OV, Mathew JP, Davis E, et al.: Mannitol and dopamine in patients undergoing cardiopulmonary bypass: a randomized clinical trial. Anesth Analg 2003; 97:1222–9
56. Nicholson ML, Baker DM, Hopkinson BR, Wenham PW: Randomized controlled trial of the effect of mannitol on renal reperfusion injury during aortic aneurysm surgery. Br J Surg 1996; 83:1230–3
57. Slogoff S, Reul GJ, Keats AS, et al.: Role of perfusion pressure and flow in major organ dysfunction after cardiopulmonary bypass. Ann Thorac Surg 1990; 50:911–8
58. Hollenberg NK, Adams DF, Mendell P, et al.: Renal vascular responses to dopamine: haemodynamic and angiographic observations in normal man. Clin Sci Mol Med 1973; 45:733–42
59. Woo EB, Tang AT, el-Gamel A, et al.: Dopamine therapy for patients at risk of renal dysfunction following cardiac surgery: science or fiction? Eur J Cardio-Thorac Surg 2002; 22:106–11
60. Marik PE: Low-dose dopamine: a systematic review. Intensive Care Med 2002; 28:877–83
61. Elliott WJ, Weber RR, Nelson KS, et al.: Renal and hemodynamic effects of intravenous fenoldopam versus nitroprusside in severe hypertension. Circulation 1990; 81:970–7

62. White WB, Halley SE: Comparative renal effects of intravenous administration of fenoldopam mesylate and sodium nitroprusside in patients with severe hypertension. Arch Intern Med 1989; 149:870–4
63. Bove T, Landoni G, Calabro MG, et al.: Renoprotective action of fenoldopam in high-risk patients undergoing cardiac surgery: a prospective, double-blind, randomized clinical trial. Circulation 2005; 111:3230–5
64. Caimmi PP, Pagani L, Micalizzi E, et al.: Fenoldopam for renal protection in patients undergoing cardiopulmonary bypass. J Cardiothorac Vasc Anesth 2003; 17:491–4
65. Oliver WC, Jr., Nuttall GA, Cherry KJ, et al.: A comparison of fenoldopam with dopamine and sodium nitroprusside in patients undergoing cross-clamping of the abdominal aorta. Anesth Analg 2006; 103:833–40
66. Zineh I, Schofield RS, Johnson JA: The evolving role of nesiritide in advanced or decompensated heart failure. Pharmacotherapy 2003; 23:1266–80
67. Mills RM, Hobbs RE: Nesiritide in perspective: evolving approaches to the management of acute decompensated heart failure. Drugs Today 2003; 39:767–74
68. de Denus S, Pharand C, Williamson DR: Brain natriuretic peptide in the management of heart failure: the versatile neurohormone. Chest 2004; 125:652–68
69. Holmes SJ, Espiner EA, Richards AM, et al.: Renal, endocrine, and hemodynamic effects of human brain natriuretic peptide in normal man. J Clin Endocrinol Metab 1993; 76:91–6
70. Jensen KT, Carstens J, Pedersen EB: Effect of BNP on renal hemodynamics, tubular function and vasoactive hormones in humans. Am J Physiol 1998; 274:F63–72
71. Jensen KT, Eiskjaer H, Carstens J, Pedersen EB: Renal effects of brain natriuretic peptide in patients with congestive heart failure. Clin Sci (Lond) 1999; 96:5–15
72. Mentzer RM, Jr., Oz MC, Sladen RN, et al.: Effects of perioperative nesiritide in patients with left ventricular dysfunction undergoing cardiac surgery: the NAPA Trial. J Am Coll Cardiol 2007; 49:716–26
73. Colucci WS, Elkayam U, Horton DP, et al.: Intravenous nesiritide, a natriuretic peptide, in the treatment of decompensated congestive heart failure. Nesiritide Study Group. N Engl J Med 2000; 343:246–53
74. Marcus LS, Hart D, Packer M, et al.: Hemodynamic and renal excretory effects of human brain natriuretic peptide infusion in patients with congestive heart failure. A double-blind, placebo-controlled, randomized crossover trial. Circulation 1996; 94:3184–9

Yannick Le Manach, MD
Pierre Coriat, MD

10 Statins in the Perioperative Period

INTRODUCTION

Statins are highly effective in lowering serum cholesterol concentrations through 3-hydroxy-3-methyl glutaryl coenzyme A (HMG-CoA) reductase inhibition, and thus are central to the primary and secondary prevention of cardiovascular disease. After a number of randomized controlled trials in nonsurgical conditions (1–5), statins are now recognized as a treatment of acute or chronic coronary artery disease (6, 7). Consequently, more than 50% of patients undergoing major vascular surgery and 80% undergoing cardiac surgery are on chronic statin therapy (8, 9). Statins also exert numerous lipid-independent effects, also call pleiotropic effects (meaning that these effects were not expected during the drug development), as a result of their ability to inhibit inflammatory response, reduce thrombosis, enhance fibrinolysis, decrease platelet reactivity, inhibit cell growth, reduce ischemic-reperfusion injury, and restore endothelial function (10–12). These beneficial effects result predominantly from the modulation of the complex interplay between the pathological triad of inflammation, dynamic obstruction, and thrombosis (12). This triad is integral to surgical stress response and central postoperative outcome.

BENEFITS OF STATINS

Lipid-Dependent Effects

Low-density lipoprotein (LDL) cholesterol are oxidized by free radicals and are linked to atherothrombosis and its associated deleterious effects.

Advances in Cardiovascular Pharmacology, edited by Philippe R. Housmans, MD, PhD and Gregory A. Nuttall, M.D.
Lippincott Williams & Wilkins, Baltimore © 2008.

TABLE 10–1. Clinical pharmacokinetics of statins

	Atorvastatin	Fluvastatin	Fluvastatin XL	Lovastatin	Pravastatin	Rosuvastatin	Simvastatin
Tmax (h)	2–3	0.5–1	4	2–4	0.9–1.6	3	1.3–2.4
Cmax (ng/mL)	27–66	448	55	10–20	45–55	37	10–34
Bioavailability (%)	12	19–29	6	5	18	20	5
Metabolism	CYP3A4	CYP2C9	CYP2C9	CYP3A4	Sulfation	CYP2C9, 2C19	CYP3A4
$T_{1/2}$ (h)	15–30	0.5–2.3	4.7	2.9	1.3–2.8	20.8	2–3
LDL-c							
Average Reduction (%)	49	27	35	37	29	53	37

Based on a 40mg dose except for Fluvastatin XL (80 mg)
Adapted from Bellosta et al.[15], Law et al.[14], James et al.[16] and Scharnagl et al.[17]

Reduction of LDL cholesterol concentration is one of the primary objectives of chronic cardiovascular disease prevention. Numerous non-statin therapies have been developed, such as bile acid sequestrants or fibrates, but only a few effects have been observed on mortality (13). Statins inhibit HMG-CoA, which is central to cholesterol metabolism, and induce a more significant reduction of LDL cholesterol concentration, which is associated with a reduction of the mortality in primary and secondary prevention of cardiovascular diseases. Nevertheless, because the power of each molecule differs, this capacity to reduce LDL cholesterol, and so mortality, is not comparable from one statin to the others. Indeed, a meta-analysis (14) showed a 53% reduction in LDL cholesterol with rosuvastatin 40 mg/d and a 55% reduction with atorvastatin 80 mg/d, whereas pravastatin and fluvastatin produced smaller reductions in LDL cholesterol (Table 10–1). This property of statins must be considered during the preoperative visit, since the risk-benefit balance is not the same with normal doses and with high doses. Furthermore, the pharmacokinetic properties of each statin (Table 10–1) are different and also should be considered.

Lipid-Independent Effects

The results of randomized trials initially suggested that statins induce a greater reduction in the risk of cardiovascular events than that expected with the magnitude of reduction in LDL cholesterol alone. Retrospectively, this observation appears to be not so clear during chronic statin therapy (18). But several lipid-independent effects have been described, most of the observed effects occurring earlier than the lowering of LDL cholesterol levels (Table 10–2) (19). In fact, if the reduction of the LDL cholesterol plasma level appears to be the main mechanism of the observed benefit of the statins during a stable period (18), the lipid-independent effects seem to have a particular importance during unstable periods, as postoperative period or acute coronary syndrome (20).

Inhibition of HMG-CoA by statins inhibits the generation of isoprotenoids (geranyl-geranyl pyrophosphate and farnesyl pyrophosphate), which bind to Rho signaling proteins, thereby preventing translocation to active sites. Rho activates nuclear factor-κB (NF-κB), which promotes a number of inflammatory responses and reduces endothelial nitric oxide (NO) synthetase (e-NOS). Therefore, statins exhibit direct anti-inflammatory effects by inhibiting Rho effects. These effects result in a rapid increase in NO bioavailability, which is observed as early as 3 hours after oral administration of atorvastatin (21), resulting in improved vasodilating (22) (reflected in improved flow-mediated dilatation) and antithrombotic properties of the vasculature (23). Statins also reduce the expression of endothelin, thus favoring vasodilatation. And more than the ability to restore the vasodilation of the atherosclerotic microcirculation (24, 25), a short-term statin treatment is able to correct the vascular hyporeactivity induced by LPS injection in a healthy human (26).

Statin therapy is associated with a significant reduction in variables linked to inflammation, including a reduction in acute-phase proteins (C-reactive protein and myeloperoxidase); reduced expression of adhesion molecules (e.g., ICAM-1, E-selectin) on the surface of endothelial cells; reduced inflammatory cytokines, including interleukins (IL-1, IL-6, and IL-8), which can activate inflammatory cells and platelets; and increased anti-inflammatory cytokines (e.g., IL-10). Statins also inhibit angiotensin II-induced reactive oxygen species production through downregulation of angiotensin-1 receptors and inhibition of activation of Rac, (member of the Rho GTPase family) that contributes to NAD(P)H-oxidase activation (27). These anti-inflammatory and endothelial-enhancing effects may increase the stability of the vulnerable atheromatous plaques and improve microcirculatory flow. Such beneficial effects are associated with a reduction in risk for periprocedural myocardial infarction, for example after coronary intervention.

Statins improve markers of coagulation by both endothelium-dependent and nonendothelium-dependent mechanisms (28). Statins increase endothelial thrombomodulin expression and reduce tissue factor expression on endothelial cells, thus favoring a nonthrombotic state of the endothelium. Statins reduce the circulating levels of von Willebrand fac-

Table 10–2. Mechanisms of the effects of statins

	HMG CoA reductase Dependant		
	Cholesterol Dependant	*Cholesterol Independant*	**HMG CoA reductase Independent**
MECHANISMS	↓ LDL-c plasma levels ↓ oxidized LDL-c	↓ Isoprenoid synthesis and down regulation of Rho GTPase family	
EFFECTS			
Vasomotricity		↑ NO bioavailability	
Coagulation	↓ Platelet activation	↑ TM expression ↓ Tissue Factor expression ↑ tPA/PAI-1 ratio ↓ Coagulation Factors	Inactivation of factor Va
Inflammation	↓ Foam cell formation ↓ Macrophage number ↓ expression of adhesion molecules	↓ Binding of lymphocytes to ICAM-1 ↓ Inflammatory cytokine production (IL1; IL6 and IL8) ↓ MCP-1 expression	Direct binding to the lymphocytes function antigen
Other		↓ Atrial Natriuretic Factor (ANF) ↓ Myosin Light Chain (MLC-2)	

LDL-c: *low density lipoprotein cholesterol*; TM: *Thrombomodulin*; tPA: *tissue plasminogen activator*; PAI: *Plasminogen activator inhibitor*; ICAM-1: *Intercellular adhesion molecule*

tors and tend to alter the balance between plasminogen activator inhibitor and tissue plasminogen activator in favor of thrombolysis. Moreover, the anti-inflammatory actions of statins also may indirectly act on coagulation and thrombosis. Statins also have systemic effects on coagulation (factors V, VII, and XII) via poorly understood mechanisms (12, 29).

Statins also may play an important role in the repair of damaged endothelium by accelerating re-endothelialization (30), mobilizing endothelial progenitor cells (30), and increasing cell proliferation. Lastly, statins may exert some effects that are directly, or not, mediated through HMG-CoA reductase inhibition, such as preventing lymphocytes from binding to endothelium. Indeed, statins have been shown to directly bind to receptors on the lymphocyte cell surface (HMG-CoA Reductase independent), preventing binding to the counter receptor on the endothelial surface (ICAM-1) (31); a reduction in the expression of ICAM-1 on the endothelial surface and their counter ligand on the monocyte also has been observed (32). Furthermore, the inhibition of the Rho GTPase family also has some nonvascular effects (reduction expression of atrial natriuretic factor (ANF) and myosin light chain (MLC)-2 in the heart) (33), which suggests other beneficial cardiac effects of the statins.

Thus, the beneficial pleiotropic effects of statins predominantly include inhibiting inflammatory response, reducing thrombosis, enhancing fibrinolysis, decreasing platelet reactivity, inhibiting cell growth, and restoring microcirculation vasoreactivity. These anti-inflammatory and endothelial-enhancing effects of statins culminate in a protective effect readily evident in the setting of ischemia-reperfusion injury (29, 34, 35). In this regard, a number of preclinical models demonstrate that statins reduce the magnitude of tissue destruction (infarct volume), tissue dysfunction, and organ failure in models of myocardial, cerebral, intestinal, and renal ischemia-reperfusion injury. Interestingly, statins also protect organs distant to the locus of ischemia-reperfusion injury, with statins reducing the severity of acute lung injury following an intestinal ischemia-reperfusion insult and reducing coronary dysfunction in a swine model of respiratory infection. Increasing evidence that statins reduce the incidence and magnitude of myocardial infarction following coronary interventions (36), decrease renal dysfunction (37), and improve long-term vasculopathy after transplantation (38) provides the clinical correlate. Moreover, an endothelial dysfunction independently predicts postoperative cardiac events (39), whereas statins are able to rapidly restore this function, suggesting the possibility of a beneficial mechanism during the perioperative period (21).

Dose-Dependent Effects

Epidemiological studies demonstrate that coronary heart disease is correlated with LDL cholesterol plasma levels without threshold below which risk is null (cardiac risk increases exponentially with increasing LDL cholesterol plasma levels) (40). This finding has contributed to the effective introduction of statins in patients with coronary artery disease and normal LDL cholesterol plasma levels (41), and to the intensification of chronic statin therapy in patients with high LDL cholesterol levels. Several clinical trials have demonstrated the additional benefit of such strategy for high-risk patients during stable periods (42–44).

Most of the lipid-independent effects are present for each statin, but the magnitude of these effects remains different and linked to the obtained reduction of LDL cholesterol plasma levels. Indeed, the better-understood mechanism involves intermediary metabolites of cholesterol, and so the stronger is the HMG-COa inhibition and the more important are the lipid-independent effects. Although the pleiotropic effects are observed in absence of hypercholesterolemia (19, 21), it appears that these effects are dose dependent and that the better marker of the magnitude of these effects (or of the HMG-COa inhibition) is the LDL cholesterol plasma level reduction. Thus the ability of each statin to reduce LDL cholesterol plasma (Table 10–1) seems to be correlated to the beneficial vascular effects and also to the muscular adverse effects. Larosa et al. (44), comparing atorvastatin 10 mg/d versus 80 mg/d in patients with stable coronary heart disease, observed a 22% relative reduction in risk after 5 years.

Several studies have compared the effect of high dose to normal dose during unstable period. Ray et al. (20) have demonstrated (PROVE IT-TIMI 22) in patients with acute coronary syndrome, that intensive statin therapy (atorvastatin, 80 mg) reduces short-term death, myocardial infarction, and rehospitalization for recurrent acute coronary syndrome compared to a standard therapy (pravastatin, 40 mg). This study shows that intensive statins leads to a relative risk reduction of 28% within 30 days after an acute coronary syndrome. These observed benefits were not noted after ileal bypass surgery, which is also associated with a dramatic early reduction in LDL cholesterol plasma level but without statins (45). Thus, Ray et al. (20) conclude that the observed benefit during this unstable period could be due to the pleiotropic effect of statins.

PERIOPERATIVE USE OF STATINS

Several studies involving a large number of patients have shown that the perioperative use of statins could be beneficial. In this way, the use of statins during the perioperative period is promising. Although two meta-analyses confirm this association (46, 47), we have to consider that most of the studies are not randomized (except the study of Durazzo et al. (48) in vascular surgery, and those of Christensen (49) and Patti et al. (50) in cardiac surgery), and that we have to be cautious with rapid conclusions. Indeed, considering the most recent history about the use of β-blockers during the perioperative period of noncardiac surgery, we need large randomized studies to make a definite conclusion.

Cardiac Risk After Cardiac Surgery

One of the first studies about statin and cardiac surgery was a randomized study of 77 patients that evaluated whether preoperative lipid control using simvastatin (20 mg) reduced the risk of postoperative thrombocytosis. Christenson (49) concluded that a preoperative therapy with statins for 4 weeks lowers the risk for thrombotic complications.

Pan et al. (9) retrospectively investigated the influence of preoperative statin therapy on adverse outcomes after primary coronary artery bypass graft surgery on 1663 patients and found that, after adjusting for demographic and clinical differences, preoperative statin therapy was associated with an approximate 50% reduction in mortality, but there was no association between statin therapy and the occurrence of atrial fibrillation or myocardial infarction. Dotani et al. (51) found similar results showing that statin therapy was associated with significant decreases in cardiac mortality. They also retrieved a significant association with unstable angina and arrhythmias at both 60 days and 1 year.

Hindler et al. (47) included 5 studies in their meta-analysis (9, 49, 51–53) and 2 abstracts; 1 of these studies was a prospective randomized controlled trial (49). Postoperative mortality was significantly lower (1.9% vs 3.1%) in patients undergoing cardiac surgery who received preoperative statin therapy than in those who did not. But no significant differences were observed between groups with regard to postoperative cardiac arrhythmia, or stroke.

More recently, Patti et al. (50) conducted a randomized study to assess the effect of statins on the incidence of postoperative atrial fibrillation. They included 200 patients undergoing elective cardiac surgery with cardiopulmonary bypass, without previous statin treatment or history of atrial fibrillation, and randomized them to atorvastatin (40 mg/d) or placebo starting 7 days before operation. The preoperative treatment with statins significantly reduced the incidence of postoperative atrial fibrillation after elective cardiac surgery with cardiopulmonary bypass and shortened hospital stay.

Cardiac Risk after Noncardiac Surgery

Although not randomized, several studies of cardiac risk after noncardiac surgery should be considered. First, Poldermans et al. (54) observed that the perioperative mortality rate among patients treated with statins was reduced 4.5-fold compared to patients without any statins. This large effect on short-term mortality was also retrieved on the long-term mortality (55). Moreover, this effect was independent from the effect of the β-blockers on long-term mortality (56). Probably because patients were included between 1991 and 2001, only 9% of these patients were preoperatively treated with statins in this population, suggesting that the indications of chronic statin therapy could be not comparable with the actual ones, and that the results of these studies may not represent the effect on all vascular populations.

In another retrospective study conducted on 1163 patients undergoing vascular surgery, O'Neil-Callahan et al. (57) also observed a protective effect of statins against cardiac morbidity. Forty-five percent of the patients included were preoperatively treated with statins.

More recently, in a retrospective cohort study of 780,591 patients who underwent noncardiac surgery, Lindenauer et al. (58) observed the potential effect of statins in reducing the risk of postoperative death. In this population undergoing all types surgery, 9% of the patients were preoperatively treated with statins, and the effect was particularly important in the most severe patients.

In the only randomized study in noncardiac surgery, Durazzo et al. (48) demonstrated that short-term treatment with 20 mg atorvastatin once a day for 45 days, irrespective of their serum cholesterol concentration, significantly reduces the incidence of major adverse cardiovascular events after vascular surgery. In this small randomized study, the incidence of cardiac events was more than 3 times higher with placebo (26%) compared with atorvastatin (8%) (48). Despite this promising finding, the trial was small and the treatment effect (69% relative risk reduction) is not consistent with the results from other randomized controlled trials conducted in nonsurgical conditions.

The meta-analysis from Hindler et al. (47) included more than 5000 vascular patients from 1 prospective cohort study (59), 1 randomized placebo controlled double-blind clinical trial (48), and 5 retrospective studies (54, 57, 60–62). The authors observed that preoperative statin therapy compared with no therapy produced mortality rates of 59% following vascular surgery (1.7% vs 6.1%).The same meta-analysis suggested that statins and β-blockers might produce independent and additive effects on cardiovascular risk (47).

To date only one study has explored the dose effect of statin during the perioperative period (63). This prospective study demonstrated that higher doses of statins and lower LDL cholesterol plasma level are significantly associated with a lower incidence of postoperative cardiac events after major vascular surgery. The authors conclude that additional risk reduction could be achieved by achieving LDL cholesterol plasma level <80 mg/dL. But several limitations have to be considered in this study: The nonrandomized design of the study remains a major concern, precluding definite conclusion. Furthermore, the dose of statins was obtained using the maximum recommended therapeutic dose (MRTD) according to the US Food and Drug Administration (FDA). With this method, atorvastatin and rosuvastatin were considered as equivalent. This is not relevant with the previously known effects of these two drugs (14). This promising strategy definitively needs further studies to confirm its effectiveness.

Thus, patients receiving preoperative statin therapy exhibit 30%–44% lower rates of mortality and of acute coronary syndromes than do patients who do not take statins at the time of surgery. However, these findings are based on observational cohort studies, most of which were retrospective in design. In most of these studies, dose and duration of statin use was not reported, and safety data were not adequately reported. Moreover, some potential biases are present in the design of these retrospective studies. Lindenauer et al. (58) considered patients who did not receive statins at postoperative day 1 as untreated, and thus a deleterious effect of statin withdrawal might have contributed to the global beneficial effect that they observed.

The few randomized studies available, even pooled together, should be considered as underpowered in obtaining a definite conclusion (64). Kapoor et al. (46) concluded in their meta-analysis, which did not separate cardiac or noncardiac surgery, that it is reasonable to advocate that statins be started preoperatively in eligible patients who would require statin therapy for medical reasons independent of the proposed operation; however, they also considered that it is premature to advocate its use for patients who do not have established coronary artery disease, at least until evidence is available from a randomized study. Hindler et al. (47) were more cautious, indicating the limitations of such a meta-analysis (i.e., possible publication bias, poor information on postoperative continuation of statins, lack of information on the minimum required duration of preoperative statin therapy, and marked differences in pharmacokinetic properties of the available statins).

Thus, at present, there is a strong need for randomized, controlled studies of perioperative statin therapy, some of which are now underway (from the trial registries: NCT00375518; ISRCTN83738615; ISRCTN47637497). These further studies should: (1) confirm the benefit of the introduction of a statin before surgery; (2) stratify the patients who could benefit from this preoperative treatment; (3) determine the optimal dose of statins regarding to the preoperative risk of the patients.

COMPLICATIONS ASSOCIATED WITH STATINS USE

The most important adverse effects associated with chronic statin therapy are myopathy and an asymptomatic increase in hepatic transaminases, both of which occur infrequently. Withdrawal of a chronic statin therapy does not seem to be associated with any relevant clinical effect during a stable period. Conversely, accumulating facts suggest morbidity withdrawal occurs during an unstable period.

Transaminases Elevation

Liver transaminase elevations were observed during the initial post-marketing surveillance of statins. Most elevations occur within the first 3 months of therapy; its incidence is 0.5% –5% (65, 66) and is dose dependent (67, 68). Indeed, Bradford et al. (69) reported that the 2-year incidence of transaminase elevation with lovastatin therapy was 0.1% for 20 mg/d and 1.9% for 80 mg/d. Nevertheless, whether transaminase elevation constitutes true hepatotoxicity has not been determined. Moreover, the incidence of clinically significant transaminase elevation (>3x ULN) were not significantly increased compared to placebo in the large statins trials (65). Practically, modest transaminase elevations (<3x ULN) are not thought to represent a contraindication to initiating, continuing, or advancing statin therapy. The occurrence of liver failure specifically due to statin remains exceedingly rare, if it even exists. (FDA reports only 30 cases of liver failure associated to statins.) Furthermore, if current labeling for all statins requires baseline measurements of transaminase, many liver experts do not agree with it. Cholestasis or active liver diseases are listed as absolute contraindication of statins, but no evidence exists to support it. Only a few case reports are available about some perioperative transaminase elevations associated with a statin therapy. Thus, no conclusion can be drawn about this adverse effect during the perioperative period, except that it seems to be poorly clinically relevant.

Statins-Induced Myopathy

During Nonsurgical Period

The ability of statins to induce clinically relevant myopathy under some circumstances is well established. The most frequent complaint is nonspecific muscle aches, which is not generally associated with an increase in creatine kinase (CK). Duration of statin therapy before the onset of myopathy varies from 1 week to more than 2 years (70). The American College of Cardiology/American Heart Association clinical advisory on the use and safety of statins (71) defined 4 syndromes:

1. Statin Myopathy (any muscle complaints related to these drugs);
2. Myalgia (muscle complaints without serum CK elevations);
3. Myositis (muscle symptoms with CK elevations);
4. Rhabdomyolysis (markedly elevated CK levels, with an elevated creatinine level consistent with pigment-induced nephropathy).

Cerivastatin, which is no longer on the market, was the primary cause of this complication (3.16 events/million prescriptions) (72). In contrast, the risk of statin-induced rhabdomyolysis ranges from 0 to 0.19 events/million prescriptions for the other commonly used statin (72, 73). Furthermore, the risk for rhabdomyolysis is associated with factors linked to increased serum statin concentrations, such as small body size, advanced age, renal or hepatic dysfunction, diabetes, hypothyroidism, and use of drugs that interfere with statin metabolism, such as antifungal agents, calcium-channel blockers, and amiodarone (Table 10–2) (15). Induction or inhibition of CYP450 isoenzymes (Table 10–1) is the most important cause of drug interactions (15, 74). Indeed, with the exception of pravastatin, which is transformed enzymatically in the liver cytosol, all statins undergo extensive microsomal metabolism by the cytochrome P450 (CYP) isoenzyme systems. Most of the drugs currently available in clinical practice (lovastatin, simvastatin, and atorvastatin) are biotransformed in the liver primarily by the CYP450 3A4 system (75). Fluvastatin is metabolized primarily by the CYP2C9 enzyme, with CYP3A4 and CYP2C8 contributing to a lesser extent (74). Rosuvastatin remains not extensively metabolized, but has some interaction with the CYP2C9 enzyme (76). Because the incidences of myopathy are dose dependent, and these interactions modulate the plasma levels of statin, particular attention must be paid when high doses of statins are used.

A recent meta-analysis (46) noted that CK activity (>10 times the upper limit of normal) occurred slightly more frequently in patients treated with statins than in patients who received a placebo (0.17% vs 0.13%, respectively). These results have been retrieved by a second meta-analysis (77). Nevertheless, we must take into account that many statin trials disclose that eligible patients with muscle complaints, previous adverse responses to cholesterol-lowering therapy, or even a mild asymptomatic elevation of CK (>1.5–6.0 times the upper limit of normal) are not randomized (2, 5, 44, 78). On the basis of the complete exclusion criteria, up to 75% of the screened participants in statin trials are not randomized and excluded. Thus, the exclusion of these patients before randomization may lead to biased reports on the frequency of occurrence of side effects with statin use. The FDA reported only 42 deaths attributable to statins (i.e., 1/million person years).

The mechanisms of statin-induced muscle injury remain unclear; however, mitochondrial dysfunction, altered P-450 metabolism, or inhibition of cell signalling pathways have been hypothesized (64). This statin-mediated adverse effect is rare and does not outweigh the beneficial effects of statins in the vast majority of patients. Furthermore, minimal data are available regarding the frequency of less-serious events such as muscle pain and weakness, which may affect 1%–5% of patients. However, these nonsevere adverse effects could alter the compliance to chronic statin therapy and must be taken into account.

During the Perioperative Period

The most serious potential perioperative side effect of statin therapy is rhabdomyolysis. However, to date, few perioperative studies have assessed its incidence. Several case reports describe severe postoperative rhabdomyolysis after surgery in patients treated with statins (79–84), but the causal link between the preoperative statin therapy and the observed muscular events has not been demonstrated at all. In an underpowered prospective study, Schouten et al. (59) did not observe any significant increase in the risk of perioperative myopathy in patients receiving statins. Although no definitive conclusion can be drawn, this study confirms that findings obtained outside the perioperative period may not be valid since the incidence of increased CK during the perioperative period (810%) (85) is markedly higher than the rates reported in medical trials. Moreover, because of the low frequency of statins-induced myopathy, very large studies are required to definitely conclude. Although further randomized trials are needed to evaluate perioperative statin safety, it would appear that the beneficial impact of statin therapy on the tremendous socioeconomic costs of perioperative morbidity and mortality largely outweigh their potential risks in the vast majority of patients.

Statins Withdrawal

The withdrawal of some cardiovascular drugs, such as β-blockers and nitrates, can exert pronounced rebound symptoms. In vitro, it has been shown that abrupt withdrawal of statins results in an overshoot translocation and activation of Rho, causing downregulation of e-NOS production below baseline levels (86). Whereas rapid improvement in endothelial function has been noted after initiation of statins, within 1 day of cessation of therapy, endothelial-dependent blood flow returned to below baseline values (19, 87). NO dependence of this withdrawal effect was demonstrated in a mouse model where statin withdrawal suppressed e-NOS production within 2 days (88). A more rapid effect was observed in cultured rat aortic vascular smooth muscle, where washout of statins produced a rebound increase above control levels of angiotensin II-mediated phosphorylation of $ERK_{1/2}$ and p38 MAPK (89).

In knockout mice, it has been shown that NAD(P)H-oxidase plays a central role in mediating the statin withdrawal mechanism (90). In patients, withdrawal of atorvastatin 10 mg/d is associated with an increased plasma level of sVCAM-1 and a decreased level of tPA when compared to untreated patients (91). Furthermore Li et al. (92) have demonstrated that discontinuation of statin therapy could induce a rebound phenomenon of inflammatory response (IL6 and CRP) in patients with hypercholesterolemia during stable period. Similar results were retrieved by Chu et al. (93) with *soluble* CD40 *liguand* and by Lee et al. (94) with *hs*CRP.

These results confirm that after withdrawal of statin, some effects can be curtailed within days, and these effects are observed without any elevation of serum cholesterol level. Conversely, some effects appear late after withdrawal, thus a platelet hyperactivation state following statin withdrawal has been described (95). The timing of this effect suggests that the raising of LDL cholesterol plasma levels after statins discontinuation is the main mechanism.

Statins Withdrawal During Nonsurgical Periods

In stable cardiac patients included in a randomized controlled trial (washout out period of the TNT study (44)), an underpowered study (96) suggests that a short-term discontinuation of statins is not associated with an increased risk of acute coronary syndromes (96, 97). In contrast, multiple reports suggest that statin withdrawal during unstable periods is associated with an increased risk of adverse cardiac events (98). For example, patients with acute coronary syndrome, in whom statins were discontinued, had an almost 3-fold higher cardiac event rate than patients continuing treatment (98, 99). This observation was more recently confirmed in a large retrospective study demonstrating a 2-fold increased mortality rate among patients who discontinued statins (100). Furthermore, in these patients, statin withdrawal was associated with a higher rate of complications than patients who had never been treated with statins.

Ischemic stroke is also an unstable period, and Blanco et al. (101) have shown in a randomized study that statin withdrawal for the first 3 days after admission was associated with a 4.7 (1.5– 14.9)-fold increase in the risk of death or dependency.

Statins Withdrawal During Perioperative Period

During perioperative periods, patients are prone to be submitted to chronic statin therapy withdrawal. Indeed it is commonly accepted that no essential therapies have to be interrupted to avoid potential interactions with anesthetic agents. Because statins are administered orally and the pleiotropic effects of statins are not readily appreciated, statin withdrawal for several days following surgery was common practice within our institution. After considering recent clinical and experimental reports describing the adverse effects associated with statin withdrawal, we examined our vascular surgery database (8). We observed that patients on long-term statin therapy who experienced statin withdrawn postoperatively were at increased risk for a postoperative cardiac event, despite multivariate risk adjustment. In contrast with previous reports by other groups, our analysis specifically investigated the effect of postoperative statin withdrawal with increased cardiac morbidity compared to early re-administration and compared to no use of statins (8). Using propensity score matched patients, the odds ratio associated with the use of statins to predict postoperative myocardial infarction was 2.1 (95% confidence interval (CI): 1.1–3.8) in the discontinuation group and 0.38 (95% CI: 0.15–0.98) in the continuation group (a relative risk reduction of 5.4; 95% CI: 1.2–25.3) (8). This finding suggests that postoperative withdrawal could dramatically reduce the perioperative protective effect of statins. In contrast, when statins were resumed early in the postoperative period, a protective effect against cardiac morbidity was demonstrated compared with patients not receiving statin therapy.

In similar conditions, Schouten et al. (102) observed that statin discontinuation was associated with an increased risk of postoperative myocardial infarction (OR: 4.6; 95% confidence interval (CI): 2.2–20.1). And interestingly, extended-release fluvastatin was associated with fewer perioperative cardiac events compared to other statins, including atorvastatin (but not rosuvastatin). This observation suggests that drugs with longer half-life could be more adapted to the perioperative period. Because atorvastatin and rosuvastatin are the most powerful (16) and have the longer half-life (15) (Table 10–1), we probably need further comparative studies to conclude that extended release forms are better for the perioperative period. These further studies would provide information about the pharmacokinetic of statins after surgeries associated with an interruption of the intestinal transit (i.e., biodisponibility of statins when administered via naso-gastric tube) or after hemorrhagic surgery (i.e., after major vascular surgery).

More recently, some studies have suggested that this potential deleterious effect could occur in other perioperative situations. Collard et al. (103) have shown that in cardiac surgery, preoperative statin therapy was associated with a significant reduction in early cardiac mortality, and that an early postoperative statin discontinuation was associated with increased in-hospital mortality. Besides, similar results have been retrieved in patients with bacteriema (104).

To conclude, discontinuation of statin therapy in humans leads to a proinflammatory, prothrombotic state with impaired endothelium function. During unstable periods (stroke, acute coronary syndrome, postoperative period, bacteriema) abrupt discontinuation of statin therapy significantly increases morbidity and/or mortality, whereas in stable vascular patients, discontinuation may be safe.

CONCLUSIONS AND PERSPECTIVES

Statins increasingly are used in patients with cardiovascular disease because the results of primary and secondary prevention studies show that they reduce the risk for myocardial infarction and stroke. In addition to their lipid-lowering properties, statins have other beneficial (pleiotropic) effects, including antioxidant, anti-inflammatory, plaque-stabilizing actions, and improved endothelial function. Moreover, accumulating data suggest that patients receiving preoperative statin therapy have a lower risk of postoperative death and acute coronary syndromes. However, further research is needed to determine whether untreated patients presenting for surgery should receive perioperative statin therapy.

These beneficial effects of statin therapy need to be compared in prospective studies to the risk for acute postoperative cardiac events associated with the pro-inflammatory and pro-thrombotic environment following surgery (105). This is especially true following vascular surgery where extensive tissue trauma and ischemia-reperfusion injury trigger an inflammatory and pro-thrombotic response secondary to platelet activation, increased fibrinogen levels, a temporary shutdown of fibrinolysis, and high circulating levels of catecholamines and stress hormones. Apart from β-blockers (106, 107), few treatments are readily available to decrease the risk for postoperative cardiovascular complications, including death.

In fact, utilizing a pharmaco-economic analysis of the existing prospective perioperative studies, Biccard et al. (108) suggested that perioperative β-blockade and statin therapy could result in cost savings through a reduction in major perioperative cardiovascular complications in patients with an expected perioperative major cardiovascular complication rate exceeding 10% following elective major noncardiac surgery. They reported a similar number-needed-to-treat (NNT = 19) to prevent major cardiovascular complications (including death) in high-risk patients for perioperative β-blocker and statin therapy but cautioned against the potentially harmful adverse effects of β-blockers in patients with a lower risk for cardiovascular events. Statin therapy may thus represent one of the most effective perioperative therapeutic regimens available for reducing the risk of postoperative cardiovascular complications in high-risk surgical patients since the introduction of β-blockers into the operative setting.

Furthermore, physicians need to be educated about the potential risks associated with discontinuation of statin therapy in the postoperative period, as underlined in the most recent ACC/AHA recommendations (109). Finally, although rare, patients at highest risk for the serious adverse effect of statins (i.e., rhabdomyolysis) should be more precisely identified in the future. In the meantime, we urge that serious consideration be given to the incorporation and maintenance of statin therapy as a perioperative strategy to improve postoperative outcome in the population of patients at increased risk of a major adverse cardiovascular event.

References

1. Randomised trial of cholesterol lowering in 4444 patients with coronary heart disease: the Scandinavian Simvastatin Survival Study (4S): Lancet 1994; 344:1383–9
2. MRC/BHF Heart Protection Study of cholesterol lowering with simvastatin in 20,536 high-risk individuals: a randomised placebo-controlled trial. Lancet 2002; 360:7–22
3. Major outcomes in moderately hypercholesterolemic, hypertensive patients randomized to pravastatin vs usual care: The Antihypertensive and Lipid-Lowering Treatment to Prevent Heart Attack Trial (ALLHAT-LLT). JAMA 2002; 288:2998–3007
4. Sever PS, Dahlof B, Poulter NR, et al.: Prevention of coronary and stroke events with atorvastatin in hypertensive patients who have average or lower-than-average cholesterol concentrations, in the Anglo-Scandinavian Cardiac Outcomes Trial-Lipid Lowering Arm (ASCOT-LLA): a multicentre randomised controlled trial. Lancet 2003; 361:1149–58
5. Shepherd J, Blauw GJ, Murphy MB, et al.: Pravastatin in elderly individuals at risk of vascular disease (PROSPER): a randomised controlled trial. Lancet 2002; 360:1623–30
6. Fraker TD, Jr., Fihn SD, Gibbons RJ, et al.: 2007 chronic angina focused update of the ACC/AHA 2002 guidelines for the management of patients with chronic stable angina: a report of the American College of Cardiology/American Heart Association Task Force on Practice Guidelines Writing Group to develop the focused update of the 2002 guidelines for the management of patients with chronic stable angina. J Am Coll Cardiol 2007; 50:2264–74
7. Anderson JL, Adams CD, Antman EM, et al.: ACC/AHA 2007 guidelines for the management of patients with unstable angina/non ST-elevation myocardial infarction: a report of the American College of Cardiology/American Heart Association Task Force on Practice Guidelines (Writing Committee to Revise the 2002

Guidelines for the Management of Patients With Unstable Angina/Non ST-Elevation Myocardial Infarction): developed in collaboration with the American College of Emergency Physicians, the Society for Cardiovascular Angiography and Interventions, and the Society of Thoracic Surgeons: endorsed by the American Association of Cardiovascular and Pulmonary Rehabilitation and the Society for Academic Emergency Medicine. Circulation 2007; 116:e148–304

8. Le Manach Y, Godet G, Coriat P, et al.: The impact of postoperative discontinuation or continuation of chronic statin therapy on cardiac outcome after major vascular surgery. Anesth Analg 2007; 104:1326–33
9. Pan W, Pintar T, Anton J, et al.: Statins are associated with a reduced incidence of perioperative mortality after coronary artery bypass graft surgery. Circulation 2004; 110:II-45–9
10. Takemoto M, Liao JK: Pleiotropic effects of 3-hydroxy-3-methylglutaryl coenzyme A reductase inhibitors. Arterioscler Thromb Vasc Biol 2001; 21:1712–9
11. Davignon J: Beneficial cardiovascular pleiotropic effects of statins. Circulation 2004; 109:III-39–43
12. Ray KK, Cannon CP: The potential relevance of the multiple lipid-independent (pleiotropic) effects of statins in the management of acute coronary syndromes. J Am Coll Cardiol 2005; 46:1425–33
13. Bucher HC, Griffith LE, Guyatt GH: Systematic review on the risk and benefit of different cholesterol-lowering interventions. Arterioscler Thromb Vasc Biol 1999; 19:187–95
14. Law MR, Wald NJ, Rudnicka AR: Quantifying effect of statins on low density lipoprotein cholesterol, ischaemic heart disease, and stroke: systematic review and meta-analysis. Br Med J 2003; 326:1423
15. Bellosta S, Paoletti R, Corsini A: Safety of statins: focus on clinical pharmacokinetics and drug interactions. Circulation 2004; 109:III-50–7
16. Jones P, Kafonek S, Laurora I, Hunninghake D: Comparative dose efficacy study of atorvastatin versus simvastatin, pravastatin, lovastatin, and fluvastatin in patients with hypercholesterolemia (the CURVES study). Am J Cardiol 1998; 81:582–7
17. Scharnagl H, Vogel M, Abletshauser C, et al.: Efficacy and safety of fluvastatin-extended release in hypercholesterolemic patients: morning administration is equivalent to evening administration. Cardiology 2006; 106:241–8

18. Robinson JG, Smith B, Maheshwari N, Schrott H: Pleiotropic effects of statins: benefit beyond cholesterol reduction? A meta-regression analysis. J Am Coll Cardiol 2005; 46:1855–62
19. Laufs U, Wassmann S, Hilgers S, et al.: Rapid effects on vascular function after initiation and withdrawal of atorvastatin in healthy, normocholesterolemic men. Am J Cardiol 2001; 88:1306–7
20. Ray KK, Cannon CP, McCabe CH, et al.: Early and late benefits of high-dose atorvastatin in patients with acute coronary syndromes: results from the PROVEIT-TIMI 22 trial. J Am Coll Cardiol 2005; 46:1405–10
21. Omori H, Nagashima H, Tsurumi Y, et al.: Direct in vivo evidence of a vascular statin: a single dose of cerivastatin rapidly increases vascular endothelial responsiveness in healthy normocholesterolaemic subjects. Br J Clin Pharmacol 2002; 54:395–9
22. O'Driscoll G, Green D, Taylor RR: Simvastatin, an HMG-coenzyme A reductase inhibitor, improves endothelial function within 1 month. Circulation 1997; 95:1126–31
23. Brandes RP: Statin-mediated inhibition of Rho: only to get more NO? Circ Res 2005; 96:927–9
24. Ludmer PL, Selwyn AP, Shook TL, et al.: Paradoxical vasoconstriction induced by acetylcholine in atherosclerotic coronary arteries. N Engl J Med 1986; 315:1046–51
25. Treasure CB, Klein JL, Weintraub WS, et al.: Beneficial effects of cholesterol-lowering therapy on the coronary endothelium in patients with coronary artery disease. N Engl J Med 1995; 332:481–7
26. Pleiner J, Schaller G, Mittermayer F, et al.: Simvastatin prevents vascular hyporeactivity during inflammation. Circulation 2004; 110:3349–54
27. Wassmann S, Laufs U, Baumer AT, et al.: Inhibition of geranylgeranylation reduces angiotensin II-mediated free radical production in vascular smooth muscle cells: involvement of angiotensin AT1 receptor expression and Rac1 GTPase. Mol Pharmacol 2001; 59:646–54
28. Undas A, Brummel-Ziedins KE, Mann KG: Statins and blood coagulation. Arterioscler Thromb Vasc Biol 2005; 25:287–94
29. Endres M, Laufs U: Effects of statins on endothelium and signaling mechanisms. Stroke 2004; 35:2708–11
30. Walter DH, Rittig K, Bahlmann FH, et al.: Statin therapy accelerates reendothelialization: a novel effect involving mobilization and incorporation of bone marrow-derived endothelial progenitor cells. Circulation 2002; 105:3017–24
31. Weitz-Schmidt G, Welzenbach K, Brinkmann V, et al.: Statins selectively inhibit leukocyte function antigen-1 by binding to a novel regulatory integrin site. Nat Med 2001; 7:687–92

32. Rezaie-Majd A, Prager GW, Bucek RA, et al.: Simvastatin reduces the expression of adhesion molecules in circulating monocytes from hypercholesterolemic patients. Arterioscler Thromb Vasc Biol 2003; 23:397–403
33. Laufs U, Kilter H, Konkol C, et al.: Impact of HMG CoA reductase inhibition on small GTPases in the heart. Cardiovasc Res 2002; 53:911–20
34. Wolfrum S, Jensen KS, Liao JK: Endothelium-dependent effects of statins. Arterioscler Thromb Vasc Biol 2003; 23:729–36
35. Halcox JPJ, Deanfield JE: Beyond the laboratory: clinical implications for statin pleiotropy. Circulation 2004; 109:II-42–8
36. Merla R, Reddy NK, Wang FW, et al.: Meta-analysis of published reports on the effect of statin treatment before percutaneous coronary intervention on periprocedural myonecrosis. Am J Cardiol 2007; 100:770–6
37. Khanal S, Attallah N, Smith DE, et al.: Statin therapy reduces contrast-induced nephropathy: an analysis of contemporary percutaneous interventions. Am J Med 2005; 118:843–9
38. Wenke K, Meiser B, Thiery J, et al.: Simvastatin initiated early after heart transplantation: 8-year prospective experience. Circulation 2003; 107:93–7
39. Gokce N, Keaney JF, Jr., Hunter LM, et al.: Risk stratification for postoperative cardiovascular events via noninvasive assessment of endothelial function: a prospective study. Circulation 2002; 105:1567–72
40. Grundy SM, Cleeman JI, Merz CN, et al.: Implications of recent clinical trials for the National Cholesterol Education Program Adult Treatment Panel III Guidelines. J Am Coll Cardiol 2004; 44:720–32
41. Chen Z, Peto R, Collins R, et al.: Serum cholesterol concentration and coronary heart disease in population with low cholesterol concentrations. BMJ 1991; 303:276–82
42. Nissen SE, Tuzcu EM, Schoenhagen P, et al.: Effect of intensive compared with moderate lipid-lowering therapy on progression of coronary atherosclerosis: A randomized controlled trial. JAMA 2004; 291:1071–80
43. Cannon CP, Braunwald E, McCabe CH, et al.: Intensive versus moderate lipid lowering with statins after acute coronary syndromes. N Engl J Med 2004; 350:1495–504
44. LaRosa JC, Grundy SM, Waters DD, et al.: Intensive lipid lowering with atorvastatin in patients with stable coronary disease. N Engl J Med 2005; 352:1425–35
45. Buchwald H, Varco RL, Matts JP, et al.: Effect of partial ileal bypass surgery on mortality and morbidity from coronary heart disease in

patients with hypercholesterolemia. Report of the Program on the Surgical Control of the Hyperlipidemias (POSCH). N Engl J Med 1990; 323:946–55
46. Kapoor AS, Kanji H, Buckingham J, et al.: Strength of evidence for perioperative use of statins to reduce cardiovascular risk: systematic review of controlled studies. Br Med J 2006; 333:1149
47. Hindler K, Shaw AD, Samuels J, et al.: Improved postoperative outcomes associated with preoperative statin therapy. Anesthesiology 2006; 105:1260–72
48. Durazzo AE, Machado FS, Ikeoka DT, et al.: Reduction in cardiovascular events after vascular surgery with atorvastatin: a randomized trial. J Vasc Surg 2004; 39:967–76
49. Christenson JT: Preoperative lipid-control with simvastatin reduces the risk of postoperative thrombocytosis and thrombotic complications following CABG Eur J Cardiothorac Surg 1999; 15:394–9
50. Patti G, Chello M, Candura D, et al.: Randomized trial of atorvastatin for reduction of postoperative atrial fibrillation in patients undergoing cardiac surgery: results of the ARMYDA-3 (Atorvastatin for Reduction of MYocardial Dysrhythmia After cardiac surgery) study. Circulation 2006; 114:1455–61
51. Dotani MI, Elnicki DM, Jain AC, Gibson CM: Effect of preoperative statin therapy and cardiac outcomes after coronary artery bypass grafting. Am J Cardiol 2000; 86:1128–30
52. Clark LL, Ikonomidis JS, Crawford FA, Jr., et al.: Preoperative statin treatment is associated with reduced postoperative mortality and morbidity in patients undergoing cardiac surgery: an 8-year retrospective cohort study. J Thorac Cardiovasc Surg 2006; 131:679–85
53. Ali IS, Buth KJ: Preoperative statin use and outcomes following cardiac surgery. Int J Cardiol 2005; 103:12–8
54. Poldermans D, Bax JJ, Kertai MD, et al.: Statins are associated with a reduced incidence of perioperative mortality in patients undergoing major noncardiac vascular surgery. Circulation 2003; 107:1848–51
55. Kertai MD, Boersma E, Westerhout CM, et al.: Association between long-term statin use and mortality after successful abdominal aortic aneurysm surgery. Am J Med 2004; 116:96–103
56. Kertai MD, Boersma E, Westerhout CM, et al.: A combination of statins and beta-blockers is independently associated with a reduction in the incidence of perioperative mortality and nonfatal myocardial infarction in patients undergoing abdominal aortic aneurysm surgery. Eur J Vasc Endovasc Surg 2004; 28:343–52
57. O'Neil-Callahan K, Katsimaglis G, Tepper MR, et al.: Statins decrease perioperative cardiac complications in patients undergo-

ing noncardiac vascular surgery: the Statins for Risk Reduction in Surgery (StaRRS) study. J Am Coll Cardiol 2005; 45:336–42

58. Lindenauer PK, Pekow P, Wang K, et al.: Lipid-lowering therapy and in-hospital mortality following major noncardiac surgery. JAMA 2004; 291:2092–9
59. Schouten O, Kertai MD, Bax JJ, et al.: Safety of perioperative statin use in high-risk patients undergoing major vascular surgery. Am J Cardiol 2005; 95:658–60
60. Abbruzzese TA, Havens J, Belkin M, et al.: Statin therapy is associated with improved patency of autogenous infrainguinal bypass grafts. J Vasc Surg 2004; 39:1178–85
61. Kennedy J, Quan H, Buchan AM, et al.: Statins are associated with better outcomes after carotid endarterectomy in symptomatic patients. Stroke 2005; 36:2072–6
62. Ward RP, Leeper NJ, Kirkpatrick JN, et al.: The effect of preoperative statin therapy on cardiovascular outcomes in patients undergoing infrainguinal vascular surgery. Int J Cardiol 2005; 104:264–8
63. Feringa HH, Schouten O, Karagiannis SE, et al.: Intensity of statin therapy in relation to myocardial ischemia, troponin T release, and clinical cardiac outcome in patients undergoing major vascular surgery. J Am Coll Cardiol 2007; 50:1649–56
64. Kersten JR, Fleisher LA: Statins: The next advance in cardioprotection? Anesthesiology 2006; 105:1079–80
65. Farmer JA, Torre-Amione G: Comparative tolerability of the HMG-CoA reductase inhibitors. Drug Saf 2000; 23:197–213
66. Bays H: Statin safety: an overview and assessment of the data—2005. Am J Cardiol 2006; 97:6C–26C
67. Bradford RH, Shear CL, Chremos AN, et al.: Expanded Clinical Evaluation of Lovastatin (EXCEL) study results. I. Efficacy in modifying plasma lipoproteins and adverse event profile in 8245 patients with moderate hypercholesterolemia. Arch Intern Med 1991; 151:43–9
68. Hsu I, Spinler SA, Johnson NE: Comparative evaluation of the safety and efficacy of HMG-CoA reductase inhibitor monotherapy in the treatment of primary hypercholesterolemia. Ann Pharmacother 1995; 29:743–59
69. Bradford RH, Shear CL, Chremos AN, et al.: Expanded Clinical Evaluation of Lovastatin (EXCEL) study results: two-year efficacy and safety follow-up. Am J Cardiol 1994; 74:667–73
70. Hamilton-Craig I: Statin-associated myopathy. Med J Aust 2001; 175:486–9

71. Pasternak RC, Smith SC, Jr., Bairey-Merz CN, et al.: ACC/AHA/NHLBI clinical advisory on the use and safety of statins. Circulation 2002; 106:1024–8
72. Thompson PD, Clarkson P, Karas RH: Statin-associated myopathy. JAMA 2003; 289:1681–90
73. Sethi M, Collard C: Perioperative statin therapy: are formal guidelines and physician education needed? Anesth Analg 2007; 104:1322–24
74. Corsini A, Bellosta S, Baetta R, et al.: New insights into the pharmacodynamic and pharmacokinetic properties of statins. Pharmacol Ther 1999; 84:413–28
75. Thummel KE, Wilkinson GR: In vitro and in vivo drug interactions involving human CYP3A Annu Rev Pharmacol Toxicol 1998; 38:389–430
76. White CM: A review of the pharmacologic and pharmacokinetic aspects of rosuvastatin. J Clin Pharmacol 2002; 42:963–70
77. Kashani A, Phillips CO, Foody JM, et al.: Risks associated with statin therapy: a systematic overview of randomized clinical trials. Circulation 2006; 114:2788–97
78. Shepherd J, Cobbe SM, Ford I, et al.: Prevention of coronary heart disease with pravastatin in men with hypercholesterolemia. West of Scotland Coronary Prevention Study Group. N Engl J Med 1995; 333:1301–7
79. Blaison G, Weber JC, Sachs D, et al.: Rhabdomyolysis caused by simvastatinin a patient following heart transplantation and cyclosporine therapy. Rev Med Interne 1992; 13:61–3
80. Forestier F, Breton Y, Bonnet E, Janvier G: Severe rhabdomyolysis after laparoscopic surgery for adenocarcinoma of the rectum in two patients treated with statins. Anesthesiology 2002; 97:1019–21
81. Corpier CL, Jones PH, Suki WN, et al.: Rhabdomyolysis and renal injury with lovastatin use. Report of two cases in cardiac transplant recipients. JAMA 1988; 260:239–41
82. Rosenberg AD, Neuwirth MG, Kagen LJ, et al.: Intraoperative rhabdomyolysis in a patient receiving pravastatin, a 3-hydroxy-3-methylglutaryl coenzyme A (HMG CoA) reductase inhibitor. Anesth Analg 1995; 81:1089–91
83. Alvarez JM, Rawdanowicz TJ, Goldstein J: Rhadbdomyolysis after coronary artery bypass grafting in a patient receiving simvastatin. J Thorac Cardiovasc Surg 1998; 116:654–5
84. Weise WJ, Possidente CJ: Fatal rhabdomyolysis associated with simvastatin in a renal transplant patient. Am J Med 2000; 108:351–2
85. Bertrand M, Godet G, Fleron MH, et al.: Lumbar muscle rhabdomyolysis after abdominal aortic surgery. Anesth Analg 1997; 85:11–5.

86. Gertz K, Laufs U, Lindauer U, et al.: Withdrawal of statin treatment abrogates stroke protection in mice. Stroke 2003; 34:551–7
87. Taneva E, Borucki K, Wiens L, et al.: Early effects on endothelial function of atorvastatin 40 mg twice daily and its withdrawal. Am J Cardiol 2006; 97:1002–6
88. Laufs U, Endres M, Custodis F, et al.: Suppression of endothelial nitric oxide production after withdrawal of statin treatment is mediated by negative feedback regulation of rho GTPase gene transcription. Circulation 2000; 102:3104–10
89. Tristano AG, Castejon AM, Castro A, Cubeddu LX: Effects of statin treatment and withdrawal on angiotensin II-induced phosphorylation of p38 MAPK and ERK1/2 in cultured vascular smooth muscle cells. Biochem Biophys Res Commun 2007; 353:11–7
90. Vecchione C, Brandes RP: Withdrawal of 3-hydroxy-3-methylglutaryl coenzyme A reductase inhibitors elicits oxidative stress and induces endothelial dysfunction in mice. Circ Res 2002; 91:173–9
91. Lai WT, Lee KT, Chu CS, et al.: Influence of withdrawal of statin treatment on proinflammatory response and fibrinolytic activity in humans: an effect independent on cholesterol elevation. Int J Cardiol 2005; 98:459–64
92. Li JJ, Li YS, Chu JM, et al.: Changes of plasma inflammatory markers after withdrawal of statin therapy in patients with hyperlipidemia. Clin Chim Acta 2006; 366:269–73
93. Chu CS, Lee KT, Lee MY, et al.: Effects of atorvastatin and atorvastatin withdrawal on soluble CD40L and adipocytokines in patients with hypercholesterolaemia. Acta Cardiol 2006; 61:263–9
94. Lee KT, Lai WT, Chu CS, et al.: Effect of withdrawal of statin on C-reactive protein. Cardiology 2004; 102:166–70
95. Puccetti L, Pasqui AL, Pastorelli M, et al.: Platelet hyperactivity after statin treatment discontinuation. Thromb Haemost 2003; 90:476–82
96. McGowan MP: There is no evidence for an increase in acute coronary syndromes after short-term abrupt discontinuation of statins in stable cardiac patients. Circulation 2004; 110:2333–5
97. Stone NJ: Stopping statins. Circulation 2004; 110:2280–2
98. Heeschen C, Hamm CW, Laufs U, et al.: Withdrawal of statins increases event rates in patients with acute coronary syndromes. Circulation 2002; 105:1446–52
99. Heeschen C, Hamm CW, Laufs U, et al.: Withdrawal of statins in patients with acute coronary syndromes. Circulation 2003; 107:e27e
100. Spencer FA, Fonarow GC, Frederick PD, et al.: Early withdrawal of statin therapy in patients with non-ST-segment elevation myocardial infarction: national registry of myocardial infarction. Arch Intern Med 2004; 164:2162–8

101. Blanco M, Nombela F, Castellanos M, et al.: Statin treatment withdrawal in ischemic stroke: a controlled randomized study. Neurology 2007; 69:904–10
102. Schouten O, Hoeks SE, Welten GM, et al.: Effect of statin withdrawal on frequency of cardiac events after vascular surgery. Am J Cardiol 2007; 100:316–20
103. Collard CD, Body SC, Shernan SK, et al.: Preoperative statin therapy is associated with reduced cardiac mortality after coronary artery bypass graft surgery. J Thorac Cardiovasc Surg 2006; 132:392–400
104. Kruger P, Fitzsimmons K, Cook D, et al.: Statin therapy is associated with fewer deaths in patients with bacteraemia. Intensive Care Med 2006; 32:75–9
105. Samama CM, Thiry D, Elalamy I, et al.: Perioperative activation of hemostasis in vascular surgery patients. Anesthesiology 2001; 94:74–8
106. Mangano DT, Layug EL, Wallace A, et al.: Effect of atenolol on mortality and cardiovascular morbidity after noncardiac surgery. N Engl J Med 1996; 335:1713–21
107. Boersma E, Poldermans D, Bax JJ, et al.: Predictors of cardiac events after major vascular surgery: role of clinical characteristics, dobutamine chocardiography, and β-blocker therapy. JAMA 2001; 285:1865–73
108. Biccard B, Sear J, Foëx P: The pharmaco-economics of peri-operative statin therapy. Anaesthesia 2005; 60:1059–63
109. Fleisher LA, Beckman JA, Brown KA, et al.: ACC/AHA 2007 Guidelines on Perioperative Cardiovascular Evaluation and Care for Noncardiac Surgery: Executive Summary: A Report of the American College of Cardiology/American Heart Association Task Force on Practice Guidelines (Writing Committee to Revise the 2002 Guidelines on Perioperative Cardiovascular Evaluation for Noncardiac Surgery): Developed in Collaboration With the American Society of Echocardiography, American Society of Nuclear Cardiology, Heart Rhythm Society, Society of Cardiovascular Anesthesiologists, Society for Cardiovascular Angiography and Interventions, Society for Vascular Medicine and Biology, and Society for Vascular Surgery. Circulation 2007; 116:1971–96

John P. Abenstein, MSEE, MD
Daniel R. Brown, MD, PhD, FCCM

11 Perioperative Glycemic Control

Diabetes mellitus (DM) is a disease whose hallmark is hyperglycemia. It is, in fact, several syndromes of abnormal carbohydrate metabolism. Diabetes is associated with varying degrees of impaired secretion and resistance to the action of insulin. The prevalence of diabetes is increasingly common, affecting nearly 10% of Americans and about 33% of cardiac surgery patients. Multiple studies have shown that as many as one-third of those with DM do not know they have the disease. The American Diabetes Association estimates that 12–25% of hospitalized adult patients have DM. If the number of obese Americans continues to increase, the incidence of diabetes could double in the next 20 years.

Patients with DM have a mortality rate 4–5 times higher than nondiabetic patients secondary to complications of the disease, which include multiorgan atherosclerosis, hypertension, nephropathy, neuropathy, and increased rates of multiple postoperative complications (1–3). Diabetics are much more likely to undergo surgical procedures as compared to those without the disease (1, 4). Studies have shown that hyperglycemia is a predictor of adverse outcomes in surgical and critical care patients (5–9). This pattern also is seen in cardiac surgery patients. Diabetic patients undergoing coronary artery bypass procedures have increased morbidity and mortality (10–12). This is thought to be secondary to a variety of factors, including a higher incidence of poor left ventricular function, dysfunctional endothelium, diffuse coronary disease, and abnormal clotting function (13).

Advances in Cardiovascular Pharmacology, edited by Philippe R. Housmans, MD, PhD and Gregory A. Nuttall, M.D.
Lippincott Williams & Wilkins, Baltimore © 2008.

Data now show tight glycemic control is associated with improved outcomes in hospitalized patients. These improved outcomes are also seen in cardiac surgery patients (14). This chapter will discuss the classification and treatment of diabetes mellitus, the anesthetic and surgical implications of diabetes, and recent studies of glycemic control and outcomes in surgical and critical care patients.

CLASSIFICATION OF DIABETES

There are two classifications of diabetes: type 1 and type 2, based on the etiology of the disease rather than age of onset or type of treatment (15). Pancreatic β cells are destroyed in type 1 diabetes, leading to insulin deficiency. This is usually an autoimmune process, although there is a subset of these patients who are classified as idiopathic type 1 DM because they have no identifiable antibodies. Although type 1 diabetes is most commonly seen in children and young adults, older patients with newly diagnosed DM may have islet cell antibodies and would therefore be diagnosed with type 1 diabetes. Patients with type 1 diabetes require insulin therapy; otherwise they will develop diabetic ketoacidosis (DKA).

The other variant of DM, type 2, is found in about 90% of all diabetic patients. Type 2 DM is characterized by variable degrees of insulin deficiency and resistance. There are no diagnostic tests specifically for type 2 diabetes. Ketoacidosis is infrequently seen in these patients. However, some patients may develop DKA secondary to other systemic illness, such as severe infection. Type 2 DM may also be secondary to drugs and/or chemicals (e.g., corticosteroids) or be seen during pregnancy.

Diagnosis

The American Diabetes Association (ADA) defines diabetes mellitus in a patient with a fasting (8 hours) plasma glucose level >126 mg/dL (normal is <100 mg/dL), symptoms of DM (i.e., polydipsia, polyuria, unexplained weight loss) and a random glucose level >200 mg/dL, or a plasma glucose value >200 mg/dL 2 hours after an oral glucose challenge (75 g glucose dissolved in water) (16). A fasting plasma glucose level between 100–125 mg/dL is defined as "impaired" glucose control. Abnormalities in insulin secretion and/or action are currently thought to lie along a continuum. Patients with impaired fasting glucose levels are thought to be at high likelihood to eventually progress to diabetes. Of note, patients with increased fasting glucose levels and body mass indexes appear to be at greater risk for hyperglycemia during times of stress such as the perioperative period.

Pharmacologic Treatment

A lack of glycemic control that leads to the development and progression of microvascular complications (retinopathy, nephropathy, and neuropathy) has been suggested in studies of type 1 and type 2 diabetic patients (17, 18). The effect of improved glycemic control and macrovascular (peripheral vascular and cardiac) complications is less clear. As stated above, glucose management in type 1 diabetic patients relies on supplementation of insulin. Medical therapy of type 2 diabetes often begins with diet modification, exercise, and oral medications, starting with either metformin or a sulfonylurea. If there is inadequate glycemic control, then combined therapy with other oral agents or the addition of insulin is indicated.

Common Oral Preparations (19) (Short-acting agents typically are held the day of surgery; longer acting agents are held up to 2–3 days prior to surgery.)

Sulfonylureas (First generation: tolbutamide, acetohexamide, tolazamide, chlorpropamide; Second generation: glyburide, glipizide, glimepiride). Increases release of endogenous insulin and enhances insulin receptor function by binding to ATP-dependent K^+ channels in pancreatic β cells; variable duration of action, typically less than 24 hours but chlorpropamide up to 72 hours.

Biguanides (metformin). Mechanism not completely understood but decreases hepatic glucose output and increases insulin action. Avoided in patients with renal or hepatic compromise due to association with development of lactic acidosis.

Thiazolidinediones (rosiglitazone, pioglitazone). Increases peripheral glucose uptake and decreases gluconeogenesis via unclear mechanisms.

Meglitinides (repaglinide, nateglinide). Stimulates insulin secretion by binding to ATP-dependent K^+ channels in pancreatic β cells.

Alpha-glucosidase inhibitors (acarbose, miglitol). Decreases GI digestion and absorption of saccharides and thereby glucose synthesis (no need to hold preoperatively).

Pharmacology of Insulin

In the hospital setting, insulin is the primary medication for the treatment of hyperglycemia, particularly during the perioperative period and in the intensive care unit (ICU). The physiologic response to injected animal insulin in a patient with type 1 diabetes was first described in 1922. In 1955, insulin was the first protein to be fully sequenced. The insulin molecule consists of 51 amino acids arranged in two chains: an A chain (21 amino acids) and a B chain (30 amino acids) that are linked by 2 disulfide bonds (20). Proinsulin, a single-chain 86 amino acid peptide, is an insulin precursor produced in pancreatic β cells and packaged into granules. Proinsulin is cleaved into insulin and secreted by the β cells when stimulated by glucose and other factors.

After excretion, insulin is distributed to the tissues where it binds to insulin receptors found on the cell surface. Insulin promotes the cellular uptake of glucose into fat and skeletal muscle and inhibits hepatic glucose output, thus lowering the blood glucose.

Today, most insulin used is either human or an analog of human insulin. When human insulin, produced by recombinant DNA techniques, became available in the 1980s, the use of animal insulin declined dramatically. Beef insulin and beef-pork insulin are no longer commercially available, although the US Food and Drug Administration (FDA) may allow for the personal importation of beef insulin from a foreign country if a patient cannot be treated with human or pork insulin.

The development and production of analogs to human insulin with recombinant DNA techniques has allowed for the structure of the insulin molecule to be modified in order to alter the pharmacokinetics (e.g., altering absorption). Modified human insulins have safety and efficacy profiles comparable to human insulin (21). Insulin lispro and aspart are similar to human insulin, except insulin lispro is 1.5-fold more potent in binding to the IGF-1 receptor.

Commercially available human insulins are virtually free of contaminants and contain <1 ppm of proinsulin (also referred to as "purified"). Side effects of insulin, such as local or systemic hypersensitivity, lipodystrophy, and antibody production causing insulin resistance, are rarely seen with human insulin (20). In the United States, all insulins are available in the concentration of 100 units/ml (U-100). Regular human insulin (Humulin R, Lilly) is also available in a more concentrated preparation of 500 units/ml (U-500). U-500 is used for rare cases of extreme insulin resistance, where very large doses of insulin are required, or for specific institutional demands, such as large number of insulin infusion bags being produced by a pharmacy.

Pharmacokinetics of Insulin

Insulin administered subcutaneously (SC) is absorbed directly into the bloodstream. The absorption of human insulin after SC absorption is the rate limiting step, and is inconsistent with the coefficients of variation of T50% (time for 50% of the insulin dose to be absorbed) varying ~25% within an individual and up to 50% between patients (20, 22). The variability of the absorption of insulin is related to differences of blood flow at the site of injection. When regular insulin is injected in the subcutaneous tissues of the abdomen, absorption is about twice as fast as other sites, secondary to differences in subcutaneous blood flow. Anesthesia alters the absorption rate of insulin because of its affect on SC blood flow. Insulin lispro and insulin aspart appear to have less variation in absorption rates (23).

Circulating insulin is distributed in equilibrium between free insulin and insulin bound to IgG antibodies (20). The presence of insulin antibodies can delay the onset of insulin activity, reduce the peak concentration of free insulin, and prolong the biologic half-life of insulin (24).

The liver and kidney metabolize insulin. The liver eliminates about 60% of excreted insulin (insulin delivered through portal vein blood flow) and the kidneys about 40%. However, in the case of exogenously administered insulin the kidney metabolizes about 60% and the liver the remaining 40% because insulin in not delivered directly to the portal vein (25). Renal dysfunction will reduce the clearance of insulin and prolong its effect, but renal function needs to be significantly decreased before this becomes clinically relevant (26).

Intravenous insulin has, by definition, virtually instantaneous uptake. The half-life of insulin is about 8 minutes, so a single IV injection of insulin will be eliminated in about 30 minutes (27, 28). The rapid elimination of IV insulin requires a continuous infusion in order to maintain a constant serum level. Insulin infusions are the mainstay of acute management of hyperglycemia in the hospital setting.

Various strategies for the management of the diabetic patient who has fasted prior to surgery have been described. None has been shown to be the preferred technique. A common recommendation is to reduce the morning dose of insulin by one-half. Those with implanted insulin pumps should have their pump discontinued and placed on a constant infusion immediately preoperatively. Whatever strategy is used, it is imperative to determine plasma glucose immediately preoperatively and at regular intervals during the perioperative period. These results should be used to guide the anesthesiologist in treating the patient with insulin and/or glucose. In general, the magnitude and type of drug therapy, anticipated duration of reduced caloric intake, and magnitude of procedural-related stress need to be weighed when determining patient-specific recommendations.

END-ORGAN DYSFUNCTION IN DIABETIC PATIENTS

Diabetes is a progressive disease that, over time, leads to multi-organ dysfunction. The anesthesiologist must determine the status of various diabetes-related comorbidities of the surgical patient. As noted previously, up to one-third of patients who are diabetic are unaware of their disease. When elevated preoperative serum glucose is found in a supposedly nondiabetic patient, the physician should re-evaluate the patient in terms of risk and anesthetic plan. The focus of the preoperative evaluation should include:

Cardiovascular Disease. Diabetes is the most common metabolic disease associated with cardiovascular disease. Diabetics are at increased risk for hypertension, coronary artery disease, diastolic dysfunction, congestive heart failure, peripheral vascular, and cerebrovascular disease. Diabetics may have significant coronary disease, including previous myocardial infarction, without symptoms (e.g., silent ischemia). American College of Cardiology guidelines for perioperative cardiovascular evaluation list diabetes as an "intermediate" clinical predictor for coronary artery disease along with mild angina pectoris, prior myocardial infarction, prior or compensated congestive heart failure, and renal insufficiency (29). The use of β-adrenergic blockade in diabetic patients has been controversial because of concerns that these drugs could worsen glucose intolerance. Recent studies have shown no increase in hypoglycemic episodes in diabetic patients receiving β-blockers. In addition, the cardiovascular benefits of β-blocker therapy are greater in diabetics as compared to nondiabetic patients. β-adrenergic blockade is appropriate therapy, when indicated, for patient with diabetes (30, 31).

Renal Disease. Diabetics commonly develop renal dysfunction. Diabetes is the leading cause of renal failure. Angiotensin converting enzyme inhibitors have been shown to decrease albuminuria and progression of renal dysfunction in diabetic patients. The renal status of a diabetic patient must be considered when the anesthesiologist is determining the anesthetic plan (e.g., avoid nephrotoxic medications, dosing of drugs dependent on renal excretion).

Other. Diabetics often have peripheral and autonomic neuropathies. Any neurologic deficits should be documented prior to surgery and extra care should be taken when positioning these patients. These patients are at increased risk for ischemic injury secondary to peripheral vascular disease. In addition, some may not notice pressure points due to their neuropathy. Autonomic neuropathy may blunt the compensatory cardiovascular response to hypotension, thus predisposing these patients to hemodynamic lability. Autonomic neuropathy also may cause gastroparesis and increases the risk of pulmonary aspiration. In patients with chronic hyperglycemia, nonenzymatic glycosylation of proteins and abnormal collagen cross-linking may result in decreased joint mobility. Decreased mobility in the temporomandibular and cervical spine joints may contribute to challenging airway management.

ACUTE GLYCEMIC COMPLICATIONS

Hyperglycemia with metabolic alterations and hypoglycemia are serious medical conditions. Hyperglycemia is associated with both diabetic ketoacidosis (DKA) and a nonketotic hyperosmolar state (NKHS) (32). The stress of surgery and severe illness may alter glycometabolic regulation, contributing to disruption of glucose homeostasis. The perioperative period is often associated with a relative decrease in insulin secretion and an increase in insulin resistance. Commonly, pathology that precipitates severe alterations in glucose regulation requires surgical intervention.

Diabetic Ketoacidosis

DKA is a life-threatening complication of hyperglycemia (reported mortality 5–10%) seen predominantly in type 1 diabetic patients. DKA results from insulin deficiency and is characterized by hyperglycemia, dehydration, hyperosmolarity, and an increased anion gap secondary to production of ketones. Precipitating factors include infection, surgical stress, trauma, or lack of insulin. Ketone production frequently results in hyperventilation with large tidal volumes (Kussmaul breathing), "fruity" breath, and nausea and vomiting. Management is focused on identifying and treating precipitating factors, volume resuscitation, glycometabolic control, and electrolyte replacement. Fluid deficits secondary to osmotic diuresis, lack of oral intake, emesis, and insensible losses from sweating and hyperventilation are frequently large (>5 liters). Dehydration may result in hypotension and pre-renal stress on an already compromised renal system. Hyperkalemia is frequently present as a result of acidemia-related extracellular potassium shifts as well as tissue catabolism. With treatment, potassium levels often plummet secondary to the cellular reuptake of potassium and aggressive replacement therapy should be anticipated.

Patients should be carefully monitored for signs of volume overload and hyperkalemia in the setting of renal failure. While a sodium deficit is frequently present, the measured sodium may be falsely low due to hyperglycemia and hypertriglyceridemia. Corrected sodium concentrations in the hyperglycemic patient may be estimated by adding 1.5–2.0 mEq/L to the measured sodium value per 100 mg/dL glucose over 100 mg/dL. Other electrolytes, especially phosphorus and magnesium, often are depleted and should be determined frequently and replaced as indicated. A glucose infusion should be started as plasma glucose approaches 200 mg/dL to avoid potential overcorrection of hyperglycemia. Intravenous insulin should be continued until serum ketones are cleared and the acidemia resolved. Patients are at risk for cerebral edema and subsequent intracranial hypertension. Careful monitoring of neurologic status is warranted. Bicarbonate administration is not routine due to concerns of worsening intracellular acidosis, leftward shift of the oxyhemoglobin dissociation curve and increased hyperosmolarity.

Guidelines for DKA Management

- Routine monitors plus arterial access (for hemodynamic monitoring and frequent blood sampling) and central venous access (for volume and electrolyte replacement)
- Aggressive crystalloid replacement (1–3 L in the first hour) starting with 0.9% saline and adjusting free water content of subsequent fluids based on sodium determinations, with subsequent volume replacement individualized to patient response
- Intravenous regular insulin infusion titrated by serial plasma glucose determinations adding a glucose infusion as glucose values approach 200 mg/dL
- Supplementation of potassium, phosphorus and magnesium as guided by serial plasma determinations

Non-Ketotic Hyperosmolar States

NKHS occur predominantly in type 2 diabetic patients during periods of stress such as infection or other illness. Compared to patients with DKA, NKHS patients are typically more dehydrated, hyperosmolar, and hyperglycemic. Neurologic alterations are usually present and may include confusion, coma, seizures, and/or focal neurological deficits. While patients with NKHS lack the acidemia from ketone production, severe dehydration may result in significant hypotension leading to lactic acidosis. Thrombotic events may occur due to hypovolemia, hyperviscosity and hypotension. Volume resuscitation is the mainstay of treatment. As with DKA, 0.9% saline is a reasonable choice for initial resuscitation with the subsequent free water composition of fluid guided by serial sodium determinations. Due to the greater hyperglycemia and hyperosmolarity seen in NKHS patients, they may be at increased risk for developing cerebral edema. More gradual (>24 hours) correction of hyperglycemia and hyperosmolarity is recommended along with frequent neurologic evaluation.

Hypoglycemia

Hypoglycemia is commonly defined in adults as a plasma glucose <50 mg/dL. Altered mental status, which may progress to coma and death, and physiologic responses to increased serum catecholamines are how hypoglycemia is commonly detected. In the perioperative environment, the ability to recognize the signs of hypoglycemia is often compromised. One must have a high index of suspicion for hypoglycemia. When caring for diabetic patients, particularly when hypoglycemic agents are used, frequent measurements of serum glucose must be taken and used to guide therapy. Hypoglycemia may develop due to residual effects of long-acting insulins, overaggressive antidiabetic treatment, or decreased caloric intake. Treatment consists of glucose administration and correction of the precipitating cause. Since the response to glucose administration is quite variable, following initial treatment (50 mL of 50% glucose in adults), serial glucose determinations should be made and a glucose infusion considered based on the patient's response.

Metabolic Response to Anesthesia and Surgery

Surgical intervention triggers a significant stress response in patients. This response is mediated by the neuroendocrine system with an increase in sympathetic tone and the release of catecholamines, glucagon, and cortisol. Nondiabetic patients generally, but not always, are able to maintain normoglycemia by secreting insulin to counterbalance the increase in serum glucose as part of the stress response. Diabetic patients frequently are unable to compensate for the stress response, and therefore can have a significant increase in their serum glucose. They require intervention to exogenously meet their insulin requirements during the perioperative period (33).

Anesthetics also impact glucose metabolism through their impact on sympathetic tone. Inhalation agents appear to suppress the secretion of insulin, which can result in glucose dysregulation and hyperglycemia (34, 35). This dysregulation of glucose metabolism can lead to much worse hyperglycemia in diabetic patients and can increase the risk of DKA or NKHS. Regional anesthetics are effective in blocking the increase in sympathetic tone while the block is in place. However, the increase in sympathetic tone is still seen postoperatively with the concomitant glucose dysregulation and hyperglycemia. There are no data to suggest improved perioperative outcomes of diabetic patients who receive regional anesthesia, as compared to general anesthesia, for their operative procedure (36, 37).

GLYCEMIC CONTROL IN THE CRITICALLY ILL AND DURING THE PERIOPERATIVE PERIOD

Glycemic control in critically ill and surgical patients is a hotly debated topic among anesthesiologists, surgeons, intensivists, and endocrinologists. Data support an association between hyperglycemia and increased morbidity and mortality in both surgical and medical patients. Hyperglycemia induces an osmotic diuresis, impairs leucocyte function, increases cardiovascular tone, decreases gastric motility, impairs wound healing, increases the generation of free radicals and proinflammatory

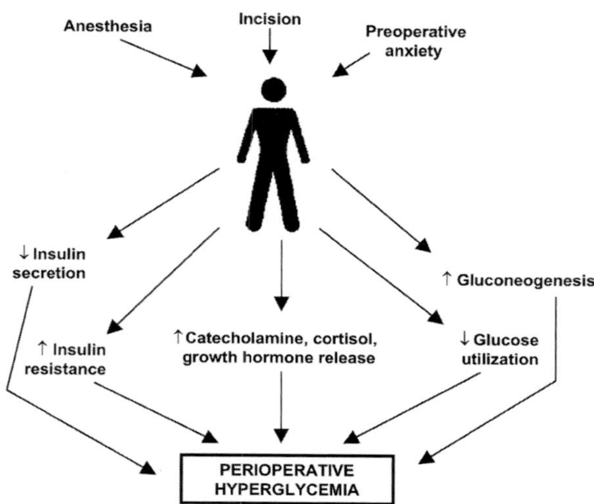

FIGURE 11–1. Physiologic response to severe stress and surgery. From Talbot TR: Diabetes mellitus and cardiothoracic surgical site infections. Am J Infect Control 2005; 33:353–9

cytokines, and increases circulating free fatty acids that are associated with myocardial damage and arrhythmias (Figure 11–1) (38).

A retrospective review of adult medical and surgical inpatients reported worse outcomes in hyperglycemic patients (5). Hyperglycemia was a common finding, present in 38% of patients, and was associated with an 18-fold increase in in-hospital mortality, a longer length of stay, more subsequent nursing home care, and a greater risk of infection. Hyperglycemia in specific disease states also has been shown to be a marker of poor outcomes. A systematic review of 26 studies in adult stroke patients concluded that hyperglycemia is associated with increased mortality and greater risk of poor functional recovery in survivors (39). The same investigators reached similar conclusions when reviewing the association between hyperglycemia and outcomes in patients with myocardial infarctions (40). Hyperglycemia with myocardial infarction was associated with increased risk of congestive heart failure and cardiogenic shock in patients without diabetes and in-hospital mortality in patients with and without diabetes.

The retrospective association of hyperglycemia and adverse outcomes has been followed by a number of prospective studies. The DIGAMI study followed diabetic patients admitted with acute myocardial infarction and randomly assigned patients to intensive insulin therapy with intravenous insulin compared to routine antidiabetic therapy (41). Intensive insulin therapy was shown to be associated with signifi-

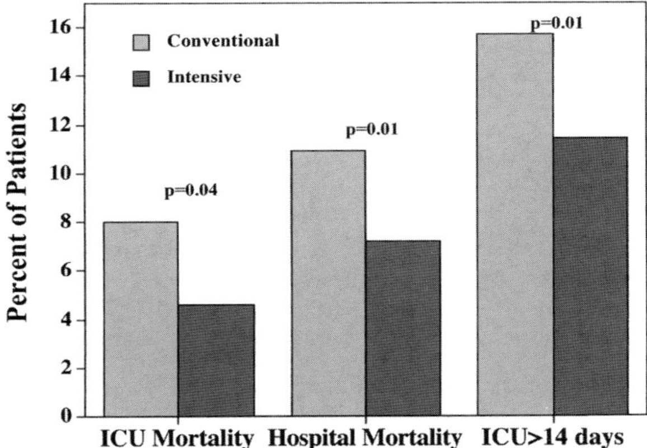

FIGURE 11–2. Outcomes of conventional and intensive glucose control in critical care patients. From Beilman GJ: New strategies to improve outcomes in the surgical intensive care unit. Surg Infect (Larchmt) 2004; 5:289–300

cantly reduced long-term mortality (i.e., determined at over 3 years average length of follow-up).

A prospective, randomized trial in critically ill adult patients comparing intensive intravenous insulin therapy with conventional therapy was conducted by Van den Berghe and colleagues (7). In this trial, patients were randomized to intensive insulin therapy (glucose 80–110 mg/dL) or conventional therapy (treat for glucose >215 mg/dL, maintain 180–200 mg/dL). The trial was stopped early due to a significant reduction in ICU mortality in the intensive insulin therapy group (4.6% vs. 8.0%, $p < 0.04$). This improvement was greater in patients receiving intensive care of more than 5 days (10.6% vs. 20.2%, $p = 0.005$). The in-hospital mortality rate was 7.2% vs. 10.9% ($p = 0.01$) for all patients and 16.8% vs. 26.3% ($p = 0.01$) for patients receiving intensive care of more than 5 days (Figure 11–2). In addition to decreased mortality, significant reductions in sepsis (decrease of 46%), were also observed. The vast majority of the patients in this study were postsurgical with more than 60% admitted following cardiac surgery. Other investigators have suggested favorable outcomes in postcardiac surgery patients with improved glycemic control. A report of more than 3500 diabetic patients undergoing coronary artery bypass grafting showed improved glycemic control and an absolute and risk-adjusted decrease in mortality of 57% and 50%, respectively, and decreased infectious complications following institution of an intravenous insulin management strategy (42).

Further investigations have been designed to determine whether the improvement in outcomes seen in cardiac and surgical patients was

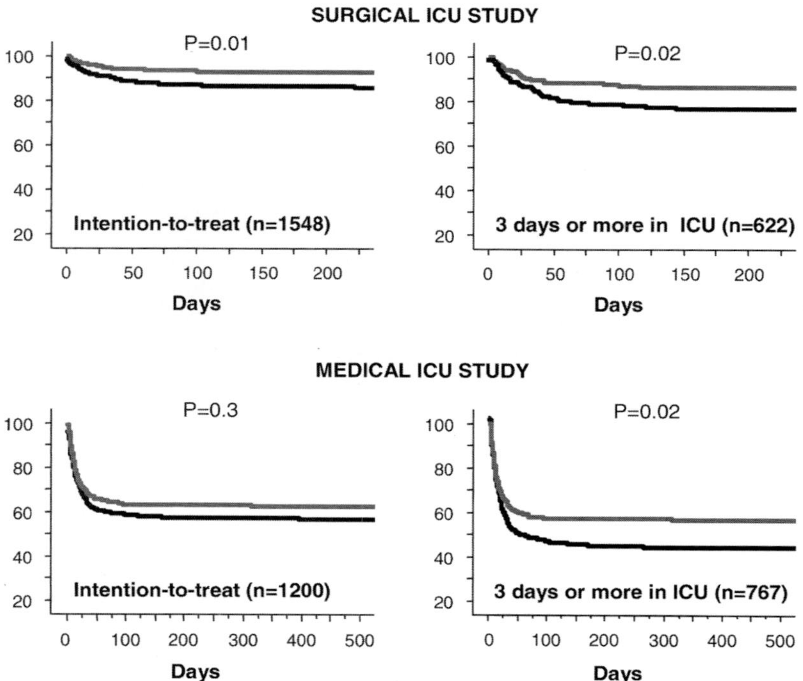

FIGURE 11–3. Kaplan-Meier curves for in-hospital survival for surgical and medical ICU patients (7,45). The effect of tight glycemic control on intensive care patients is shown for the intention-to-treat group and for patients whose ICU stay was three or more days. From Vanhorebeek I, Langouche L, Van den Berghe G: Tight blood glucose control with insulin in the ICU: facts and controversies. Chest 2007; 132:268–78

more broadly applicable. A retrospective study of an adult ICU with a mixed medical and surgical population showed an association between hyperglycemia and mortality (43). A subsequent study by the same author reported the effect of instituting an intensive glucose management protocol in critically ill patients in the same ICU (44). Intensive glucose management significantly improved glycemic control and was associated with decreased mortality, organ dysfunction, and length of stay in the ICU. More recently, Van Den Berghe and colleagues conducted a prospective, randomized trial similar in design to their earlier trial (7) but in critically ill medical patients, and reported reduced morbidity among all patients secondary to reduction in renal failure, time on the ventilator, and decreased ICU length-of-stay. While there was no difference in mortality when assessed by an intent-to-treat analysis, the authors did report reduced mortality in those treated for three or more days (43.0% vs. 52.5%, p = 0.009) (Figure 11–3) (45).

A growing body of literature includes intraoperative glycemic control in the study design. A retrospective study of more than 6000 cardiac surgery patients reported high peak serum glucose during cardiopulmonary bypass to be an independent risk factor for death and morbidity in diabetic, as well as nondiabetic, patients (46). Other investigators have reported perioperative, including intraoperative, hyperglycemia to be a predictor of adverse patient outcomes in cardiac surgery (47, 48), carotid endarterectomy (49), and infrainguinal arterial bypass patients (50).

To date, there are limited prospective data comparing outcomes in patients receiving intensive intraoperative insulin therapy to conventional intraoperative glucose management (51). Gandhi and colleagues prospectively randomized 400 cardiac surgery patients to receive intensive or conventional glycemic management intraoperatively followed by intensive postoperative glycemic management. While they were able to achieve a significant difference in mean intraoperative glucose concentrations, they reported no difference in a composite 30-day endpoint of death or major morbidity. Interestingly, there were more deaths and strokes in the intensive intraoperative treatment group.

Protocols

Based on data outlined above and subsequent quality metrics proposed by a variety of groups, perioperative physicians frequently strive for tighter glycemic control in their patients. Insulin infusions are the most effective technique in achieving this goal. Tight glycemic control through an insulin infusion is a routine practice in many operative suites and intensive care units. Many protocols for delivery of intravenous insulin in these settings have been published, although none has been shown to be superior (7, 42, 44). An intraoperative insulin protocol also has been validated in cardiac surgery patients (51). Successful implementation of these protocols relies on frequent determinations of plasma glucose to guide titration of the insulin infusion. In addition, since the response to insulin varies from patient-to-patient and in a patient over time, protocols should allow for variable insulin administration for a given glucose determination (changing the "sliding scale"). A protocol for treatment of hypoglycemia also should be incorporated into any algorithms for insulin administration.

Unanswered Questions

If tighter glycemic control is desired, what glucose level should be targeted? Should intensive glycemic control be attempted in all patients? Pathophysiologic reasoning suggests that avoiding hyperglycemia would be beneficial, though this must be weighed against the risks of hypoglycemia. An international multidisciplinary consensus conference was held in 2001 and a position statement on inpatient diabetes and metabolic control developed (52). In addition to critically ill patients, the consensus statement recommended intravenous insulin therapy during the perioperative and perinatal period. The following guidelines were proposed as upper limits for glycemic targets: ICU patients <110 mg/dL; Non-ICU patients <110 mg/dL preprandial, < 180 mg/dL maximum; Perinatal patients <100 mg/dL. However, data published following these recommendations have questioned the low recommended targets. An international study currently underway aims to compare targets of 81–108 mg/dL to 144–180 mg/dL in critically ill patients (53). Other questions remain. For non-diabetic patients found to be hyperglycemic during the perioperative period, how will we ensure that this information is communicated to primary physicians so that appropriate diabetic testing can occur and, if indicated, treatment initiated?

CONCLUSION

Diabetes is the most commonly encountered endocrine disease and is associated with multiorgan pathology that often impacts anesthesia management. Acute hyperglycemic is often present in patients during the perioperative period and perioperative physicians need to be aware of the pathophysiology and required therapy. In addition, anesthesiologists need to be aware of emerging data linking poor outcomes with perioperative hyperglycemia. The management strategy for hyperglycemic patients has changed in many intensive care units and anesthetic practice will likely need to change as well. While many questions remain unanswered, anesthesiologists will likely be asked by surgeons, proceduralists, intensivists, and perhaps regulating agencies to achieve improved glycemic control.

References

1. Edelson GW, Fachnie JD, Whitehouse FW: Perioperative management of diabetes. Henry Ford Hosp Med J 1990; 38:262–5
2. Salomon NW, Page US, Okies JE, et al.: Diabetes mellitus and coronary artery bypass. Short-term risk and long-term prognosis. J Thorac Cardiovasc Surg 1983; 85:264–71
3. Thourani VH, Weintraub WS, Stein B, et al.: Influence of diabetes mellitus on early and late outcome after coronary artery bypass grafting. Ann Thorac Surg 1999; 67:1045–52
4. Root HF: Preoperative medical care of the diabetic patient. Postgrad Med 1966; 40:439–44

5. Umpierrez GE, Isaacs SD, Bazargan N, et al.: Hyperglycemia: an independent marker of in-hospital mortality in patients with undiagnosed diabetes. J Clin Endocrinol Metab 2002; 87:978–82
6. Pomposelli JJ, Baxter JK, 3rd, Babineau TJ, et al.: Early postoperative glucose control predicts nosocomial infection rate in diabetic patients. JPEN JParenter Enteral Nutr 1998; 22:77–81
7. van den Berghe G, Wouters P, Weekers F, et al.: Intensive insulin therapy in the critically ill patients. N Engl J Med 2001; 345:1359–67
8. Finney SJ, Zekveld C, Elia A, Evans TW: Glucose control and mortality in critically ill patients. JAMA 2003; 290:2041–7
9. Clement S, Braithwaite SS, Magee MF, et al.: Management of diabetes and hyperglycemia in hospitals. Diabetes Care 2004; 27:553–91
10. Carson JL, Scholz PM, Chen AY, et al.: Diabetes mellitus increases short-term mortality and morbidity in patients undergoing coronary artery bypass graft surgery. J Am Coll Cardiol 2002; 40:418–23
11. Cohen Y, Raz I, Merin G, Mozes B: Comparison of factors associated with 30-day mortality after coronary artery bypass grafting in patients with versus without diabetes mellitus. Israeli Coronary Artery Bypass (ISCAB) Study Consortium. Am J Cardiol 1998; 81:7–11
12. Szabo Z, Hakanson E, Svedjeholm R: Early postoperative outcome and medium-term survival in 540 diabetic and 2239 nondiabetic patients undergoing coronary artery bypass grafting. Ann Thorac Surg 2002; 74:712–9
13. Jacoby RM, Nesto RW: Acute myocardial infarction in the diabetic patient: pathophysiology, clinical course and prognosis. J Am Coll Cardiol 1992; 20:736–44
14. Lazar HL, Chipkin SR, Fitzgerald CA, et al.: Tight glycemic control in diabetic coronary artery bypass graft patients improves perioperative outcomes and decreases recurrent ischemic events. Circulation 2004; 109:1497–502
15. Genuth S, Alberti KG, Bennett P, et al.: Follow-up report on the diagnosis of diabetes mellitus. Diabetes Care 2003; 26:3160–7
16. Diagnosis and classification of diabetes mellitus. Diabetes Care 2005; 28 Suppl 1:S37–42
17. The effect of intensive treatment of diabetes on the development and progression of long-term complications in insulin-dependent diabetes mellitus. The Diabetes Control and Complications Trial Research Group. N Engl J Med 1993; 329:977–86
18. Intensive blood-glucose control with sulphonylureas or insulin compared with conventional treatment and risk of complications in patients with type 2 diabetes (UKPDS 33). UK Prospective Diabetes Study (UKPDS) Group. Lancet 1998; 352:837–53

19. Krentz AJ, Bailey CJ: Oral antidiabetic agents: current role in type 2 diabetes mellitus. Drugs 2005; 65:385–411
20. Binder C, Brange J: Insulin chemistry and pharmacokinetics. In: Jr DP, Sherwin R, eds. Ellenberg's and Rifkin's Diabetes Mellitus. 6th ed. Stamford, CT: Appleton and Lange; 2002
21. Kurtzhals P, Schaffer L, Sorensen A, et al.: Correlations of receptor binding and metabolic and mitogenic potencies of insulin analogs designed for clinical use. Diabetes 2000; 49:999–1005
22. Koda-Kimble M, Carlisle B: Diabetes mellitus. In: Koda-Kimble M, Young L, eds. Applied Theraputics, The Clinical Use of Drugs. 7th Ed. ed. Philadelphia, PA: Lippincott, William, and Wilkins; 2001:48–1.
23. ter Braak EW, Woodworth JR, Bianchi R, et al.: Injection site effects on the pharmacokinetics and glucodynamics of insulin lispro and regular insulin. Diabetes Care 1996; 19:1437–40
24. Francis AJ, Hanning I, Alberti KG: The influence of insulin antibody levels on the plasma profiles and action of subcutaneously injected human and bovine short acting insulins. Diabetologia 1985; 28:330–4
25. Nolte M, Karam J: Pancreatic hormones and antidiabetic drugs. In: Katzung B, ed. Basic and Clinical Pharmacology Stamford, CT: Appleton and Lang; 2001:711
26. Rabkin R, Ryan MP, Duckworth WC: The renal metabolism of insulin. Diabetologia 1984; 27:351–7
27. Hipszer B, Joseph J, Kam M: Pharmacokinetics of intravenous insulin delivery in humans with type 1 diabetes. Diabetes Technol Ther 2005; 7:83–93
28. Ravis WR, Comerci C, Ganjam VK: Pharmacokinetics of insulin following intravenous and subcutaneous administration in canines. Biopharm Drug Dispos 1986; 7:407–20
29. Eagle KA, Berger PB, Calkins H, et al.: ACC/AHA guideline update for perioperative cardiovascular evaluation for noncardiac surgery-executive summary: a report of the American College of Cardiology/ American Heart Association Task Force on Practice Guidelines (Committee to Update the 1996 Guidelines on Perioperative Cardiovascular Evaluation for Noncardiac Surgery). J Am Coll Cardiol 2002; 39:542–53
30. Bangalore S, Parkar S, Grossman E, Messerli FH: A meta-analysis of 94,492 patients with hypertension treated with beta blockers to determine the risk of new-onset diabetes mellitus. Am J Cardiol 2007; 100:1254–62
31. Sawicki PT, Siebenhofer A: beta blocker treatment in diabetes mellitus. J Intern Med 2001; 250:11–7

32. Magee MF, Bhatt BA: Management of decompensated diabetes. Diabetic ketoacidosis and hyperglycemic hyperosmolar syndrome. Crit Care Clin 2001; 17:75–106
33. McCowen KC, Malhotra A, Bistrian BR: Stress-induced hyperglycemia. Crit Care Clin 2001; 17:107–24
34. Lattermann R, Schricker T, Wachter U, et al.: Understanding the mechanisms by which isoflurane modifies the hyperglycemic response to surgery. Anesth Analg 2001; 93:121–7
35. Desborough JP, Jones PM, Persaud SJ, et al.: Isoflurane inhibits insulin secretion from isolated rat pancreatic islets of Langerhans. Br J Anaesth 1993; 71:873–6
36. Coursin DB, Connery LE, Ketzler JT: Perioperative diabetic and hyperglycemic management issues. Crit Care Med 2004; 32:S116–25
37. Rehman HU, Mohammed K: Perioperative management of diabetic patients. Curr Surg 2003; 60:607–11
38. Das UN: Insulin: an endogenous cardioprotector. Curr Opin Crit Care 2003; 9:375–83
39. Capes SE, Hunt D, Malmberg K, et al.: Stress hyperglycemia and prognosis of stroke in nondiabetic and diabetic patients: a systematic overview. Stroke 2001; 32:2426–32
40. Capes SE, Hunt D, Malmberg K, Gerstein HC: Stress hyperglycaemia and increased risk of death after myocardial infarction in patients with and without diabetes: a systematic overview. Lancet 2000; 355:773–8
41. Malmberg K, Norhammar A, Wedel H, Ryden L: Glycometabolic state at admission: important risk marker of mortality in conventionally treated patients with diabetes mellitus and acute myocardial infarction: long-term results from the Diabetes and Insulin-Glucose Infusion in Acute Myocardial Infarction (DIGAMI) study. Circulation 1999; 99:2626–32
42. Furnary AP, Gao G, Grunkemeier GL, et al.: Continuous insulin infusion reduces mortality in patients with diabetes undergoing coronary artery bypass grafting. J Thorac Cardiovasc Surg 2003; 125:1007–21
43. Krinsley JS: Association between hyperglycemia and increased hospital mortality in a heterogeneous population of critically ill patients. Mayo Clin Proc 2003; 78:1471–8
44. Krinsley JS: Effect of an intensive glucose management protocol on the mortality of critically ill adult patients. Mayo Clin Proc 2004; 79:992–1000
45. Van den Berghe G, Wilmer A, Hermans G, et al.: Intensive insulin therapy in the medical ICU. N Engl J Med 2006; 354:449–61
46. Doenst T, Wijeysundera D, Karkouti K, et al.: Hyperglycemia during cardiopulmonary bypass is an independent risk factor for mor-

tality in patients undergoing cardiac surgery. J Thorac Cardiovasc Surg 2005; 130:1144

47. Ouattara A, Lecomte P, Le Manach Y, et al.: Poor intraoperative blood glucose control is associated with a worsened hospital outcome after cardiac surgery in diabetic patients. Anesthesiology 2005; 103:687–94
48. Gandhi GY, Nuttall GA, Abel MD, et al.: Intraoperative hyperglycemia and perioperative outcomes in cardiac surgery patients. Mayo Clin Proc 2005; 80:862–6
49. McGirt MJ, Woodworth GF, Brooke BS, et al.: Hyperglycemia independently increases the risk of perioperative stroke, myocardial infarction, and death after carotid endarterectomy. Neurosurgery 2006; 58:1066–73; discussion–73
50. Malmstedt J, Wahlberg E, Jorneskog G, Swedenborg J: Influence of perioperative blood glucose levels on outcome after infrainguinal bypass surgery in patients with diabetes. Br J Surg 2006; 93:1360–7
51. Gandhi GY, Nuttall GA, Abel MD, et al.: Intensive intraoperative insulin therapy versus conventional glucose management during cardiac surgery: a randomized trial. Ann Intern Med 2007; 146:233–43
52. Garber AJ, Moghissi ES, Bransome ED, Jr., et al.: American College of Endocrinology position statement on inpatient diabetes and metabolic control. Endocr Pract 2004; 10:77–82
53. Bellomo R, Egi M: Glycemic control in the intensive care unit: why we should wait for NICE-SUGAR. Mayo Clin Proc 2005; 80:1546–8
54. Talbot TR: Diabetes mellitus and cardiothoracic surgical site infections. Am J Infect Control 2005; 33:353–9
55. Beilman GJ: New strategies to improve outcomes in the surgical intensive care unit. Surg Infect (Larchmt) 2004; 5:289–300
56. Vanhorebeek I, Langouche L, Van den Berghe G: Tight blood glucose control with insulin in the ICU: facts and controversies. Chest 2007; 132:268–78

Index

Page numbers in italics denote figures; those followed by "t" denote tables.

A-HeFT trial (African American Heart Failure Trial), 84
Acarbose, 253
ACE (angiotensin-converting enzyme) inhibitors, 76–77
Acebutolol, 45–46, 46t, 55
Acetazolamide, 208–209
Acetohexamide, 253
Action potentials, 119–120
  fast, 119, 119–120
  ionic currents involved in, 115–116, 117t
  membrane, 118–121
  slow, 119, 119–120
  types of, 119, 119–120
Activated prothrombin complex concentrate (APCC), 171–172
Acute glycemic complications, 256–259
Acute heart failure
  guidelines for treatment of, 22, 23
  SURVIVE study, 25
Acute myocardial infarction
  β-blocker therapy for, 50
  levosimendan for, 26–28
Acute renal failure, after cardiac surgery, 215
Adenosine
  pharmacology of, 128–130
  as preconditioning agent, 98
African American Heart Failure Trial (A-HeFT), 84
Afterdepolarization
  delayed, 128
  early, 128, 128
Aged heart, 99–100
Agency for Healthcare Research and Quality, 62
al-Nafis, Ibn, 68
Alfentanil, 135–137, 136t
α-adrenergic receptors (α-blockers), 48–49
α-glucosidase inhibitors, 253
American College of Cardiology / American Heart Association (ACC/AHA) guidelines, 61
American Diabetes Association, 252
6-Amidino-2-naphthyl para-guanidinobenzoate. See Nafamostat
Amiodarone, 132t, 134–135
Anesthetic agents. See also specific agents by name
  antiarrhythmic drug interactions, 135–141
  diuretics and, 205–225
  electrophysiologic effects of, 135–141
  intravenous, 138–140, 139t
  local, 139t, 140–141
  metabolic response to, 259
  volatile
    antiarrhythmic drug interactions, 135–137
    cellular and clinical effects of, 135–137, 136t
    electrophysiologic effects of, 135–137
Anesthetic-induced postconditioning, 103–104, 104

Anesthetic-induced preconditioning, 96–97, 97
Angina, 98
Angiotensin-converting enzyme (ACE) inhibitors, 76–77
Anti-inhibitor coagulant complex, 171
Antiarrhythmic agents
  anesthetic interactions, 135–141
  with β-blocker properties, 56
  class I, 130–133, 131t
  class II, 132t, 133–134
  class III, 132t, 134–135
  class IV, 132t, 135
  classification of, 130
  pharmacology of, 128–135
Antidiuretic hormone, 75–76
Antifibrinolytic agents, 158
  classes of, 186
  lysine analog, 188–189, 189
  perioperative use of, 186–189
  pharmacology of, 183–204, 189–195
Aortic dissection, 50, 51
APCC. See Activated prothrombin complex concentrate
Aprotinin, 158, 186
  adverse effects of, 195
  dosing, 193–194
  perioperative use of, 187–188
  pharmacokinetics, 194
  pharmacology of, 193–195
Arrhythmias, 127–128
Arterial hypertension
  β-blocker therapy for, 50
  pulmonary, 80–83
Atenolol, 54–55
  mechanisms of action and effects of, 132t, 133–134
  pharmacologic/pharmacokinetic properties of, 45–46, 46t
Atorvastatin, 227–228, 228t
ATP-sensitive potassium (K_{ATP}) channels, 20–22
Atrial myocytes, 121, 121t
Atrioventricular node, 124
  action potentials and conduction velocities, 121, 121t
  electrophysiologic characteristics, 121, 121t
Automatic dysrhythmias, 51
Automaticity, abnormal, 127, 127
Autonomic neuropathy, 256
Autonomic regulation of cardiac electrical activity, 126–127
Autoplex® T. *See* Factor VIII inhibitor bypassing fraction
Azimilide, 132t, 134–135

BART trial (Blood Conservation using Antifibrinolytis: A Randomized Trial in High-Risk Cardiac Surgery Patients), 188, 191
Bazett's formula, 126
Beriplex® P/N. *See* Prothrombin complex concentrate (PCC)
β-adrenergic receptor agonists
  partial agonists, 46
  side effects of β_1-AR agonists, 17–18
β-adrenergic receptor antagonists (β-blockers), 43, 45–50
  alpha receptor blocking activity of, 48–49
  antiarrhythmic agents, 56
  cardioselectivity of, 46, 46t
  cardiovascular effects of, 49, 58, 58
  clinical effects of, 49–50
  current recommendations, 61–62
  first generation—nonselective, 53–54
  intrinsic sympathomimetic activity of, 46–48
  lipid solubility of, 48
  metabolic effects of, 50
  nonselective, 53–54
  oxidation phenotype of, 48
  perioperative use of, 56–61
    cardiovascular effects of, 58, 58
    effects on all-cause mortality, 59, 60
    effects on myocardial infarction, 59, 60
    evaluation of clinical efficacy of, 58–61
    rationale for, 56–57
    recommendations and remaining questions for, 61–62
  pharmacologic/pharmacokinetic properties of, 45–46, 47t
  physiologic actions in different tissues, 49–50

physiologic properties of, 45, 46t
precautions for, 52–53
properties of, 46–49
pulmonary effects of, 49
recommendations, 61–62
remaining questions, 61–62
second generation—selective β_1-AR antagonists, 54–55
side effects of, 52–53
structure activity relationships, 48
therapeutic uses of, 50–52
third generation—β-AR antagonists with additional properties, 55–56
uptitration by levosimendan, 29
β-adrenergic receptors (β-ARs), 43–45
responses elicited by stimulation of, 45, 46t
signaling, 44, 44–45
Biguanides, 253
Bisoprolol, 45–46, 46t, 55
Bleeding, from direct thrombin inhibitors
APCC effects on, 172
rVIIa to control, 170
Blood Conservation using Antifibrinolytis: A Randomized Trial in High-Risk Cardiac Surgery Patients (BART) trial, 188, 191
Blood pressure-flow autoregulation, 68–70, 69
Bumetanide, 210–213, 211t
Bupivacaine
cellular and clinical effects of, 139t, 140–141
electrophysiologic and arrhythmogenic effects of, 128, 129

Calcium (Ca^{2+})
intracellular
effects of positive inotropic agents on, 3, 3, 4
and myocardial cell shortening, 18, 18
myofilament, 19
and myogenic tone, 69–70, 70
Calcium (Ca^{2+}) channel blockers, 135
Calcium (Ca^{2+}) channels
functional roles, 117t
subtypes and effects, 116, 117t
Carbonic anhydrase inhibitors, 208–209, 211t
Cardiac cells
fast-conducting or fast-response (cardiomyocytes and specialized conducting cells), 121
slow-conducting or slow-response (nodal cells), 121
types of, 120–121
Cardiac conduction, 124–125
Cardiac electrophysiology
at cellular level, 115–121
pharmacological applications, 115–155
regulation by autonomic nervous system, 126–127
at subcellular level, 115–121
at tissue and organ levels, 122–126
Cardiac ion channels, 115–118
Cardiac ischemia, perioperative, 57–58
Cardiac memory, 91
Cardiac protection, pharmacological-induced, 95–97
Cardiac repolarization, 125–126
Cardiac risk
after cardiac surgery, 233
after noncardiac surgery, 233–235
postoperative, 57, 57t
Cardiac surgery
acute renal failure after, 215
cardiac risk after, 233
congenital, 163
desmopressin use in, 161–163
diuretic use in, 214–217
pediatric
desmopressin use in, 163
rVIIa use in, 168–169
rVIIa safety and efficacy in, 166–168
Cardiac tissue conduction, 122–126, 123
Cardiogenic shock, 28
Cardiomyocytes, 120
action potentials and conduction velocities, 121, 121t

electrophysiologic characteristics, 121, 121t
Cardioprotection
by ischemic postconditioning, 103–104
by ischemic preconditioning, 94–95
by levosimendan, 20–22, 26–28
Cardiovascular anesthesia, 205–225
Cardiovascular disease
β-blocker therapy for, 50–51
in diabetic patients, 256
Carvedilol, 56
α-blocking potency, 48–49
metabolism of, 48
pharmacologic/pharmacokinetic properties of, 45–46, 46t
Catecholamines, 26
Celiprolol, 56
pharmacologic/pharmacokinetic properties of, 45–46, 46t
pulmonary effects of, 49
Cell membrane, 115–121
Cellular proliferation, 80, 81
Cerivastatin, 237
Channelopathies, 116
Chlorpropamide, 253
Cholesterol
low-density lipoprotein (LDL), 227–228
synthesis of, 85, 85
Chronic heart failure, 22–26
Cibenzoline, 130–131, 131t, 133
CK-1827452, 11
Coagulation cascade, 185, 185–186
Conduction
cardiac, 124–125
in cardiac tissue, 122–126, 123
epicardial, 122–123, 123
Congenital cardiac surgery, 163
Congestive heart failure, 50
Connexins (Cx), 122
Coronary steal, 95
Critically ill: glycemic control in, 259–264, 261, 262
Crossbridge cycling, 3, 3, 4

DDAVP (1-deamino-8-D-arginine-vasopressin). See Desmopressin
Delayed afterdepolarization, 128
Desflurane
cellular and clinical effects of, 135–137, 136t
as preconditioning agent, 99
Desmopressin, 158–163
adverse reactions to, 159–160
applications, 160–161
in cardiac surgery, 161–163
in combination with tranexamic acid, 162
in congenital cardiac surgery, 163
contraindications to, 159–160
dosing, 159
effects of, 158–159
guidelines for use, 163
indications for, 160–161, 160t
mechanism of action, 158–159
in pediatric cardiac surgery, 163
pharmacokinetics, 159
Diabetes mellitus, 251
classification of, 252–255
definition of, 252
diagnosis of, 252
end-organ dysfunction in, 255–256
pharmacologic treatment of, 253
and preconditioning, 100, 100–101
type 1, 252
type 2, 252
Diabetic ketoacidosis, 257–258
Digitalis, 128–130
Diltiazem, 132t, 135
Diphenylhydantoine, 130–131, 131t, 133
Direct thrombin inhibitors
APCC effects on bleeding from, 172
rVIIa to control bleeding from, 170
Disopyramide, 130–131, 131t
Diuretics
in cardiac surgery, 214–217
and cardiovascular anesthesia, 205–225
classes of, 208–214
loop, 210–213
in cardiac and vascular surgery, 215
effects on electrolyte balance, 211t, 213
effects on urine excretion, 210, 211t

osmotic, 209–210
in cardiac and vascular surgery, 215
effects on electrolyte balance, 211t
effects on urine excretion, 211t
principles of use, 206–208
renal function and, 206–208
thiazide, 213–214
in vascular surgery, 214–217
vasoactive agents, 217–220
Dobutamine, 7–8
for acute heart failure, 22–24
cardiovascular effects of, 7
mechanism of action and dosage, 5t
SURVIVE study, 25, 26
Dofetilide, 132t, 134–135
Dopamine, 6–7
for diuresis, 218
mechanism of action and dosage, 5t
renal-dose, 216, 218
Dronedarone, 134
Droperidol, 140
Dynorphine, 138
Dysrhythmias, automatic, 51

EACA. See ε-aminocaproic acid
Early afterdepolarization, 128, 128
EDRF. See Endothelium-derived relaxing factor
Edrophonium, 140
Electrophysiology
cardiac
regulation by autonomic nervous system, 126–127
at tissue and organ levels, 122–126
pharmacological applications, 115–155
End-organ dysfunction, in diabetic patients, 255–256
Endocrine disorders, 51
Endothelial dysfunction, 74, 75
Endothelium, 74
Endothelium-derived relaxing factor (EDRF), 74
Enzymatic coagulation cascade, 185, 185–186
Epicardial conduction, 122–123, 123
Epinephrine, 4–6, 5t
Epoprostenol, 83
ε-aminocaproic acid (EACA), 158
adverse effects of, 190
molecular weight, 189
perioperative use of, 188–189
pH, 189
pharmacology of, 189–190
Esmolol, 55
mechanisms of action and effects of, 132t, 133–134
pharmacologic/pharmacokinetic properties of, 45–46, 46t
Ethacrynic acid, 210–213
Evolving therapies, 10–11
Exercise-induced ventricular tachycardia, 51

Factor VIII inhibitor bypassing fraction (FEIBA®) (FEIBA® VH, Autoplex® T), 171
Fenoldopam, 218–219
Fentanyl, 136t, 137–138
Fibrinolysis, 186, 187. See also Antifibrinolytic agents
Flecainide, 130–131, 131t, 133
Fluvastatin, 227–228, 228t
Fluvastatin XL, 227–228, 228t
Food and Drug Administration (FDA)
approved indications for desmopressin, 160–161, 160t
approved therapies for PAH, 80
Furosemide, 210–213
in cardiac and vascular surgery, 215
effects on urine excretion, 210, 211t

Galen, 67
Gap junctional intercellular coupling, 122
Glaucoma, 51–52
Glimepiride, 253
Glipizide, 253
Glucose control, impaired, 252
Glyburide, 253
Glycemic complications, acute, 256–259
Glycemic control, 252
in critically ill, 259–264, 261, 262
impaired glucose control, 252

intraoperative, 263
perioperative, 259–264
guidelines for, 264
protocols for, 263
unanswered questions, 263–264
Glycerin, 209

Halothane, 135–137, 136t
Harvey, William, 68
Heart disease
β-blocker therapy for, 50
ischemic, 50
preconditioning in, 99
Heart failure
acute
guidelines for treatment of, 22, 23
SURVIVE study, 25
β-blocker therapy for, 50–51
chronic, 22–26
congestive, 50
Hemostasis
enzymatic coagulation cascade, 185, 185–186
mechanisms of, 184–186
platelet adhesion and aggregation, 184, 184
regulation of, 186
Hepatic synthesis of cholesterol, 85, 85
His-Purkinje tracts, 120–121
Hydralazine
antioxidant effects of, 83, 84
and reversal of nitrate tolerance, 83–84
Hydrochlorothiazide, 213
Hypercholesterolemia, 101–103, 102
Hyperglycemia, 256–257
Hypertension
arterial, 50
β-blocker therapy for, 50
essential, 50
pulmonary, 80–83
Hyperthyroidism, 51
Hypertrophic obstructive cardiomyopathy, 50, 51
Hypoglycemia, 256–257, 258–259

Ibutilide, 132t, 134–135
Impact of Nicorandil on Angina (IONA) study, 98
Impaired glucose control, 252
Inhaled nitric oxide, 82
Inhibitors of carbonic anhydrase, 208–209
effects on electrolyte balance, 211t
effects on urine excretion, 211t
Inhibitors of sodium-chloride symport, 213–214
effects on electrolyte balance, 211t
effects on urine excretion, 211t
Inotropic therapy, 1–15
central mechanisms, 2
downstream mechanisms, 2
effects on intracellular Ca^{2+} and crossbridge cycling, 3, *3*, 4
mechanism of action and dosage, 5t
mechanisms, 2
physiology of, 2–4
SURVIVE study, 25
upstream mechanisms, 2
Insulin
pharmacokinetics of, 254–255
pharmacology of, 253–254
Intraoperative glycemic control, 263
Intravenous agents
antiarrhythmic drug interactions, 138–140
cellular and clinical effects of, 138–140, 139t
electrophysiologic effects of, 137–138
Ion channels, 115–121
cardiac, 115–118
involved in action potentials, 115–116, 117t
states, 118
structure of, 116–118
subunits, 116–118, 118
IONA (Impact of Nicorandil on Angina) study, 98
Ischemic heart disease, 50
Ischemic postconditioning, 103–104
Ischemic preconditioning, 91–92, 92
clinical potential of, 97–99
mechanisms of cardioprotection by, 94–95
Isoflurane
anesthetic-induced preconditioning by, 96
cellular and clinical effects of, 135–137, 136t
Isoproterenol, 48
Isosorbide, 209

Ketamine, 138–140, 139t
Kidney disease, in diabetic patients, 256
Kidney failure, acute, after cardiac surgery, 215
Kidney function
  and diuretic use, 206–208
  sodium transport, 206–208, 207

Labetalol, 55–56
  α-blocking potency, 48–49
  pharmacologic/pharmacokinetic properties of, 45–46, 46t
LDL (low-density lipoprotein) cholesterol, 227–228
Leapfrog Group, 62
Left ventricular failure, due to acute myocardial infarction, 26–28
Levobupivacaine, 139t, 140–141
Levosimendan, 9–10, 17–42
  for acute heart failure, 22–26, 23
  areas of interest for potential future application, 28–29
  β_1-adrenoceptor blockade uptitration by, 29
  for cardiogenic shock, 28
  cardioprotection by, 20–22, 26–28
  in combination with catecholamines, 26
  dosage, 5t, 29–30
  indications for, 22–28
  K_{ATP} channel opening by, 20–22
  mechanisms of action, 5t, 19–22
  for myocardial ischemia, 26–28
  myofilament Ca^{2+} sensitization by, 19
  opening of potassium channels by, 19–20
  perioperative administration of, 31–32
  phosphodiesterase III inhibition by, 19
  practical use of, 29–32
  prerequisites for optimal effect and safety, 29–30, 30t
  recommendation for mode of administration of, 31, 31t
  REVIVE-2 trial, 24–25, 26
  for right ventricular dysfunction, 28
  RUSSLAN study, 26–28
  safety, 30–31
  SURVIVE study, 25, 30–31
  vasodilation by, 19–20
Lidocaine
  cellular and clinical effects of, 139t, 140–141
  mechanisms of action and effects of, 130–131, 131t, 133
  pharmacology of, 130–131
Liver: cholesterol synthesis by, 85, 85
Local anaesthetics, 139t, 140–141
Loop diuretics, 210–213
  in cardiac and vascular surgery, 215
  effects on electrolyte balance, 211t, 213
  effects on urine excretion, 210, 211t
Lovastatin, 227–228, 228t
Low-density lipoprotein (LDL) cholesterol, 227–228
Lysine analogues, 186
  mechanism of action, 188–189, 189
  perioperative use of, 187–188

M-cells, 121
Magnesium, 128–130
Malpighi, Marcello, 68
Mannitol, 209–210
Marfan's syndrome, 51
Meglitinides, 253
Membrane action potential, 118–121
Memory, cardiac, 91
Metabolic response to anesthesia and surgery, 259, 260
Metformin, 253
Metolazone, 213
Metoprolol, 54
  lipid solubility of, 48
  mechanisms of action and effects of, 132t, 133–134
  oxidative metabolism of, 48
  pharmacologic/pharmacokinetic properties of, 45–46, 46t
Mexiletine, 130–131, 131t, 133
Miglitol, 253
Milrinone, 4, 5t, 8–9
Mineralocorticoid receptor antagonists, 214
Morphine
  cellular and clinical effects of, 136t, 137–138

as preconditioning agent, 98
Muscle injury, statin-induced, 237–238
Myalgia, statin-induced, 237
Myocardial cell shortening, 18, 18
Myocardial infarction
acute
β-blocker therapy for, 50
levosimendan for, 26–28
β-blocker therapy for, 50, 59, *60*
perioperative, 56, 57, 59, 60
preconditioning and, 91–92, 92
Myocardial ischemia, 26–28
Myocardial postconditioning, 103, 104–105
Myocardial preconditioning
anesthetic-induced, 96
early phase, 93–94
and infarct size, 91–92, 92
late phase, 93–94
pharmacology of, 91–113
phases of protection, 93–94, 94
physiology of, 91–113
research on, 91–93, 93
Myocardial stunning, 94
Myocytes, 121, 121t
Myogenic tone, 68–70, 70
mechanism of, 69–70, 70
normal pressure-flow autoregulation, 68–70, 69
Myopathy, statin-induced, 236–238
during nonsurgical period, 236–238
during perioperative period, 238
Myosin activators, 10–11
Myositis, with statins, 237

Nadolol, 53
additional therapeutic uses for, 52
pharmacologic/pharmacokinetic properties of, 45–46, 46t
Nafamostat
dosing, 192
pharmacology of, 192–193
Nafis, Ibn al-, 68
Nateglinide, 253
National Quality Forum, 62
Nesiritide, 219–220
Nicorandil
Impact of Nicorandil on Angina (IONA) study, 98
as preconditioning agent, 98
Nitrate tolerance, 83–84, 84
Nitric oxide, 74
inhaled, 82
Nitric oxide synthase uncoupling, 74, 75
Nitro-glycerine (NTG) tolerance, 83, 84
Nodal cells, 120
action potentials and conduction velocities, 121, 121t
electrophysiologic characteristics, 121, 121t
Non-ketotic hyperosmolar state, 258
Norepinephrine, 6
NovoSeven®. *See* Recombinant activated factor VII (rVIIa)
NTG (nitro-glycerine) tolerance, 83, 84

Octaplex®. *See* Prothrombin complex concentrate (PCC)
Opiates
antiarrhythmic drug interactions, 137–138
cellular and clinical effects of, 136t, 137–138
electrophysiologic effects of, 137–138
Oral preparations, for diabetes mellitus, 253
Osmotic diuretics, 209–210
in cardiac and vascular surgery, 215
effects on electrolyte balance, 211t
effects on urine excretion, 211t

PCC. See Prothrombin complex concentrate
Pediatric cardiac surgery
desmopressin use in, 163
rVIIa use in, 168–169
Penbutolol, 45–46, 46t, 54
Perioperative cardiac ischemia, 57–58
Perioperative glycemic control
guidelines for, 264
protocols for, 263
unanswered questions, 263–264
Perioperative myocardial infarction, 56, 57, 59, 60
Perioperative period
antifibrinolytic use during, 186–189

aprotinin use during, 187–188
β-blocker use during, 56–61
cardiovascular effects of, 58, 58
effects on all-cause mortality, 59, 60
effects on myocardial infarction, 59, 60
recommendations and remaining questions for, 61–62
ε-aminocaproic acid use during, 188–189
glycemic control during, 259–264
lysine analog use during, 187–188
statin-induced myopathy during, 238
statin use during, 102, 102–103, 232–235, 241
statin withdrawal during, 239–241
tranexamic acid use during, 188–189
Pharmacologic treatment. See also specific agents by name
of diabetes mellitus, 253
preconditioning, 97–99
Phosphodiesterase III inhibition, 19
Phosphodiesterase inhibitors
side effects of, 17–18
in therapy of pulmonary hypertension, 80–83, 81–82
Physostigmine, 140
Pindolol, 54
lipid solubility of, 48
pharmacologic/pharmacokinetic properties of, 45–46, 46t
Pioglitazone, 253
Platelet adhesion and aggregation, 184, 184
Postconditioning
anesthetic-induced, 103–104, 104
ischemic, 103–104
myocardial, 103, 104–105
Postoperative cardiac risk, 57, 57t
Potassium channels
ATP-sensitive (K_{ATP}), 20–22
functional roles, 117t
opening by levosimendan, 19–20, 20–22
subtypes and effects, 116, 117t
Potassium sparing agents, 214
Pravastatin, 227–228, 228t
Prazosin, 51
Preconditioning
of aged heart, 99–100
anesthetic, 96–97, 97
diabetes mellitus and, 100, 100–101
of diseased heart, 99
in hypercholesterolemia, 101–103, 102
ischemic, 91–92, 92
clinical potential of, 97–99
mechanisms of cardioprotection by, 94–95
myocardial
early phase, 93–94
and infarct size, 91–92, 92
late phase, 93–94
pharmacology of, 91–113
phases of protection, 93–94, 94
physiology of, 91–113
research on, 91–93, 93
pharmacological, 97–99
Procainamide, 130–131, 131t
Procoagulant agents, 157–182. See also specific agents by name
Propafenone, 130–131, 131t, 133
Propofol, 138–140, 139t
Propranolol, 53
additional therapeutic uses for, 52
for hyperthyroidism, 51
for hypertrophic cardiomyopathy, 51
lipid solubility of, 48
mechanisms of action and effects of, 132t, 133–134
metabolism of, 48
pharmacologic/pharmacokinetic properties of, 45–46, 46t
Prothrombin complex concentrate (PCC) (Beriplex® P/N, Octaplex®), 171–172
Pulmonary hypertension, 80–83
Purkinje fibers
action potentials and conduction velocities, 121, 121t
electrophysiologic characteristics, 121, 121t

QT interval, long, 126
Quinidine, 130–131, 131t

Randomized Multicenter Evaluation of Intravenous Levosimendan Efficacy (REVIVE-2) trial, 24–25, 26
Randomized Study on Safety and Effectiveness of Levosimendan in Patients with Left Ventricular Failure due to an Acute Myocardial Infarct (RUSSLAN study), 26–28
Recombinant activated factor VII (rVIIa) (NovoSeven®), 158, 163–171
  to control bleeding from direct thrombin inhibitors, 170
  costs of, 166
  dosing, 164–166
  efficacy in adult cardiac surgical patients, 166–168
  guidelines for use, 170–171
  mechanism of action, 164, 165
  non-FDA approved applications, 163, 164t
  in pediatric cardiac surgical patients, 168–169
  pharmacokinetics, 164–166
  safety in adult cardiac surgical patients, 166–168
Reentry, 128, 129
Reentry tachycardia, 51
Remifentanil
  cellular and clinical effects of, 135–137, 136t
  as preconditioning agent, 98
Renal disease, in diabetic patients, 256
Renal-dose dopamine, 216, 218
Renal failure, acute, after cardiac surgery, 215
Renal function
  and diuretic use, 206–208
  sodium transport, 206–208, 207
Repaglinide, 253
Repolarization, cardiac, 125–126
REVIVE-2 (Randomized Multicenter Evaluation of Intravenous Levosimendan Efficacy) trial, 24–25, 26
Rhabdomyolysis, with statins, 237
Right ventricular dysfunction, 28
Risk, cardiac
  after cardiac surgery, 233
  after noncardiac surgery, 233–235
Ropivacaine, 139t, 140–141
Rosiglitazone, 253
Rosuvastatin, 227–228, 228t
RUSSLAN study (Randomized Study on Safety and Effectiveness of Levosimendan in Patients with Left Ventricular Failure due to an Acute Myocardial Infarct), 26–28
rVIIa. See Recombinant activated factor VII

Safety
  levosimendan, 30–31
    prerequisites for, 29–30, 30t
    RUSSLAN study, 26–28
  rVIIa, in cardiac surgery, 166–168
  statin, 236–237
Sarcoplasmic reticulum calcium ATPase (SERCA) expression, 10
Sepsis, 28–29
SERCA (sarcoplasmic reticulum calcium ATPase) expression, 10
Sevoflurane
  cardiac protection by, 96
  cellular and clinical effects of, 135–137, 136t
  as preconditioning agent, 98–99
Shock, cardiogenic, 28
Sicilian Gambit, 130
Sildenafil (Viagra)
  as preconditioning agent, 98
  in therapy of PAH, 80–82, 81–82, 82–83
Simvastatin, 227–228, 228t
Sinoatrial node, 124
  action potentials and conduction velocities, 121, 121t
  electrophysiologic characteristics, 121, 121t
Smooth muscle tone, vascular
  pharmacological modulation of, 75–86
  physiological modulation of, 68–75

Sodium channels
functional roles, 117t
subtypes and effects, 116, 117t
voltage-gated, α-subunit, 116–118, *118*
Sodium-chloride symport inhibitors, 213–214
effects on electrolyte balance, 211t
effects on urine excretion, 211t
Sodium-hydrogen exchanger inhibitors, 98
Sodium transport, 206–208, 207
Sotalol, 134
d-Sotalol, 132t, 134–135
dl-Sotalol, 132t, 133–134
Spironolactone, 214
Statins, 227
ACC/AHA clinical advisory on use and safety of, 236–237
benefits of, 227–232, 241
clinical pharmacokinetics of, 227–228, 228t
complications associated with use, 236–241
dose-dependent effects of, 231–232
in hypercholesterolemia, 101–103, 102
lipid-dependent effects of, 227–231, 230t
lipid-independent effects of, 228–231, 230t
mechanisms of effects of, 228–229, 230t
muscle injury induced by, 237–238
myopathy induced by, 236–238
perioperative use of, 102, 102–103, 232–235, 241
pleiotropic effects of, 84–86, 85
as preconditioning agents, 98, 101–103, 102
preoperative use of, 235
transaminases elevation with, 236
Statins withdrawal, 238–241
during nonsurgical periods, 239
during perioperative period, 239–241
risks of, 242
Stress, severe, 259–260, 260
Stunning, myocardial, 94
Sufentanil, 136t, 137–138
Sulfonylureas, 253
Supraventricular arrhythmias, 50
Supraventricular tachyarrhythmias, 51
Surgery
cardiac
acute renal failure after, 215
cardiac risk after, 233
congenital, 163
desmopressin use in, 161–163
diuretic use in, 214–217
pediatric, 163, 168–169
rVIIa use in, 166–168, 168–169
cardiac risk after, 233–235
diuretic use in, 214–217
metabolic response to, 259
noncardiac, 233–235
physiologic response to, 259–260, 260
vascular, 214–217
Survival of Patients with Acute Heart Failure in Need of Intravenous Inotropic Support (SURVIVE) study, 25, 30–31
Sympathetic nervous system, 71–74
Sympathetic neuroeffector junction, 71–73, 71–74

Tachyarrhythmias, supraventricular, 51
Tachycardia, 128, 128
β-blocker therapy for, 51
reentry, 51
ventricular
β-blocker therapy for, 51
exercise-induced, 51
mechanism of, 128, 129
Terazosin, 51
Thiazide diuretics, 213–214
Thiazolidinediones, 253
Thiopental, 138–140, 139t
Thrombin inhibitors, direct
APCC effects on bleeding from, 172
rVIIa to control bleeding resulting from, 170
Timolol, 53–54
oxidative metabolism of, 48
pharmacologic/pharmacokinetic properties of, 45–46, 46t
Tissue conduction, cardiac, 122–124, 123

Tolazamide, 253
Tolbutamide, 253
Torsade de pointes tachycardia, 134
Torsemide, 210–213
Tranexamic acid (TXA), 158
  adverse effects of, 192
  BART trial, 191
  in combination with desmopressin, 162
  dosing, 191
  perioperative use of, 188–189
  pharmacology of, 190–192
Trans-4-aminomethylcyclohexane-1-carboxylic acid. See Tranexamic acid (TXA)
Transaminases, 236
Triggered activity, 128, 128
TXA. See Tranexamic acid

UK14,304, 71–74, 72–73
Urea, 209

V-HeFT. See Veterans Heart Failure Trials
Vascular smooth muscle tone
  pharmacological modulation of, 75–86
  physiological modulation of, 68–75
Vascular surgery, 214–217
Vascular tone modulators, 67–90
Vasoactive agents, 217–220
Vasodilation
  cGMP pathway mediation of, 80, 81
  by levosimendan, 19–20
  NTG-induced, 83, 84
Vasoplegia, 75–79, 77–79
Vasoplegic syndrome, 75–80
Vasopressin, 75–80, 77–79
Vaughan-Williams Classification system, 51, 130
Vecuronium bromide, 140
Ventricular myocytes, 121, 121t
Ventricular tachycardia
  exercise-induced, 51
  mechanism of, 128, 129
Verapamil, 132t, 135
Veterans Heart Failure Trials (V-HeFT), 83–84
Viagra. See Sildenafil
Volatile anesthetics
  antiarrhythmic drug interactions, 135–137
  cardioprotective effects of
    as postconditioning agents, 105
    as preconditioning agents, 96–97, 98–99
  cellular and clinical effects of, 135–137, 136t
  electrophysiologic effects of, 135–137
Voltage-gated sodium channels, α-subunit, 116–118, *118*

Withdrawal, statin, 238–241, 242
Wolff-Parkinson-White syndrome, 140